HANDBOOK OF HEAD AND NECK IMAGING

HANDBOOKS IN RADIOLOGY SERIES

Other Volumes in This Series

Genitourinary and Gastrointestinal Radiology
STEPHEN R. ELL, M.D., PH.D.

Neuroradiology
ANNE G. OSBORN, M.D.

Nuclear Medicine
FREDERICK L. DATZ, M.D.

Interventional Radiology and Angiography
MYRON M. WOJTOWICZ, M.D.

Skeletal Radiology
B.J. MANASTER, M.D., PH.D.

HANDBOOK OF HEAD AND NECK IMAGING

H. RIC HARNSBERGER, M.D.
Professor of ENT/Neuroradiology
Director, Neuroradiology Section
University of Utah Medical Center
Salt Lake City, Utah

SECOND EDITION

with 209 illustrations

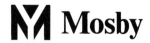 **Mosby**

St. Louis   Baltimore   Berlin   Boston   Carlsbad   Chicago   London   Madrid
Naples   New York   Philadelphia   Sydney   Tokyo   Toronto

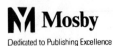
Mosby

Dedicated to Publishing Excellence

Executive Editor: Susan M. Gay
Senior Managing Editor: Lynne Gery
Project Manager: Linda Clarke
Production: York Production Services
Manufacturing Manager: Theresa Fuchs

SECOND EDITION
Copyright © 1995 by Mosby–Year Book, Inc.

Previous edition copyrighted 1990

Printed in the United States of America.
Composition by York Production Services.
Printing/binding by Malloy Lithographing.

Mosby–Year Book, Inc.
11830 Westline Industrial Drive
St. Louis, Missouri 63146

Library of Congress Cataloging in Publication Data

Harnsberger, H. Ric.
   Handbook of head and neck imaging / H. Ric Harnsberger. —2nd ed.
     p.   cm.—(Handbooks in radiology series)
   Rev. ed. of: Head and neck imaging. c1990.
   Includes bibliographical references and index.
   ISBN 0–8151–4233–1
   1. Head—Imaging.   2. Neck—Imaging.   I. Harnsberger, H. Ric.
Head and neck imaging.   II. Title.   III. Title: Head and neck
imaging.   IV. Series.
   [DNLM: 1. Head—radiography—handbooks.   2. Neck—radiography—
handbooks.   3. Diagnostic Imaging.   WE 39 H291ha   1995]
   RC936.H27   1995
   617.5'1'0757—dc20
   DNLM/DLC
   for Library of Congress   94–35225
                                                                        CIP

98   99   /   9   8   7   6   5

To Jungle J (64?) and the 3 D's, from whence comes
the joy and excitement in life which pushed me through to
the end of this book project.

To my parents, Doris and Hutch,
a wellspring of love and support without limit.

To Julian Maack, Medical Illustrator Extraordinaire and philosopher,
thanks for the incredible drawings.

Introduction

GLOBAL ORGANIZATION

The overall organization of the second edition of *Handbook of Head and Neck Imaging* has not substantially changed from the first edition. Two new chapters have been added: "The Perivertebral Space" (Chapter 7) and "Cystic Masses of the Head and Neck: Rare Lesions with Characteristic Radiologic Features" (Chapter 10). Many of the chapters have been strengthened by information from the last four years' literature, multiple additional figures, and references through the first half of 1994.

The *Handbook of Head and Neck Imaging* has been constructed to function as a ready reference for the radiologist confronted by the everyday imaging issues in this field. It is also an introductory work for residents and fellows interested in delving into the anatomy and pathology of the extracranial head and neck. Emphasis is placed on the anatomic foundations of the head and neck region, because the anatomy does not change, no matter the imaging modality used to study it.

It has been my experience that the biggest deterrent to quality imaging in the head and neck region is a useful approach to its anatomy. With this in mind, I have undertaken to subdivide the head and neck by major anatomic subunits. Part I covers the anatomy and pathology in the suprahyoid and infrahyoid neck, including the oral cavity and larynx. Part III on imaging of the face focuses on the orbit and sinonasal region. Part IV encompasses all issues regarding skull base and cranial nerve imaging. Only Part II on imaging of primary and nodal squamous cell carcinoma breaks from the anatomic orientation to look at the imaging issues surrounding the most predominant malignancy of the extracranial head and neck, squamous cell carcinoma.

PART I: IMAGING OF THE SUPRAHYOID AND INFRAHYOID NECK

The handbook begins with an anatomy-based discussion of the deep core tissues of the area of the head and neck from the hyoid bone to the skull base, referred to as the suprahyoid neck. The aim of Chapters 1 to 7 is to provide the imager a useful method for the dividing of these deep core tissues such that it can be applied to analysis of lesions found in this area. In Chapter 1, "Introduction to the Suprahyoid Neck," the anatomic basis for dividing up this area into fascia-defined spaces is presented. The old terms "nasopharynx" and "oropharynx," which are still used in the discussion of squamous cell carcinoma, are replaced by these spaces (parapharyngeal, pharyngeal mucosal, masticator, parotid, carotid, retropharyngeal, and perivertebral), which can be used as a basis for analysis of any lesion found in this area of the extracranial head and neck.

After the global anatomy is presented in Chapter 1, the appearance of masses in each of these fascia-defined spaces is illustrated as a group so that the reader can refer to this section to determine the space of origin of any mass in the deep core tissues of the suprahyoid neck. Once the space of origin of a mass is identified, the chapter dealing with this specific space can be consulted for differential diagnosis list and a discussion of these statistically common lesions in the space.

Chapters 2 to 7 present each of the spaces of the deep core tissues of the suprahyoid neck individually, with discussion of fascial definition, extent, and contents. A space-specific differential diagnosis is presented, along with the clinical presentation, histopathologic findings, and radiologic characteristics of the statistically common lesions of each space.

Chapter 8 covers the more anterior oral cavity and emphasizes the mucosal, sublingual, and submandibular spaces. These oral cavity spaces can be used to construct unique differential diagnosis lists. For each space the unique clinical, pathologic and radiologic features of diseases are reviewed.

Chapter 9, "The Infrahyoid Neck, Normal Anatomy and Pathology of the Head and Neck from the Hyoid Bone to the Clavicles" is one of the largest chapters of the handbook. This chapter covers the anatomy of the infrahyoid neck by individual space. The clinical, pathologic, and radiologic features of diseases in these spaces are discussed. Many of the suprahyoid neck spaces traverse into the infrahyoid neck. Consequently these spaces are revisited in this chapter.

Chapter 10, "Cystic Masses of the Head and Neck: Rare Lesions with Characteristic Radiologic Features," diverges from the space-oriented discussion which has characterized the first nine chapters to look at specific cystic neck masses regardless of space of origin. In this chapter the characteristic appearances of these lesions are emphasized so that these rare lesions will become familiar to all radiologists interested in this area.

Chapter 11, "The Larynx and Hypopharynx," focuses specifically on the larynx and hypopharynx. The anatomy and pathology of these two anatomic areas are sufficiently interlinked to justify unifying this discussion into one chapter.

PART II: IMAGING OF PRIMARY AND NODAL SQUAMOUS CELL CARCINOMA

Part II covers imaging of primary and nodal squamous cell carcinoma. In this discussion the classic descriptive terms "nasopharynx" and "oropharynx" are utilized to discuss mucosal surfaces where primary squamous cell carcinoma arise. Chapter 12, "Squamous Cell Carcinoma: Primary Tumor Staging and Follow-up," focuses on the broader issues of staging primary tumor. Sections on perineural tumor spread, tumor recurrence, unknown primary tumor search, and radiation therapy port planning are all included. The discussion of CT vs MR in the staging of squamous cell carcinoma is emphasized, and suggested CT and MR protocols are included. The most current T (primary tumor) stages from the American Joint Commission on Cancer handbook are summarized and translated into radiologic terms in this chapter.

Chapter 13, "Squamous Cell Carcinoma: Nodal Staging," delves intensively into the clinical and radiologic issues of nodal staging of squamous cell carcinoma. An in-depth discussion of the normal nodal lymph node chains in the neck is followed by the radiologic criteria used to stage malignant adenopathy in the neck in the setting of known squamous cell carcinoma. American Joint Commission on Cancer guidelines are summarized in radiologic terms in the tables.

PART III: IMAGING OF THE FACE

Part III on imaging of the face is confined to the anatomic areas of the orbit (Chapter 14) and the sinonasal region (Chapter 15). The orbital chapter is divided up by major anatomic area as possible. These subdivisions include the globe, optic nerve and sheath, conal-intraconal area and extraconal area. A section on congenital-pediatric lesions is also included.

The sinonasal region chapter has been significantly expanded to include an in-depth discussion of the normal anatomy and imaging issues surrounding the use of coronal sinus CT in the evaluation of patients with sinusitis. Multiple additional figures illustrate the classic obstructive inflammatory patterns and the relevant mucociliary drainage anatomy. In addition, there is a new section in this chapter concerning the development of sinuses and congenital lesions in and around the sinonasal area.

PART IV: IMAGING OF THE SKULL BASE AND CRANIAL NERVES

The volume concludes with five chapters in Part IV covering imaging of the skull base and cranial nerves. This portion of the book begins with Chapter 16, "The Skull Base," which focuses on the normal bony and foraminal anatomy of the skull base. Chapter 17, "The Temporal Bone: External, Middle, and Inner Ear Segments," discusses the anatomy and imaging issues of the temporal bone area. This chapter is divided into external, middle, and inner ear segments with the anatomy and pathology of each of these three portions of the temporal bone discussed from this perspective.

Chapters 18 and 19 cover the complex anatomy and pathology of "The Upper Cranial Nerves" and "The Lower Cranial Nerves," respectively. Multiple additional drawings have been added to these two chapters to help you with the job of relearning your cranial nerve anatomy.

The book concludes with Chapter 20, "Sensorineural Hearing Loss with Emphasis on the Cerebellopontine Angle and Inner Ear." The central acoustic pathway from its origins in the cochlea to its termination in the superior temporal gyrus is discussed in segments. Multiple new drawings are provided to enhance your anatomic understanding of this area.

H. Ric Harnsberger, M.D.

Contents

I
Imaging of the
Suprahyoid and Infrahyoid Neck

1

Introduction to the Suprahyoid Neck

CRITICAL IMAGING QUESTIONS: SUPRAHYOID NECK

1. Name the three layers of deep cervical fascia and the spaces they define.
2. Describe an approach to analyzing and interpreting masses of the suprahyoid neck.
3. Which space in the suprahyoid neck is the *key space* in the evaluation of deep facial masses? Why is this space the critical space of the suprahyoid neck?
4. When a midline mass is found in the posterior oropharynx, the displacement of what structure helps to define whether the mass is in the retropharyngeal or perivertebral space?

Answers to these questions are found in the text beside the question number (Q#) in the margin.

SUPRAHYOID NECK

A. Introduction

1. General comments.
   a. In this book the extracranial head and neck have been divided at the hyoid bone into two distinct regions, termed the *suprahyoid neck* and the *infrahyoid neck* (Fig. 1-1). The hyoid bone has been chosen as the line of division, because the fascial attachments to it functionally cleave the neck into these two regions.
   b. The region of the extracranial head and neck from the skull base to the hyoid bone is referred to as the suprahyoid neck. The remaining neck from the hyoid bone to the cervicothoracic junction is the infrahyoid neck.
      1) Previously, the suprahyoid neck was discussed in terms of the nasopharynx, oropharynx, and oral cavity, because squamous cell carcinoma was staged along these lines. Chapter 12 follows these traditional divisions in its discussion of staging of squamous cell carcinoma (SCCa); in this context these traditional pharyngeal subdivisions remain extremely useful.
      2) Because the spaces of the suprahyoid neck as defined by the deep cervical fascia cut across the boundaries of the nasopharynx and oropharynx, however, the involvement of these fascia by diseases other than SCCa is poorly described using the more traditional pharyngeal subdivisions.
      3) Instead, a spatial radiologic analysis of deep facial lesions is presented as a practical alternative to the nonfascially oriented pharyngeal subdivisions of nasopharynx and oropharynx, which gives the radiologist a useful method for analyzing nonsquamous lesions of the deep face.
         a) This spatial orientation is most useful in analyzing the axial CT and MRI scans viewed by us all on a day-to-day basis.
      4) In this discussion the oral cavity is excluded, but it is considered in Chapter 8 as a unique region of the suprahyoid neck. This is because the spaces of the oral cavity (sublingual and submandibular spaces) are confined to the oral cavity and do not display the same craniocaudad extent seen in the deep facial spaces.
   c. Masses of the suprahyoid neck generally are now imaged either with CT or MRI before surgical intervention. Each method has its own strengths and weaknesses, but the ability of MRI to differentiate tumor–muscle interfaces, skull base and intracranial invasion, as well as perineural tumor spread gives it an edge over CT in the suprahyoid neck for the majority of cases when a mass is being eval-

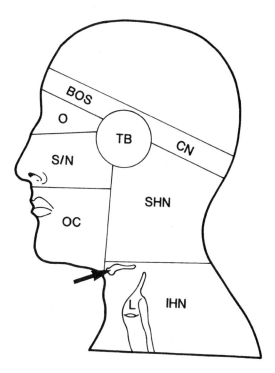

Fig. 1-1   The "head and neck man." In teaching and writing about the extracranial head and neck area the discussion is usually divided by the major anatomic regions shown in this drawing. The suprahyoid neck (*SHN*) represents the deep core tissues posterior to the sinonasal (*S/N*) and oral cavity (*OC*) areas. Below the level of the hyoid bone (*arrow*) the infrahyoid neck (*IHN*) can be seen. A distinct area within the infrahyoid neck is the larynx (*L*). *BOS*, Base of skull; *CN*, cranial nerves; *O*, orbit; *TB*, temporal bone.

uated. In the infrahyoid neck where fat is more plentiful, CT and MRI are comparable insofar as the information they provide.

d. This chapter principally focuses on the normal anatomy of the suprahyoid neck. The three layers of deep cervical fascia are used to delineate the individual spaces between the skull base and the hyoid bone. Once the spaces are defined and their critical contents enumerated, a description of how to determine the space of origin of a mass found in the deep face is presented.

e. As an introduction to the suprahyoid neck, this chapter presents a great deal of information. The chapters that follow discuss each of the spaces in greater detail, allowing the reader to digest the material more fully. In follow-up chapters a thorough discussion of unique, space-specific, differential diagnoses is presented.

2. Radiologic evaluation of lesions in the deep spaces of the suprahyoid neck.
   a. When a mass of the suprahyoid neck is suspected by the clinician, three questions are posed to the radiologist at the time of CT or MRI.
      1) Where is the mass (what *space* is it in)?
      2) What important neurovascular structures are in the vicinity of the mass?
      3) What is the likely pathologic diagnosis to be found at surgery?
   b. To answer these questions the radiologist needs a rational approach to analyzing masses of the suprahyoid neck. Such an approach is built on normal spatial anatomy coupled with pattern recognition of the radiographic appearance of a mass in each of the major spaces of the suprahyoid neck.
   c. This chapter begins with a careful review of the anatomy of the spaces of the suprahyoid neck. Following this, the radiologic features that identify a mass as primary to a specific space are presented. Space-specific differential diagnoses can be found in the subsequent chapters describing individual spaces of the suprahyoid neck.

B. The normal suprahyoid neck; the old way.

1. In the past the suprahyoid neck was divided into three areas, termed *nasopharynx, oropharynx,* and *oral cavity* (Fig. 1-2). This method of subdivision is effective when the primary concern is radiologic staging of SCCa, because the primary tumor in each of these areas have different routes of spread, nodal dissemination patterns, and prognosis. These terms are ineffective when nonsquamous lesions are under investigation, because nonsquamous masses spread within fascia-defined spaces.
2. Inasmuch as the terms nasopharynx, oropharynx, and oral cavity are still essential to the staging of SCCa, students of the head and neck must be familiar with them. This discussion of the suprahyoid neck begins using the traditional pharyngeal subdivision terminology.
3. Nasopharynx (Fig. 1-2).
   a. The nasopharynx sits atop the upper aerodigestive tract as a midline, tubular structure functioning as a conduit for air and secretions from the nose and sinuses.
   b. Boundaries of the nasopharynx.
      1) Anterior: Posterior nasal cavity at the nasal choana.
      2) Posterosuperior: Lower clivus, upper cervical spine, and prevertebral muscles.

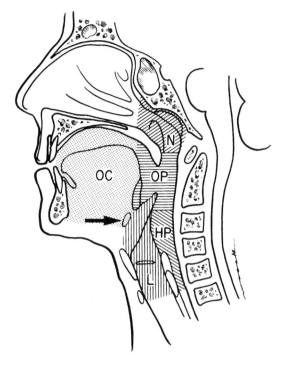

Fig. 1-2   Normal upper aerodigestive tract. This sagittal drawing of upper aerodigestive tract illustrates its major subdivisions: the nasopharynx (*N*), oropharynx (*OP*), oral cavity (*OC*), hypopharynx (*HP*), and larynx (*L*). Only the most cephalad aspect of the larynx and hypopharynx is above the hyoid bone (*arrow*). This traditional method of subdivision for the upper aerodigestive tract follows along the lines of the primary sites in the extracranial head and neck where squamous cell carcinoma is found. This traditional terminology remains central to the staging issued in squamous cell carcinoma of the upper aerodigestive tract.

      3) Inferior: Divided from the oropharynx by a horizontal line drawn along the hard and soft palates.

      4) Lateral wall: Composed of the torus tubarius (cartilaginous eustachian tube), the eustachian tube orifice, and the mucosa of the lateral pharyngeal recess (fossa of Rosenmüller).

   c) Nasopharyngeal carcinoma is the most common malignant lesion seen in the nasopharynx. Staging of this tumor is discussed in Chapter 12.

4. Oropharynx (Fig. 1-2).

   a. The oropharynx is the region of the upper aerodigestive tract that is visible posteriorly through the open mouth. Newcomers to the field of head and neck imaging frequently confuse the oral cavity with the oropharynx. Using these terms interchangeably demonstrates a basic lack of understanding that tends to unnerve referring clinicians.

   b. Boundaries.
   1) Anterior: A ring of structures separates the oropharynx from the oral cavity. This ring includes the circumvallate papillae of the tongue, the anterior tonsillar pillars, and the soft palate. The lingual tonsil is in the oropharynx and not the oral cavity.
   2) Posterior: Superior and middle constrictor muscles.
   3) Inferior: Separated from the larynx by the epiglottis and glossoepiglottic fold and from the hypopharynx by the pharyngoepiglottic fold.
   4) Superior: The soft palate forms the roof of the oropharynx.
   c. Staging of oropharyngeal SCCa is presented in Chapter 12.
5. The exact contents of the nasopharynx, oropharynx, and oral cavity depends on how much of the adjacent deep tissues are included. In the past these areas were subdivided into medial, lateral, and posterior compartments as a mechanism for discussion of the contents and the diseases that affect this region.
   a. Inasmuch as the term *compartment* has little practical application to the surgeon operating in the deep face, it is dispensed with in favor of surgically and pathologically defined *spaces* of the suprahyoid neck. Table 1-1 compares the old compartmental terminology with the newer, spatial terminology.

C. Normal spaces of the suprahyoid neck: a new look.

1. The spaces of the suprahyoid neck were originally described by anatomists in the nineteenth century as they dissected the layers of the deep cervical fascia.

Table 1-1   Compartments versus Spaces of the Suprahyoid Neck

Compartment	Space
Medial	Pharyngeal mucosal space (PMS)
Lateral	Parapharyngeal space (PPS)
	Masticator space (MS)
	Parotid space (PS)
	Carotid space (CS)
Posterior	Retropharyngeal space (RPS)
	Danger space (DS)
	Perivertebral space (PVS)

2. These spaces were rediscovered in the twentieth century by surgeons dissecting abscess pockets confined within the spaces of the suprahyoid neck.

3. Over the years a confusing array of terms have been used to describe the deep cervical fascia and the spaces they define.

  a. The following is a practical summation of the anatomic and surgical literature regarding the fascia and spaces of the suprahyoid neck. It is aimed at providing a working terminology for the physician in this field.

4. Deep cervical fascia.

  a. Three layers of deep cervical fascia exist throughout the extracranial head and neck, encompassing the anatomic structures of both the suprahyoid and infrahyoid necks.

  b. In the suprahyoid neck these three layers cleave the region into the deep spaces of the face.

Q #1

  c. In the suprahyoid neck the layers of deep cervical fascia are:

  1) Superficial layer (investing fascia).
  2) Middle layer (buccopharyngeal fascia).
  3) Deep layer (prevertebral fascia).

  d. The spaces defined by the three layers of deep cervical fascia include:

  1) Parapharyngeal space (PPS; see Chapter 2).
  2) Pharyngeal mucosal space (PMS; see Chapter 2).
  3) Masticator space (MS; see Chapter 3).
  4) Parotid space (PS; see Chapter 4).
  5) Carotid space (CS; see Chapter 5).
  6) Retropharyngeal space (RPS; see Chapter 6).
  7) Perivertebral space (PVS; see Chapter 7).

  e. Chapters 2 through 7 discuss the contents, differential diagnosis, and imaging issues specific to each space.

  f. All but two of the spaces are *true fascia-enclosed spaces;* that is, they are completely circumscribed by the three layers of deep cervical fascia. Exceptions are the parapharyngeal space and the pharyngeal mucosal space. These two spaces have complex fascial borders with multiple fascia constituting the space margins.

  1) The parapharyngeal space has complex borders made up of the superficial layer of deep cervical fascia along the deep margin of the masticator and parotid spaces anterolaterally, the middle layer medially, and all three layers in the carotid sheath posteriorly (Figs. 1-3 to 1-6).
  2) The pharyngeal mucosal space is bounded by the middle layer of deep cervical fascia along its posterolateral margin. On its "airway" side, however, there is no fascia (Figs. 1-3 to 1-6).

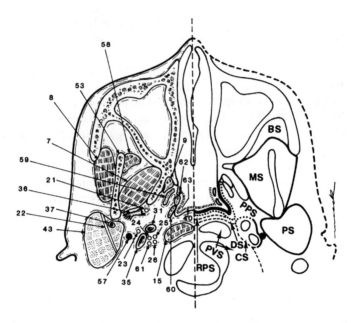

Fig. 1-3 Axial view of the normal anatomy of the midnasopharynx. *Left,* Critical anatomy of the region. Note that the darkest curvilinear line on the right (the pharyngobasilar fascia) is only seen in the most cephalad portion of the nasopharynx, where it connects the superior constrictor muscle to the skull base. The pharyngobasilar fascia is within the pharyngeal mucosal space at this level. *Right,* Three layers of deep cervical fascia and the spaces they define. See page 27 for the key to numbered and lettered structures. (From Harnsberger HR: CT and MRI masses of the deep face. *Curr Probl Diagn Radiol* 16:141–173, 1987. Used by permission.)

5. The transaxial and coronal relationships of the fascia and spaces of the suprahyoid neck are illustrated in Figs. 1-3 to 1-7. In each figure the fascia and spaces are shown on the right and the critical contents on the left. Table 1-2 summarizes the contents of each of these spaces.
   a. Note in the coronal drawing (Fig. 1-7), that no horizontal fascia separates the nasopharynx from the oropharynx. Instead, spaces (e.g., parapharyngeal and masticator spaces) are contiguous from the nasopharyngeal to the oropharyngeal area without fascial interruption.
      1) The deep facial spaces abut the skull base at their cranial end, as defined by Fig. 1-8. This strategic interaction between the spaces and skull-base apertures is fully discussed in Chapter 16.

Table 1-2   Critical Contents of the Deep Spaces of the Suprahyoid Head and Neck

Parapharyngeal space (PPS)	Retromandibular vein
Fat	External carotid and internal maxillary
Branches of cranial nerve V_3	arteries
Internal maxillary artery	Intraparotid lymph nodes
Ascending pharyngeal artery	
Pharyngeal venous plexus	**Carotid space (CS)**
	Internal carotid artery
Pharyngeal mucosal space (PMS)	Internal jugular vein
Lymphoid tissue (adenoids, faucial and	Cranial nerves IX through XII
lingual tonsils)	Sympathetic plexus
Superior, middle constrictor muscles	Lymph nodes (deep cervical chain)
Salpingopharyngeus muscle	
Pharyngobasilar fascia	**Retropharyngeal space (RPS)**
Levator palatini muscle*	Fat
Torus tubarius aspect of the eustachian	Lateral retropharyngeal nodes
tube (defined as the projecting pos-	(of Rouviere)
terior lip of the pharyngeal opening	Medial retropharyngeal nodes
of the eustachian tube)*	
	Danger Space (DS)
Masticator space (MS)	Fat
Lateral pterygoid muscle	
Medial pterygoid muscle	**Perivertebral space (PVS)**
Masseter muscle	Prevertebral component
Temporalis muscle	Prevertebral muscles
Inferior alveolar nerve (branch of cra-	Vertebral artery
nial nerve V_3)	Vertebral vein
Ramus and body of mandible	Scalene muscles
	Brachial plexus
Parotid space (PS)	Phrenic nerve
Parotid gland	Paraspinal component
Facial nerve	Paraspinal muscles

*Originates outside PMS from lateral skull base.

    2) The three-dimensional relationships of these spaces in the craniocaudal direction is depicted in Fig. 1-9.

    3) The two most important interactions of the deep spaces and the skull base are the parotid space-stylomastoid foramen-cranial nerve VII and the masticator space-foramen ovale-cranial nerve V_3.

  b. Also observe the relatively central location of the parapharyngeal space as it relates to the surrounding pharyngeal mucosal, masticator, parotid, and carotid spaces. This central location is extremely

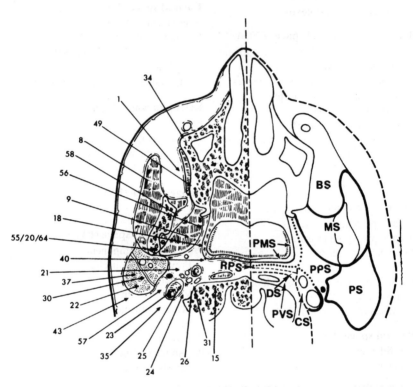

Fig. 1-4   Axial view of the normal anatomy of the low nasopharynx through the level of the soft palate. *Left,* Critical contents of spaces. *Right,* Three layers of deep cervical fascia and spaces. See page 27 for the key to numbered and lettered structures. (From Harnsberger HR: CT and MRI masses of the deep face. *Curr Probl Diagn Radiol* 16:141–173, 1987. Used by permission.)

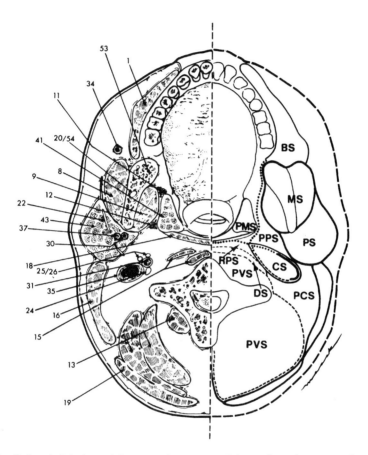

Fig. 1-5   Axial view of the normal anatomy of the midoropharynx. *Left,* Critical contents of spaces. *Right,* Three layers of deep cervical fascia and spaces. See page 27 for the key to numbered and lettered structures. (From Hardin CW, Harnsberger HR, Osborn AG, et al: CT in the evaluation of the normal and diseased oral cavity and oropharynx. *Semin Ultrasound CT MR* 7:131–153, 1986. Used by permission.)

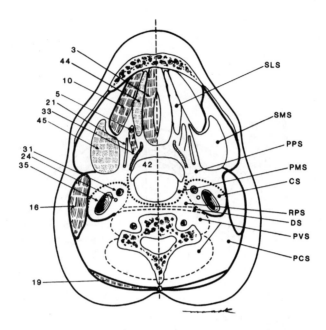

Fig. 1-6 Axial view showing the normal anatomy of the low oropharynx. *Left,* Critical contents of spaces. *Right,* Three layers of deep cervical fascia and spaces. See page 27 for the key to numbered and lettered structures.

important in determining the space of origin of a mass in the suprahyoid neck.

D. Radiographic evaluation of masses of the deep face.

1. Method of mass analysis.
   a. When a mass is identified in the suprahyoid neck, the principal question that must be answered is: what is the space of origin of the mass?

Q #2
   b. To answer this question it is necessary to understand the basic spatial anatomy and terminology of the suprahyoid neck, as already described. The mass is given a space of origin by considering its center (relative to the parapharyngeal space) and its displacement pattern (of the parapharyngeal space) (Fig. 1-10).
   c. What emerges from repeated use of this method is pattern recognition of the appearance of a mass in each individual space.

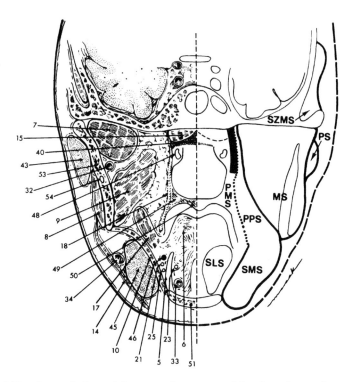

Fig. 1-7   Coronal view of the normal anatomy of the deep face. This vantage point best delineates the craniocaudad extent of the deep facial spaces, especially the pharyngeal mucosal, parapharyngeal, and masticator spaces. Note that no horizontal fascia divide the deep spaces. As a result, infection and tumor spread in either a cranial or caudal direction without obstructing fascial barriers. *Left,* Critical contents of spaces. *Right,* Three layers of deep cervical fascia. See page 27 for the key to numbered and lettered structures. (From Hardin CW, Harnsberger HR, Osborn AG, et al: CT in the evaluation of the normal and diseased oral cavity and oropharynx. *Semin Ultrasound CT MR* 7:131–153, 1986. Used by permission.)

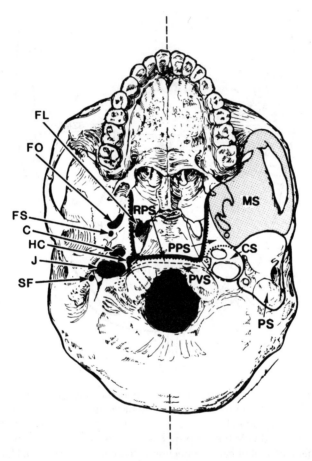

Fig. 1-8   The skull base seen from below, depicting the interaction of the spaces of the deep face and the skull-base foramen. On the left are the important apertures, while on the right are the deep spaces abutting the skull base. *Heavy line*, pharyngobasilar fascia; *light line*, superficial layer of deep cervical fascia; *dotted line*, middle layer, deep cervical fascia; *dashed line*, deep layer, deep cervical fascia. Foramina/canals: *C*, carotid canal; *FL*, foramen lacerum; *FO*, foramen ovale; *FS*, foramen spinosum; *HC*, hypoglossal canal; *J*, jugular foramen; *SF*, stylomastoid foramen. Spaces: *CS*, carotid space; *MS*, masticator space; *PPS*, parapharyngeal space; *PVS*, perivertebral space, prevertebral portion; *RPS*, retropharyngeal space. (From Osborn AG, Harnsberger HR, Smoker WRK: Base of skull imaging. *Semin Ultrasound CT MR* 7:91–106, 1986. Used by permission.)

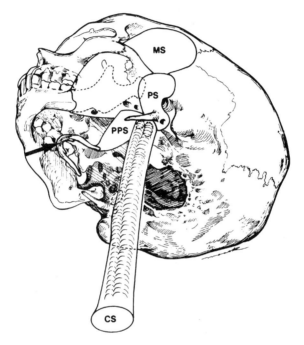

Fig. 1-9   Oblique view of the major deep facial spaces as seen from below. This figure provides a three-dimensional sense for the spaces of the suprahyoid neck, especially in the craniocaudad dimension.   Note that of the spaces included in the drawing, only the carotid space traverses both the suprahyoid and the infrahyoid neck. The perivertebral and retropharyngeal spaces (not shown) also traverse the entire neck. *CS,* Carotid space; *MS,* Masticator space; *PPS,* parapharyngeal space; *PS,* parotid space; *arrow,* hyoid bone.

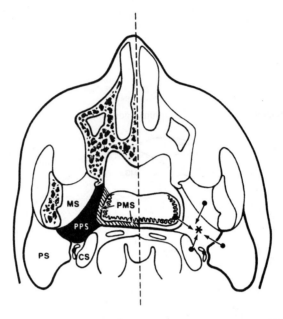

Fig. 1-10 Axial view of the midnasopharynx shows the center (*black dots*) of the four main deep fascial spaces and the displacement pattern that would occur relative to the parapharyngeal space (*PPS; asterisk*) if a mass was present in any of these spaces. The PPS is the central space on each side of the core tissues of the deep face. Although almost no disease process begins in the PPS primarily, its central location and conspicuity on CT and MR imaging make it a vital space to recognize. *CS,* Carotid space; *MS,* masticator space; *PMS,* pharyngeal mucosal space; *PS,* parotid space.

    d. Once the space of origin is assigned, the unique, space-specific, differential diagnosis is matched with the radiologic features of the mass.

    e. This approach often yields a short list of diagnostic possibilities. At worst this method provides the surgeon with a precise understanding of the space occupied by the mass and an awareness of the critical adjacent neurovascular structures.

Q #3

    f. Figs. 1-11 to 1-14 demonstrate the major appearance of masses in the four spaces of the deep face that encircle the parapharyngeal space.

       1) Note that for the spaces surrounding the parapharyngeal space (pharyngeal mucosal, masticator, parotid, and carotid spaces), the center is defined relative to the parapharyngeal space (Table 1-3).

Table 1-3   Strategic Location of the Parapharyngeal Space

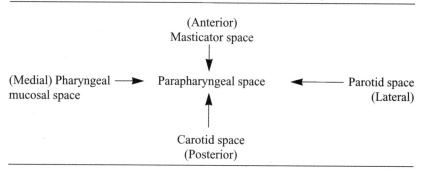

```
                         (Anterior)
                       Masticator space
                             │
                             ▼
(Medial) Pharyngeal  ──▶  Parapharyngeal space  ◀──────  Parotid space
mucosal space                ▲                            (Lateral)
                             │
                             │
                       Carotid space
                       (Posterior)
```

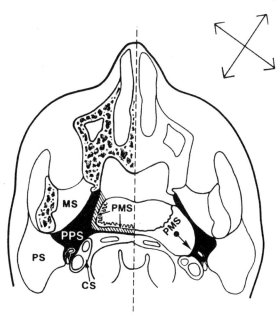

Fig. 1-11   Axial view of the midnasopharynx shows the center (*black dot*) and the displacement pattern of a mass primary to the pharyngeal mucosal space (*PMS*). Note that the center is medial to the laterally displaced parapharyngeal space (*PPS*). Also note the vector of spread (*arrow*) of the mass from medial to lateral. The most common lesion primary to the PMS is squamous cell carcinoma. (From Harnsberger HR: CT and MRI masses of the deep face. *Curr Probl Diagn Radiol* 16:141–173, 1987. Used by permission.)

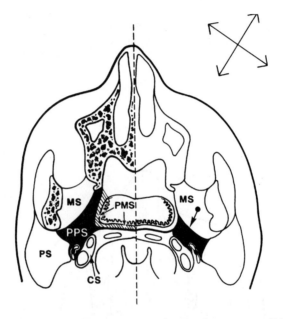

Fig. 1-12   Axial view of a mass primary to the masticator space (MS) demonstrates the center (*black dot*) of the lesion to be anterior to the posteriorly displaced parapharyngeal space (PPS). Note the mass vector of spread (*arrow*) from anterior to posterior. The most common lesions of the MS are odontogenic abscess and sarcomatous tumors. (From Harnsberger HR: CT and MRI masses of the deep face. *Curr Probl Diagn Radiol;* 16:141–173, 1987. Used by permission.)

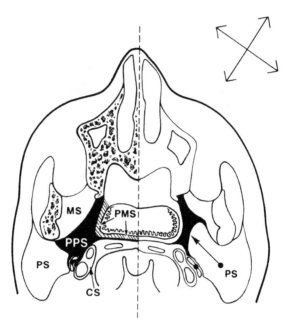

Fig. 1-13   Axial view of a mass primary to the deep aspect of the parotid space (*PS*) shows the center (*black dot*) of the lesion to be lateral to the medially displaced parapharyngeal space (*PPS*). Note the mass vector of spread (*arrow*) from lateral to medial and the associated widening of the stylomandibular notch. Benign mixed tumor and mucoepidermoid carcinoma are the most common benign and malignant tumors found in the PS.   (From Harnsberger HR: CT and MRI masses of the deep face. *Curr Probl Diagn Radiol* 16:141–173, 1987. Used by permission.)

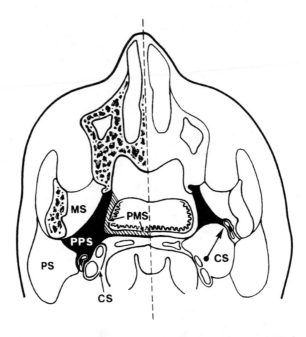

Fig. 1-14   Axial view of a mass primary to the carotid space (*CS*) demonstrates the center (*black dot*) of the lesion to be posterior to the anteriorly displaced parapharyngeal space (*PPS*). Note the mass vector of spread (*arrow*) from posterior to anterior and in the more cephalad carotid space lesions, the styloid process is lifted anterolaterally. Paraganglioma and schwannoma are the two most commonly encountered tumors of the CS. (From Harnsberger HR: CT and MRI masses of the deep face. *Curr Probl Diagn Radiol* 16:141–173, 1987. Used by permission.)

    2) Also observe that the displacement pattern of each specific space is also defined by the mass effect of the lesion on the parapharyngeal space (Fig. 1-10).

Q #4

  g. Figs. 1-15 to 1-18 show the important features of masses in the two midline spaces of the suprahyoid neck (the retropharyngeal and perivertebral spaces). The relationship of the mass to the prevertebral muscles is the pivotal radiologic feature defining the space of origin within these two spaces (Table 1-4).

    1) In the case of a retropharyngeal space mass that fills the whole space (Fig. 1-15), the prevertebral muscles are displaced posteriorly.

    2) A mass in the prevertebral portion of the perivertebral space displaces the prevertebral muscles anteriorly (Fig. 1-16).

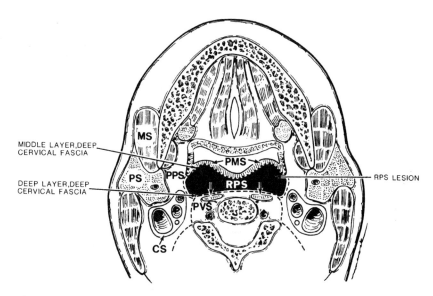

MIDDLE LAYER,DEEP
CERVICAL FASCIA

DEEP LAYER,DEEP
CERVICAL FASCIA

MS

PMS

PS   PPS   RPS

PVS

CS

RPS LESION

Fig. 1-15   Axial view of a mass primary to the entire retropharyngeal space
(*RPS*) at the level of the low oropharynx illustrating the "bow-tie" shape of this
space when diseased. The relationship to the parapharyngeal space is no longer
important in the case of lesions of the posterior midline spaces. Instead, the characteristic shape and anterior location relative to the prevertebral muscles define
the space of origin as the RPS. RPS lesions involving the entire space are most
commonly abscesses that have broken out of RPS suppurative nodes and extranodal squamous cell carcinoma.

Table 1-4   The Prevertebral Muscles Help to Define the Location of a Mass in the Posterior Midline Spaces

(Anterior)

Retropharyngeal space mass

↓

Prevertebral muscles

↑

Perivertebral space mass

(Posterior)

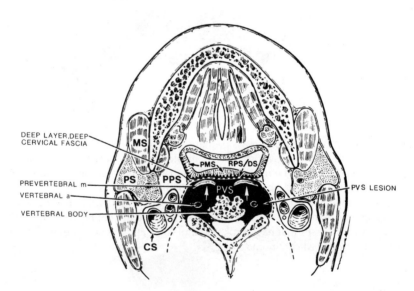

Fig. 1-16   Axial view of a mass primary to the prevertebral portion of the perivertebral space (*PVS*) at the level of the low oropharynx demonstrating the lesion to be posterior to the elevated prevertebral muscles (*white arrows*). Note the involvement of the adjacent vertebral body, which is often seen in PVS lesions. By far the two most common lesions seen in the PVS are abscesses from vertebral body osteomyelitis and metastatic tumor that spreads from the adjacent vertebral body.

3) A mass in the paraspinal portion of the perivertebral space is easily visualized on axial imaging. The mass either arises within the
   posterior elements of the vertebral body with centrifugal displacement of paraspinal muscles (Fig. 1-17) or begins within the
   muscles themselves.
4) When the mass is in the lateral recess of the retropharyngeal
   space (i.e., is a nodal mass), the displacement pattern is only
   slightly different from a carotid space mass (Fig. 1-18). The only
   difference between a nodal mass in the retropharyngeal space
   and a mass in the carotid space is the more medial location of the
   nodal retropharyngeal space lesion. (See Chapter 6 for a more
   detailed discussion.)

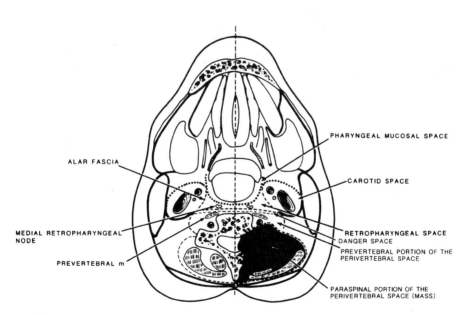

ALAR FASCIA

PHARYNGEAL MUCOSAL SPACE

CAROTID SPACE

MEDIAL RETROPHARYNGEAL NODE

PREVERTEBRAL m

RETROPHARYNGEAL SPACE
DANGER SPACE
PREVERTEBRAL PORTION OF THE PERIVERTEBRAL SPACE

PARASPINAL PORTION OF THE PERIVERTEBRAL SPACE (MASS)

Fig. 1-17   Appearance of a mass in the paraspinal portion of the perivertebral
space at the level of the low oropharynx. The mass arises from the posterior elements of the vertebral body and displaces the paraspinal muscles away from the
center. An epidural component is visible within the spinal canal.

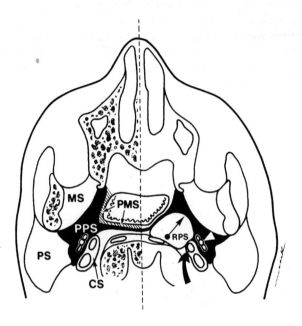

Fig. 1-18   Axial view of a mass primary to the lateral aspect of the retropharyngeal space (*RPS*) shows the center (*black dot*) of the lesion to be posteromedial to the parapharyngeal space (*PPS*). Note the mass vector of spread (*arrow*) from posteromedial to anterolateral. The difference between a mass of carotid space origin and a mass from the lateral aspect of the RPS can be subtle, but the center of the lateral RPS mass is always medial to the internal carotid artery (*curved arrow*) and does not displace the styloid process (*white arrowhead*) unless the mass is large. Inflammatory nodal disease and nodal tumors (squamous cell carcinoma, non-Hodgkin lymphoma, and other metastases) constitute the most commonly seen lesions is the lateral retropharyngeal nodal chain.

Key to Chapter 1 Figures (Figs. 1-3 to 1-7)

Muscles

1 = buccinator
2 = digastric (anterior belly)
3 = genioglossus
4 = geniohyoid
5 = hyoglossus
6 = intrinsic, of tongue
7 = lateral pterygoid
8 = masseter
9 = medial pterygoid
10 = mylohyoid
11 = palatoglossus (anterior tonsillar pillar)
12 = palatopharyngeus (posterior tonsillar pillar)
13 = paraspinal
14 = platysma
15 = prevertebral
16 = sternocleidomastoid
17 = styloglossus
18 = superior pharyngeal constrictor
19 = trapezius
58 = temporalis
59 = tensor palatini

Vessels

30 = external carotid artery
31 = internal carotid artery
32 = internal maxillary artery
33 = lingual artery
34 = facial vein
35 = jugular vein
36 = pharyngeal venous plexus
37 = retromandibular vein
64 = inferior alveolar artery

Miscellaneous

40 = adenoids
41 = faucial tonsil
42 = lingual tonsil
43 = parotid gland
44 = sublingual gland
45 = submandibular gland
46 = submandibular gland duct
47 = lingual septum
48 = cartilaginous eustachian tube

49 = soft palate
50 = uvula
62 = torus tubarius
63 = lateral pharyngeal recess (fossa of Rosenmüller)

Nerves

20 = inferior alveolar (branch of V_3)
21 = lingual (branch of V_3)
22 = facial (VII)
23 = glossopharyngeal (IX)
24 = vagus (X)
25 = hypoglossal (XII)
26 = sympathetic plexus
61 = spinal accessory

Spaces

BS = buccal space
CS = carotid space
MS = masticator space
PCS = posterior cervical space
PPS = parapharyngeal space
PS = parotid space
PVS = perivertebral space
RPS = retropharyngeal space
SLS = sublingual space
SMS = submandibular space
SZMS = suprazygomatic masticator space (temporal space, temporal fossa)

Bone

51 = hyoid
52 = body of mandible
53 = ramus of mandible
54 = mandibular canal
55 = mandibular foramen
56 = hamulus
57 = styloid process

Fascia

Deep Cervical Fascia (DCF)
_____ = superficial layer, DCF
.... = middle layer, DCF
-------- = deep layer, DCF
▬▬▬▬ = pharyngobasilar fascia

SUGGESTED READING

Babbel RW, Harnsberger HR: The parapharyngeal space: the key to unlocking the suprahyoid neck. *Semin Ultrasound CT MR* 11:444–459, 1990.

Braun IF, Hoffman JC: Computer tomography of the buccomasseteric region. I: anatomy. *AJNR* 5:605–610, 1984.

Davis WL, Harnsberger HR, Smoker WRK, et al: Retropharyngeal space: evaluation of the normal anatomy and diseases with CT and MR imaging. *Radiology* 174:59–64.

Dillon WP, Mills CM, Kjos B, et al: Magnetic resonance imaging of the nasopharynx. *Radiology* 152:731–738, 1984.

Hardin CW, Harnsberger HR, Osborn AG, et al: CT in the evaluation of the normal and diseased oral cavity and oropharynx. *Semin Ultrasound CT MR* 6:131–153, 1986.

Hardin CW, Harnsberger HR, Osborn AG, et al: Infection and tumor of the masticator space: CT evaluation. *Radiology* 157:413–417, 1985.

Harnsberger HR: CT and MRI of masses of the deep face. *Curr Probl Diagn Radiol* 16:141–173, 1987.

Harnsberger HR, Osborn AG: Differential diagnosis of head and neck lesions based on their space of origin. 1. The suprahyoid part of the neck. *Am J Roentgenol* 157:147–154, 1991.

Hollinshead WH: *Textbook of anatomy*, ed 1. New York, 1967, Harper & Row.

Hoover LA, Hanafee WN: Differential diagnosis of nasopharyngeal tumors by computed tomographic scanning. *Arch Otolaryngol* 109:43–47, 1983.

Last RJ: *Anatomy: regional and applied*, ed 6. New York, 1978, Churchill Livingstone.

McCrath P, Mills P: *Atlas of sectional anatomy: head, neck, and trunk*, Basel, 1984, S Karger AG.

Mancuso AA, Hanafee WN: *Computed tomography and magnetic resonance imaging of the head and neck*, ed 2. Baltimore, 1985, Williams & Wilkins.

Paonessa DF, Goldstein JC: Anatomy and physiology of head and neck infections (with emphasis on the fascia of the face and neck). *Otolaryngol Clin North Am* 9:561–580, 1976.

Silver AJ, Mawad ME, Hilal SK, et al: Computed tomography of the nasopharynx and related spaces. I: anatomy. *Radiology* 147:725–731, 1983.

Silver AJ, Mawad ME, Hilal SK, et al: Computed tomography of the nasopharynx and related spaces. II: pathology. *Radiology* 147:733–738, 1983.

Smoker WRK, Gentry RG: Computed tomography of the nasopharynx and related spaces. *Semin Ultrasound CT MR* 6:107–129, 1986.

Smoker WRK, Harnsberger HR: Differential diagnosis of head and neck lesions based on their space of origin. 2. The infrahyoid portion of the neck. *Am J Roentgenol* 157:155–159, 1991.

Som PM, Biller HR, Lawson W: Tumors of the parapharyngeal space: preoperative evaluation, diagnosis, and surgical approaches. *Ann Otol Rhinol Laryngol (Suppl)* 90:3–15; 1981.

Som PM, Sacher M, Stollman AL, et al: Common tumors of the parapharyngeal space: refined imaging diagnosis. *Radiology* 169:81–85, 1988.

Wong YK, Novotny GM: Retropharyngeal space: a review of anatomy, pathology, and clinical presentation. *J Otolaryngol* 7:528–536, 1978.

2

The Parapharyngeal Space and the Pharyngeal Mucosal Space

CRITICAL IMAGING QUESTIONS: PARAPHARYNGEAL SPACE AND PHARYNGEAL MUCOSAL SPACE

Parapharyngeal space:

1. If few lesions are found to originate in the parapharyngeal space, why is it so important to understand the anatomy and spatial relationship of the parapharyngeal space?

2. Using your knowledge of the location of the deep cervical fascia, how can a mass in the parapharyngeal space initially present as a submandibular space lesion?

3a. What is the one benign tumor that may be seen primarily originating within the parapharyngeal space?

3b. Why must we be certain that this benign tumor originated in the parapharyngeal space and not in the deep lobe of the parotid gland?

Pharyngeal mucosal space:

4. What radiologic features define a mass originating in the pharyngeal mucosal space?

5. What are the statistically common lesions of the pharyngeal mucosal space?

Answers to these questions are found in the text beside the question number (Q#) in the margin.

PARAPHARYNGEAL SPACE (PPS)

A. Introduction.

1. The parapharyngeal space (PPS) is the central space of the deep face, around which most of the other important spaces are situated. These surrounding spaces include the pharyngeal mucosal, masticator, parotid, carotid, and lateral retropharyngeal spaces.
2. Because the contents of the PPS are limited, few lesions actually arise in this space. Rather, most infections and tumors found in the PPS originate in one of the surrounding spaces mentioned previously.

Q#1
3. The importance of the PPS therefore is not what occurs in this space but how masses in the surrounding spaces displace the fat of the PPS (Fig. 2-1).
4. The center of a deep facial mass lesion relative to the PPS and the direction in which the mass displaces the PPS fat indicate its space of origin to the observer.

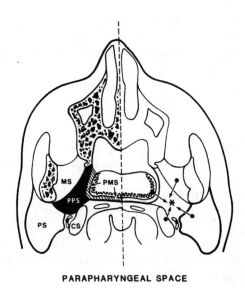

PARAPHARYNGEAL SPACE

Fig. 2-1 Axial view through the low nasopharynx emphasizing the central position held by the parapharyngeal space (*PPS; asterisk*). Although principally filled by fat alone, the PPS acts as the key to understanding the space of origin for masses of the deep face. It is displaced in a characteristic fashion by masses of the surrounding spaces (*arrows*). *CS,* Carotid space; *MS,* masticator space; *PMS,* pharyngeal mucosal space; *PS,* parotid space.

5. Because each space has its own unique differential diagnosis, identification of the space of origin for a mass lesion is the first and most important step in the analysis of CT or MRI of this area of the body. The
space-specific differential diagnosis arises from the fact that very different normal tissue types are seen in each of the spaces of the deep face.

    a. The statistically common lesions arising in these spaces come from
these space-specific tissues:

        1) Pharyngeal mucosal space: Mucosa, lymphoid tissue, minor sali-
vary glands.

        2) Masticator space: Muscles of mastication, mandible, V_3.

        3) Parotid space: Salivary tissue, lymph nodes, VII.

        4) Carotid space: Carotid artery, jugular vein, cranial nerves IX to
XII.

        5) Lateral retropharyngeal space: Lateral lymph nodes (Nodes of
Rouviere).

B. Normal anatomy.

1. Fascial margins. The fascial margins of the PPS are complex and made
up of different layers of the deep cervical fascia. (See Figs. 1-3 to 1-7.)

    a. The medial fascial margin of the PPS is made up of the middle layer
of deep cervical fascia as it curves around the lateral side of the pharyngeal mucosal space.

    b. The lateral fascial margin is formed by the medial slip of the super-
ficial layer of deep cervical fascia as it curves around the deep border of the masticator and parotid spaces.

    c. Posteriorly the PPS fascia is made up of the anterior part of the
carotid sheath, which is made up of all three layers of the deep cervical fascia.

2. Contents.

Fat.

Internal maxillary artery.

Ascending pharyngeal artery.

Pharyngeal venous plexus.

    a. The PPS has *no* mucosa, muscle, bone, nodes, or normal salivary
gland tissue within its boundaries. As a result it is unusual for a disease process to originate in the PPS.

    b. PPS fat.

        1) The fatty triangle of the PPS is easily identified on routine axial
CT and MRI. Even when a mass is present this fat can be seen as
displaced by the mass. Only when the mass is very large is the
PPS fat completely obscured.

        2) On coronal imaging the entire craniocaudal nature of the PPS is
easily identified. (See Fig. 1-7.)

    c. Pharyngeal venous plexus.
      1) At times the pharyngeal venous plexus may be very prominent and asymmetric, mimicking a vascular mass (i.e., radiologic pseudomass).
      2) Avoid misdiagnosing this pseudomass as a structural lesion that "needs to be biopsied."

3. Extent and boundaries.
    a. In the radiologic literature the term *parapharyngeal space* has been used to describe a larger area of the deep face than the fatty triangle we thus far have defined as the PPS. The carotid, medial parotid, and deep masticator spaces were included in this previous definition. Because the lumping of these pieces from adjacent spaces does not follow fascial planes and prevents formation of a unique differential diagnosis for each space, we will not pursue this older definition further. Instead we will adhere to the fascial definition of the PPS described earlier, confining it to the readily identifiable fatty triangle only.
    b. The PPS is a crescent-shaped space in the craniocaudal dimension and extends from the skull base to the superior cornu of the hyoid bone (see Fig 1-7). As a fatty tube separating the other deep facial spaces from one another, the PPS functions as an "elevator shaft" through which infection and tumor in these adjacent spaces may travel from the hyoid bone level to the skull base.

Q#2
    c. Inferiorly the PPS is not separated from the posterior aspect of the submandibular space by fascia. As a result of this open communication, lesions of the PPS may first become clinically obvious as submandibular space masses.
    d. Other PPS-bordering spaces include the masticator and parotid spaces laterally, the pharyngeal mucosal space medially, and the carotid space posteriorly. The lateral aspect of the retropharyngeal space can extend far enough to make up the posteromedial border of the PPS. (See Fig. 1-18.)

C. Imaging issues.

1. Imaging issues of the PPS are limited, because few lesions primarily arise in this space.
2. Interaction of the PPS fat with surrounding masses is the radiologic relationship used in the evaluation of deep facial lesions.
3. Only rarely does a mass actually originate in the PPS. Pleomorphic adenomas of minor salivary gland rests in the PPS, lipomas, and atypical second branchial cleft cysts are the only lesions known to originate in the PPS.

a. To say that a mass lesion originates in the PPS, fat must be identified surrounding the entire circumference of the lesion.

b. In most cases where a mass is originally thought to be in the PPS, careful inspection of a complete set of images reveals a point of attachment to one of the adjacent deep facial spaces, usually the deep lobe of the parotid.

D. Pitfalls in imaging the PPS.

1. When a lesion is discovered in the PPS, be sure that:

a. The entire PPS from skull base to hyoid bone is imaged.

b. The real space of origin for the infection or tumor is established, given that most lesions in the PPS do not originate there.

c. The lesion is not a PPS pseudomass (e.g., asymmetric pterygoid venous plexus).

2. PPS pseudomass.

a. Asymmetric pterygoid venous plexus.

1) The only pseudomass of the PPS is the asymmetric pterygoid venous plexus.

2) On enhanced CT this normal anatomic variant appears as a racemose-enhancing, high-density area along the medial border of the lateral pterygoid muscle. On MRI a contrast-enhancing area is seen in the same location on a T1-weighted fat suppressed axial image. At times only careful inspection of all imaging sequences allows for correct identification of this normal venous structure.

3) Do not mistake this normal variant as a focal vascular tumor.

E. Lesions (Table 2-1).

1. Congenital lesions.

a. Atypical second branchial cleft cyst.

1) Clinical presentation. Child or young adult with protruding parotid gland externally and bulging posterolateral pharyngeal wall internally. The mass may arise rapidly after an upper respiratory tract infection.

2) Pathologic findings. Thin-walled cyst lined with stratified squamous epithelium, with lymphoid tissue deep in the lining membrane. The fluid within is typically turbid, yellowish, and often contains cholesterol crystals. This rare type of second branchial cleft cyst projects in the PPS toward the skull base rather than downward to the mandibular angle (as in the typical second branchial cleft cyst).

3) Imaging features. A cystic mass is seen projecting from the oropharyngeal faucial tonsil deep margin up the PPS toward the

Table 2-1   Parapharyngeal Space Mass: Differential Diagnosis

Pseudomass
Asymmetric pterygoid venous plexus*

Congenital
Atypical (parapharyngeal) second branchial cleft cyst

Inflammatory
Abscess spread from adjacent deep facial spaces, especially*:
    Pharyngeal mucosal space: Adenoids, tonsils (tonsillitis)
    Parotid space: Calculus disease
    Masticator space: Odontogenic infection

Benign tumor
Pleomorphic adenoma (benign mixed tumor) of salivary gland rest in the PPS
Lipoma

Malignant tumor
Mucoepidermoid and adenoid cystic carcinoma and malignant mixed tumor of
    salivary gland rest in the PPS

Direct spread of malignant tumor from adjacent deep facial space, especially*:
    Pharyngeal mucosal space: Squamous cell carcinoma, non-Hodgkin
      lymphoma, minor salivary gland malignancy
    Masticator space: Sarcoma
    Parotid space: Mucoepidermoid carcinoma, adenoid cystic carcinoma

*More common lesion of the PPS.

skull base. On axial images the more cephalad component of the
lesion appears surrounded by the PPS fat, whereas on more caudal images it anneals to the deep margin of the faucial tonsil.

2. Inflammatory disease.
    a. PPS abscess.
        1) Clinical presentation. Symptoms depend on the space of origin
           of the infection. Pharyngitis usually precedes a pharyngeal
           mucosal space abscess that spreads to the PPS. Dental infection
           or manipulation can create masticator space infection with sub-
           sequent involvement of the PPS. Calculus disease may cause
           parotid space infection that secondarily involves the PPS.
        2) Imaging features. In the absence of penetrating trauma, PPS
           abscess will always be seen in conjunction with a second deep
           facial space infection. Search the study for the space of origin of
           the infectious process, and identify each space involved. If the
           PPS abscess abuts the skull base, carefully search the area for
           possible sites of osteomyelitis.

3) Comment.
    a) As a rule a drain must be placed in any space containing pus. The radiologist must help the surgeon in determining how many drains should be placed and the most cosmetic surgical approach to the drainage procedure.
    b) Radiologic evaluation of a suspected abscess in the head and neck region is best accomplished using CT and not MRI. CT allows the confident identification of abscess pockets but also permits identification of mandibular osteomyelitis and calculus disease. MRI may not help in identifying these important precipitating lesions.

3. Benign tumor.
  a. Pleomorphic adenoma (benign mixed tumor) of salivary tissue rest in the PPS.
    1) Clinical presentation. Posterolateral pharyngeal mass. Nonspecific clinical presentation.

Q#3a

    2) Pathologic findings. Same appearance as pleomorphic adenoma of the parotid gland but ectopic. The benign mixed tumor is the only tumor seen with any frequency originating in the PPS.
    3) Imaging features. Round to oval, well-circumscribed mass centered within the PPS. A rim of PPS fat can be seen around the periphery of the lesion. Enhanced CT usually demonstrates moderate, uniform enhancement; MR imaging shows mass intensity paralleling that of muscle.

Q#3b

    4) Comment. Before diagnosing pleomorphic adenoma as primary to the PPS, be sure that the tumor does not connect to the deep lobe of the parotid gland. This distinction is clinically important. The surgeon will approach a true PPS lesion from a submandibular or oral route, but a deep-lobe parotid tumor must be approached via a transparotid approach so that facial nerve control can be achieved at the time of surgical dissection. Facial nerve injury can occur if a deep-lobe parotid lesion is mistakenly approached from the oral or submandibular direction.

4. Malignant tumor.
  a. As noted previously, malignant tumors do not as a rule originate in the PPS; rather, these tumors break out of their space of origin and invade the PPS. The most common example of this process is seen when squamous cell carcinoma (SCCa) of the pharyngeal mucosal space (PMS) of the nasopharynx and oropharynx invades laterally into the adjacent PPS.

    b. Invasive SCCa of the PMS.

       1) Clinical presentation. Patient usually has known mucosal SCCa of the nasopharynx or oropharynx. Infrequently an "unknown primary" is present in the deep crypts of the nasopharyngeal adenoids or the oropharyngeal faucial tonsil.

       2) Imaging features. CT or MRI is used to stage the primary and nodal tumor. Tumor of the PMS is seen breaking into the PPS medially to laterally (Fig. 2-2).

       3) Comment. In this situation the more lateral PPS fat is still visible on CT or MRI, allowing the tumor to be identified as primary to the PMS.

    c. Minor salivary gland malignancy and non-Hodgkin lymphoma.

       1) Both of these tumors usually begin in the PMS and, like SCCa, invade the PPS medially to laterally.

       2) Non-Hodgkin lymphoma is found in its extranodal, extralymphatic form in the differential diagnosis of malignant lesions of

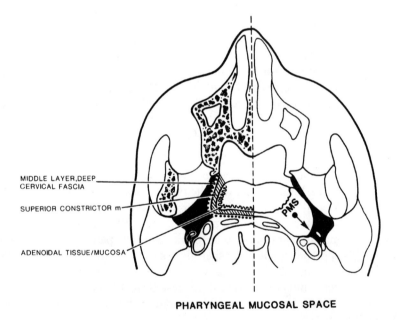

MIDDLE LAYER,DEEP CERVICAL FASCIA

SUPERIOR CONSTRICTOR m

ADENOIDAL TISSUE/MUCOSA

PMS

PHARYNGEAL MUCOSAL SPACE

Fig. 2-2   Axial view through the low nasopharynx showing the contents and fascial boundaries of the pharyngeal mucosal space (*PMS*) on the left and the appearance of a PMS mass on the right. The middle layer of deep cervical fascia (*dotted line*) encompasses the posterolateral margin of the superior constrictor muscle, defining the PMS. The center (*black dot*) of a PMS mass is medial to the parapharyngeal space (*black area*), invading the parapharyngeal space fat medially to laterally. The normal contours of the mucosal surface is disrupted by the PMS mass.

all the deep facial spaces. It is extremely rare for this lesion to occur in the PPS alone, however, without other deep facial space involvement.

PHARYNGEAL MUCOSAL SPACE (PMS)

A. Introduction.

1. This section concentrates on the radiologic features of the PMS mass.
2. A differential diagnosis of lesions originating in the PMS is presented, although by far the most common and important lesion of this space is SCCa.
3. In the discussion regarding SCCa of the PMS, both the more traditional terminology used for staging squamous lesions (nasopharynx, oropharynx, oral cavity, hypopharynx) and the spatial terminology used to evaluate deep facial masses (PPS, PMS, masticator, parotid, carotid, retropharyngeal, perivertebral spaces) are used.
   a. This section focuses on the spatial terminology. It is recommended that the reader turn to Chapter 12 after completing this section to gain an appreciation for the dual perspectives of this subject.

B. Normal anatomy.

1. Fascia (Fig. 2-2, *left*).
   a. The PMS is the area of the nasopharynx and oropharynx on the airway side of the middle layer of deep cervical fascia (buccopharyngeal fascia).
   b. Near the skull base this fascia encircles the lateral and posterior margins of the pharyngobasilar fascia, the tough aponeurosis of the superior constrictor muscle that attaches it to the skull base (Fig. 2-3. See also Fig. 1-3, *thick line*).
   c. More caudal in the nasopharynx and oropharynx, this middle layer of deep cervical fascia surrounds the superior and middle constrictor muscles themselves (See Figs. 1-4 and 1-5).
2. Contents (Fig. 2-2, *left*).
   Mucosa.
   Lymphoid tissue of Waldeyer's ring (adenoids, tonsils).
   Minor salivary glands.
   Pharyngobasilar fascia.
   Superior and middle constrictor muscles.
   Salpingopharyngeus muscle.
   Levator palatini muscle.*
   Cartilaginous end of the eustachian tube.*
   *The levator palatini muscle and the eustachian tube originate outside the PMS from the skull base.

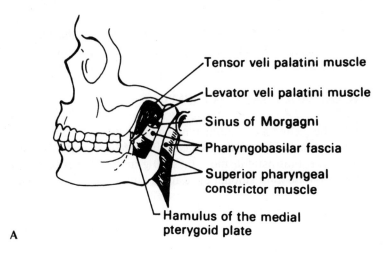

Tensor veli palatini muscle

Levator veli palatini muscle

Sinus of Morgagni

Pharyngobasilar fascia

Superior pharyngeal
constrictor muscle

Hamulus of the medial
pterygoid plate

A

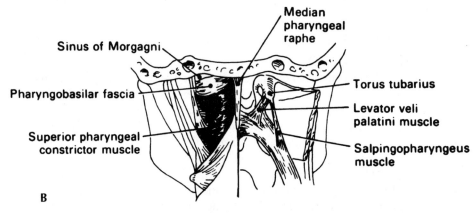

Median
pharyngeal
raphe

Sinus of Morgagni

Pharyngobasilar fascia

Torus tubarius

Levator veli
palatini muscle

Superior pharyngeal
constrictor muscle

Salpingopharyngeus
muscle

B

Fig. 2-3 **A,** Lateral view of the pharyngobasilar fascia. This fascia (aponeurosis) attaches the superior constrictor to the skull base. The gap in the upper margin of the pharyngobasilar fascia is called the *sinus of Morgagni*. Through this gap the distal eustachian tube and levator palatini muscle pass on their way into the pharyngeal mucosal space. Nasopharyngeal carcinoma tends to escape the confines of the pharyngeal mucosal space through the sinus of Morgagni, thereby accessing the skull base. **B,** Posterior view of the pharyngobasilar fascia. *Left,* The pharyngobasilar fascia can be seen attaching the superior pharyngeal constictor to the skull base. *Right,* the pharyngobasilar fascia and superior constrictor muscle have been removed, revealing the cartilaginous eustachian tube (torus tubarius) and the distal levator palatini muscle in the pharyngeal mucosal space. (From Smoker WRK, Gentry LR: CT of the nasopharynx and related spaces. *Semin Ultrasound CT MR* 7:107–130, 1986. Used by permission.)

    a. Mucosa. Exposure of the PMS mucosa to toxic substances (e.g., tobacco smoke and alcohol) is thought to be responsible for the metaplasia, and finally neoplasia, producing SCCa of the upper aerodigestive tract (excluding SCCa of the nasopharynx).

    b. Lymphoid tissue. The lymphatic tissue of Waldeyer's ring is responsible for the occurrence of non-Hodgkin lymphoma in the PMS, which is the second most common malignancy of the PMS.

        1) The volume of lymphatic tissue in the PMS gradually declines with age; thus patients older than 40 years are not expected to have a significant amount of residual lymphatic tissue. Exceptions to this rule exist, however, especially when the patient has recently had an upper respiratory tract infection.

    c. Minor salivary glands.

        1) Minor salivary glands are spread throughout the mucosa of the upper aerodigestive tract.

        2) Benign and malignant tumors may occur in these minor salivary glands, explaining why benign mixed tumors and minor salivary gland malignancy are found within the PMS.

    d. Pharyngobasilar fascia.

        1) The pharyngobasilar fascia attaches the superior constrictor muscle to the skull base (Fig. 2-3).

        2) Along the superior aspect of the posterolateral margin of this fascia is a notch called the *sinus of Morgagni*. Through this notch the levator palatini muscle and the eustachian tube pass on their way from the skull base to the PMS. The cartilaginous opening of the eustachian tube within the PMS is referred to as the *torus tubarius*.

        3) Nasopharyngeal carcinoma originating in the PMS may access the skull base through the sinus of Morgagni. This natural gap in the barrier of the pharyngobasilar fascia permits the tumor to escape the PMS to the skull base and beyond.

3. Extend and boundaries.

    a. The PMS is not completely fascia enclosed. Its posterior and lateral margins are defined by the middle layer of deep cervical fascia, but its airway side has no fascial margin.

    b. The bordering spaces of the PMS include the retropharyngeal space posteriorly and the PPS laterally.

C. Imaging issues.

Q#4

1. The first issue when evaluating any mass identified on cross-section imaging is to determine its space of origin. A mass is designated as *primary* to the pharyngeal mucosal space when:

  a. Its center is medial to the fat of the PPS (Fig. 2-2).
  b. It invades the PPS medially to laterally, displacing the fat of the PPS laterally.
  c. It disrupts the normal mucosal and submucosal architecture of the PMS.

Q#5

2. Once the mass is assigned to the PMS, the unique differential diagnosis of this space (Table 2-2) should be reviewed. The radiologic features of the mass in question should be matched to the extent possible with the known characteristics of PMS lesions.
3. Remember that the referring physician can see nearly every millimeter of the PMS surface. Freely apply this information at the time of image interpretation.
4. Much of the time the histologic diagnosis of SCCa of the mucosa of the PMS has already been made at the time of imaging. In such a circumstance the job of the imager is to provide both a primary tumor stage (T) and a nodal tumor stage (N). (See Chapter 12 for a complete discussion of the staging process.)

Table 2-2   Pharyngeal Mucosal Space: Differential Diagnosis

Pseudomass
  Asymmetric fossa of Rosenmüller
  Mucosal inflammation from infectious or radiation-induced pharyngitis

Congenital
  Tornwaldt's cyst

Inflammatory
  Adenoidal or faucial tonsil hypertrophy
  Adenoidal or faucial tonsillitis
  Adenoidal or faucial tonsil abscess
  Postinflammatory dystrophic calcification
  Postinflammatory retention cyst

Benign tumor
  Benign mixed tumor of minor salivary gland origin

Malignant tumor
  Squamous cell carcinoma
  Non-Hodgkin lymphoma
  Minor salivary gland malignancy

D. Pitfalls in imaging the PMS.

1. The most common error made when interpreting images of the PMS area is labeling normal asymmetry as tumor.
    a. The lateral pharyngeal recess (fossa of Rosenmüller) of the PMS is notoriously asymmetric. Inflammatory debris and asymmetry in the amount of lymphoid tissue can lead an unwary radiologist to the impression of mass in the PMS.
    b. To solve this problem first look at the adjacent deep spaces (PPS, retropharyngeal space). If the soft-tissue planes are maintained, the "mass" is probably not real. Next ask the referring physician if the mucosa is normal. Finally, when CT is used, a modified Valsalva maneuver will often open the collapsed recess, resolving the question of mass.
2. The variability of lymphoid tissue also can create the misimpression of mass in the PMS. Depending on the age of the patient and whether a recent upper respiratory illness has occurred, the amount of visible lymphatic tissue varies immensely.
    a. Again, preservation of the normal soft-tissue planes of the PPS and retropharyngeal space indicates that the "mass" is probably hypertrophic lymphatic tissue.
    b. With its ability to delineate the fine-detailed anatomy of the PMS, PPS, and retropharyngeal space, MRI permits the early identification of subtle invasion. If no loss of soft-tissue planes is present, especially if the levator and tensor palatini muscles are visible, the chance of missing a PMS tumor is small.

E. Common lesions.

1. Inflammatory disease.
    a. Adenoidal and tonsillar hyperplasia
        1) Clinical presentation. Nasal obstruction leading to mouth breathing, difficulty in feeding (especially in small children), noisy respiration, and snoring. Secondary eustachian tube malfunction can lead to otitis media.
        2) Pathophysiology. Hyperplasia of these organs is not in itself a disease but only the morphologic expression of marked immunobiologic activity. This overactivity results in hypertrophy of the lymphoepithelial tissue of the pharyngeal ring, most commonly the adenoid component.
        3) Imaging features. The nasopharyngeal mucosal space is full of tissue (hypertrophic adenoidal tissue) on cross-sectional imaging without violation of the middle layer of deep cervical fascia. Less commonly the oropharyngeal mucosal space is encroached

on by hypertrophic faucial tonsils. Again, no deeply invasive mass is identified.

b. Tonsillar (peritonsillar) abscess.
  1) Clinical presentation. In younger patients the first symptoms are those of tonsillitis, which include sore throat and fever. These initial symptoms resolve, but this few-day, symptom-free interval is followed by rapidly increasing difficulty in swallowing. Ear pain and trismus are also present. Protrusion of the pharyngeal wall suggests submucosal mass. The clinician will request imaging to look for "peritonsillar abscess" and possible deeper extension to the deep facial spaces.
  2) Imaging features. In most cases the abscess pocket is confined by the pharyngeal constrictor muscle to the PMS. Infrequently CT will show rupture of the PMS abscess into the adjacent PPS and beyond.
  3) Comment. Pharyngitis progressing to PMS abscess is the most common cause of secondary infection of the PPS. Ultrasonography has recently been proposed as adequate to the task of identifying peritonsillar abscess. If the patient can cooperate and the abscess is still confined by the pharyngeal constrictor muscle, ultrasonography will suffice. If deep extension is suspected, however, CT is the modality of choice.

c. Postinflammatory retention cyst (mucoceles).
  1) Clinical presentation. Superficial mass of the PMS. Usually asymptomatic. When they occur in the lateral pharyngeal recess, they may cause mechanical obstruction of the eustachian tube with resultant fluid accumulation in the middle-ear cavity.
  2) Imaging features. A well-circumscribed cystic mass of the PMS is seen. The mass is usually small (1 to 2 cm) but may become quite large if unattended. In the lateral pharyngeal recess they are usually oblong, projecting along the axis of the eustachian tube.
  3) Comment. These retention cysts are usually incidental findings on CT or MRI.

d. Postinflammatory calcification.
  1) Clinical presentation. Incidental finding.
  2) Imaging features. Seen on CT as multiple clumps of calcification in the PMS. Faucial tonsil location is the most common, although the calcific deposits also may be present in the lingual tonsil or nasopharyngeal adenoids.
  3) Comment. The patient usually has a remote history of an episode of severe pharyngitis.

2. Benign tumor.
  a. Benign mixed tumor.
    1) Clinical presentation. When small and submucosal, this tumor may be seen only as a "marble under the rug" bump. When large, it appears as a pedunculated mass pushing into the airway of the upper pharynx.
    2) Imaging features. Small benign mixed tumor will be seen best on MRI as a well-circumscribed, homogenous, soft-tissue mass in the PMS. High-resolution T1- and T2-weighted images in the axial and coronal plane clearly delineate this lesion without the need for contrast in most cases. When large, an oval to round, well-circumscribed PMS mass pedunculating into the airway of the upper pharynx is seen on CT or MRI.
    3) Comment. These lesions arise in the minor salivary glands of the PMS.
3. Malignant tumors.
  a. Squamous cell carcinoma.
    1) Clinical presentation.
      a) Most commonly seen in patients with known mucosal SCCa.
      b) Less commonly seen in patients with malignant adenopathy in the neck. CT or MRI defines the submucosal, clinically occult primary tumor.
    2) Imaging features. Infiltrating mass with its center medial to the PPS and invading the PPS fat medially to laterally. When primary to the nasopharyngeal mucosal space, there may be associated findings that include middle-ear fluid resulting from eustachian tube malfunction and cervical adenopathy, usually in the spinal accessory chain or deep cervical chain. When primary to the oropharyngeal mucosal space, spread may be seen into either the subjacent PPS or the masticator space.
    3) Comment. The CT or MRI appearance of SCCa of the PMS is identical to that of the other two malignancies of this space: non-Hodgkin lymphoma, and minor salivary gland malignancy.
  b. Non-Hodgkin lymphoma.
    1) Clinical presentation. Unlike SCCa, non-Hodgkin lymphoma often has other systemic manifestations that signal its presence. Malaise, fever, distant adenopathy, and hepatosplenomegaly differentiate this tumor clinically from SCCa. When non-Hodgkin lymphoma is confined to the head and neck area, however, it may present without systemic symptoms and appear indistinguishable from SCCa.
    2) Imaging features. CT or MRI will show PMS involvement to be the same as with SCCa. However, associated extranodal, extra-

lymphatic sites or multiple large nonnecrotic lymph nodes in atypical drainage locations may suggest the diagnosis of non-Hodgkin lymphoma.

   3) Comment. When non-Hodgkin lymphoma is found in the PMS, it is in an extranodal, lymphatic site.

  c. Minor salivary gland malignancy.

   1) Clinical presentation. No distinctive features.

   2) Imaging features. CT or MRI will show the tumor mass in the PMS to appear the same as SCCa or non-Hodgkin lymphoma.

4. Congenital PMS lesions.

  a. Tornwaldt's cyst.

   1) Clinical presentation. This lesion usually appears as an asymptomatic, incidental finding on MRI of the head (4% of head MRIs will demonstrate this lesion). When the cyst becomes infected, the patient has a nasopharyngeal mass and sepsis.

   2) Pathologic findings. Tornwaldt's cyst is a midline, congenital, epithelial-lined cyst seen in the nasopharyngeal PMS. It results from growth of notochordal remnants and is present in 4% of all autopsy specimens.

   3) Imaging features. Seen as a midline cystic mass in the upper nasopharynx, nestled between the prevertebral muscles within the pharyngeal raphe. The cyst may be a few millimeters to several centimeters in diameter. Smaller cysts are not seen on CT, whereas MRI clearly delineates the cyst in most cases.

    a) The T1 signal of Tornwaldt's cyst varies from hypointense to hyperintense, probably resulting from the amount and type of protein within the cyst.

SUGGESTED READING

Parapharyngeal Space

Babbel RW, Harnsberger HR: The parapharyngeal space: the key to unlocking the suprahyoid neck. *Semin Ultrasound CT MR* 11:444–459, 1990.

Dillon WP, Mancuso AA: *The oropharynx and nasopharynx*. In Newton TH, Hasso AN, Dillon WP, editors; *Computed tomography of the head and neck*, ed 1. New York, 1988, Raven Press.

Harnsberger HR: CT and MRI of masses of the deep face. *Curr Probl Diagn Radiol* 16:141–173, 1987.

Harnsberger HR, Osborn AG: Differential diagnosis of head and neck lesions based on their space of origin. 1. The suprahyoid part of the neck. *Am J Roentgenol* 157:147–154, 1991.

Som PM, Braun IF, Shapiro MD, et al: Tumors of the parapharyngeal space and upper neck: MR imaging characteristics. *Radiology* 164:823–829, 1987.

Som PM, Sacher M, Stollman AL, et al: Common tumors of the parapharyngeal space: refined imaging diagnosis. *Radiology* 169:81–85, 1988.

Pharyngeal Mucosal Space

Kwok P, Hawke M, Jahn AF, et al: Tornwaldt's cyst: clinical and radiologic aspects. *J Otolaryngol* 16:104–107, 1987.
Muraki AS, Mancuso AA, Harnsberger HR, et al: CT of the oropharynx, tongue base, and floor of the mouth: normal anatomy and range of variations, and applications of staging carcinoma. *Radiology* 148:725–731, 1983.
Parker GD, Harnsberger HR, Jacobs JM: The pharyngeal mucosal space. *Semin Ultrasound CT MR* 11:460–475, 1990.
Silver AJ, Mawad ME, Hilal SK, et al: CT of the nasopharynx and related space. I: anatomy. *Radiology* 147:725–731, 1983.
Silver AJ, Mawad ME, Hilal SK, et al: CT of the nasopharynx and related space. II: pathology. *Radiology* 147:733–738, 1983.

3

The Masticator Space

CRITICAL IMAGING QUESTIONS: MASTICATOR SPACE

1. What features characterize a lesion as primary to the masticator space?
2. When a tumor is found within the masticator space, what cranial nerve branch should be inspected for the possibility of perineural tumor?
3. What are the statistically common lesions of the masticator space?
4. If an abscess is found in the masticator space, where is the most likely source?

Answers to these questions are found in the text beside the question number (Q#) in the margin.

MASTICATOR SPACE (MS)

A. Normal anatomy.

1. Fascia. The superficial layer of deep cervical fascia (investing fascia) splits along the inferior mandible, creating a sling that encloses the masticator space (MS) (Figs. 3-1 and 3-2).

   a. The medial slip of this fascia runs along the deep edge of the pterygoid muscles from the inferior mandible to attach to the skull base.

      1) Curtin (1987) refers to this fascia as the *medial pterygoid fascia*.

      2) Its insertion on the skull base is medial to the foramen ovale (Fig. 3-2). This strategic location means that lesions extenting cephalad in the MS will enter the skull base through the foramen ovale.

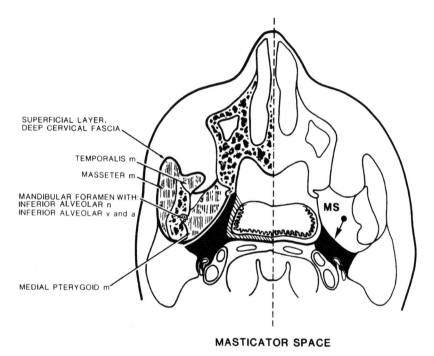

MASTICATOR SPACE

Fig. 3-1   *Left,* Superficial layer of deep cervical fascia (*dark line*) encloses the MS. The mandibular ramus is seen as the central feature of the MS, with the muscles of mastication (masseter, temporalis, medial and lateral pterygoid muscles) making up the remainder of the volume of this space. The masticator nerve (motor branch of cranial nerve V_3) innervates the muscles of the MS, and the inferior alveolar nerve (sensory branch of V_3) passes through the MS on its way to the inferior alveolar foramen. *Right,* Appearance of a masticator space (MS) mass. The center (*black dot*) is seen anterior to the parapharyngeal space (*black area*). The displacement pattern of the mass is from anterior to posterior, with bowing of the parapharyngeal space posteriorly.

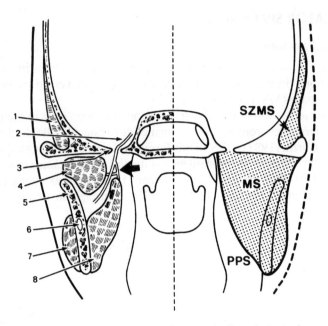

Fig. 3-2 Coronal view of the masticator space (MS). *Left,* Critical contents of the MS. Note the cephalad extent of the attachment of the temporalis muscle in the suprazygomatic portion of the MS. *1,* Temporalis muscle; *2,* mandibular division of trigeminal nerve (V_3); *3,* foramen ovale; *4,* lateral pterygoid muscle; *5,* mandibular ramus; *6,* inferior alveolar nerve; *7,* masseter muscle; *8,* medial pterygoid muscle; *heavy arrow,* masticator nerve branch of the main trunk of cranial nerve V_3. *Right,* Sling of the superficial layer of deep cervical fascia (*heavy black line*) is best demonstrated in the coronal view. Observe its origin from the inferior surface of the mandible, with its medial slip traveling up the medial pterygoid muscle to insert on the skull base just medial to the foramen ovale. The lateral slip of fascia runs up the lateral surface of the masseter muscle to attach to the zygomatic arch, then continues upward on the surface of the temporal muscle. *PPS,* parapharyngeal space; *SZMS,* suprazygomatic masticator space.

    b. The lateral slip of this fascia runs over the superficial masseter muscle to the zygomatic arch, then cephalad over the temporalis muscle to the top of the suprazygomatic MS (Fig. 3-2).

2. Contents (Figs. 3-1 and 3-2).
    Muscles of mastication.
        Masseter muscle.
        Temporalis muscle.
        Medial pterygoid muscle.
        Lateral pterygoid muscle.
    Masticator nerve branches (Proximal V_3 motor branch).

Inferior alveolar nerve (V_3 sensory branch).

Inferior alveolar vein and artery.

Ramus and posterior body of the mandible.

a. Muscles of mastication. Of the four muscles of mastication, the masseter muscle is the largest.

1) All four muscles are supplied by the masticator nerve, which is the more proximal of the two motor branches of cranial nerve V_3. (See Chapter 18 for complete coverage of the trigeminal nerve.) Because these muscles constitute the principal volume of the MS, injury or involvement by malignant tumor of cranial nerve V_3 results in motor atrophy and diminished MS volume.

2) The muscles of MS origins and insertions are shown in Table 3-1. Because of their extensive attachments to the skull base, tumor or infection can access the skull base by following the course of these muscles.

3) Malignancy in the MS muscles or an abscess in this space is clinically signalled by trismus (i.e., difficulty in opening the mouth secondary to masticator muscle spasm).

b. MS nerves. Masticator nerve branches (motor nerve to the muscles of mastication) and the inferior alveolar nerve (sensory nerve to the mandible and teeth) are the only two nerves that enter the MS. As such they provide a natural avenue for perineural tumor spread to the foramen ovale of the skull base and intracranially to Meckel's cave as well as beyond to the root entry zone of cranial nerve V at the lateral pons.

Table 3-1   Masticator Space Muscles

Muscle	Origin	Insertion
Masseter muscle	Zygomatic arch	Lateral surface of ramus, angle, posterior body of mandible
Temporalis muscle	Calvarium of the floor of suprazygomatic masticator space (temporal fossa)	Coronoid process of mandible fossa
Lateral pterygoid muscle	Two heads Masticator space surface of skull base Lateral pterygoid plate	Medial aspect of mandibular condyle
Medial pterygoid muscle	Fossa between pterygoid plates	Medial aspect of angle of mandible

    1) Comment. The combination of atrophy of the muscles of mastication, mandibular dental pain, and serous otitis media secondary to involvement of the V_3 branch to the tensor palatini muscle with eustachian tube malfunction strongly suggests malignant tumor involving the mandibular division of the trigeminal nerve.

   c. Mandible, posterior body, and ramus. The central strut of the MS is the posterior body and ramus of the mandible. Odontogenic infection and tumors of mandibular origin account for many of the lesions that arise in the MS.

   d. The parotid duct is not in the MS, but it passes just superficial to it as it courses over the masseter muscle. Lesions of the MS can involve the parotid duct by direct lateral invasion. Conversely, lesions of the parotid duct may appear clinically as arising from the MS.

3. Extent and boundaries.

   a. The MS is far more extensive craniocaudally than is commonly recognized. Coronal imaging clearly delineates the true extent of the MS (See Figs. 1-7 and 3-2). It extends from the inferior edge of the mandible below to the superior attachment of the temporalis muscle above.

   b. In the past the cephalad extension of the MS above the zygoma was referred to as the *temporal fossa* or *space*. Inasmuch as no fascia divides the temporal space from the MS space it can be viewed as the most cephalad recess of the MS space (or the suprazygomatic MS). This cephalad projection of the MS becomes extremely important when tumor or infection is being imaged, because the lesion often extends above the zygoma and may be missed if not searched for.

    1) Comment. Clinical colleagues may still refer to the suprazygomatic masticator space as the temporal fossa. As long as everyone understands that this area is contiguous to the MS below, the exact terminology is not important.

   c. The nasopharyngeal portion of the MS has been referred to as the *infratemporal fossa.* This term has been used to describe the area between the pterygopalatine fossa medially and the zygomatic arch laterally. No fascia defines the infratemporal fossa. As a result this term can be replaced by the more anatomic term *nasopharyngeal masticator space.*

    1) Comment. Again, surgical colleagues may still refer to the nasopharyngeal masticator space as the infratemporal fossa. Awareness that the same area is being described by both terms prevents miscommunication.

   d. Bordering spaces (Fig. 3-1). The anterior boundary of the MS is the buccal space (BS). The posteromedial MS borders the parapharyngeal space. Directly posterior to the MS is the parotid space.

1) Buccal space. The BS has no true fascia boundaries. As it is a region in close proximity to the MS, the BS is often involved simultaneously with the MS when infection or malignancy is present.
   a) Contents.
      Buccal fat pad.
      Facial artery and vein.
      Parotid duct (distal portion).
      Buccinator muscle.
   b) Because the BS can be easily palpated, smaller lesions of this area often are not imaged.
   c) When a malignant tumor involves this area, the most important information that can come from CT or MRI is its relationship to the distal parotid duct.

B. Imaging issues.

1. What radiographic features define a lesion as primary to the MS?

Q#1
   a. A mass is primary to the MS when:
      1) The center of the mass is anterior to the parapharyngeal space within the muscles of mastication or the mandible (Fig. 3-1, *right*).
      2) The mass invades the parapharyngeal space from anterior to posterior, displacing the parapharyngeal fat posteriorly.
   b. When the mass is clearly centered in the muscles of mastication or the mandible, identification of its MS origin is not difficult. When the lesion is large, use of these rules helps to make this identification simple.
   c. Once the mass has been localized to the MS, the unique differential diagnosis (Table 3-2) should be reviewed. Matching the radiologic features of the lesion to the statistically common lesions of the MS will often yield a short list of possible diagnoses to be suggested to the referring physician.
2. Is there perineural tumor spread along cranial nerve V_3?

Q#2
   a. Malignant tumor of the MS initially spreads cephalad toward the skull base, within the muscles of the MS, or along the mandibular division of the trigeminal nerve (V_3). The tumor gains access to the main trunk of V_3 along either the masticator nerve or the inferior alveolar nerve (Fig. 3-3).
   b. Tumor involving cranial nerve V_3 produces pain or numbness of the ipsilateral chin and jaw.

Table 3-2   Masticator Space Mass: Differential Diagnosis

Pseudotumor
   Accessory parotid gland*
   Benign masseteric hypertrophy*
   Cranial nerve V_3 denervation atrophy

Congenital
   Hemangioma
   Lymphangioma

Inflammatory
   Odontogenic abscess*
   Mandibular osteomyelitis

Benign tumor
   Osteoblastoma
   Leiomyoma
   Neural sheath tumor (neurofibroma, schwannoma)

Malignant tumor
   Sarcoma*
      Soft tissue
      Chondrosarcoma
      Osteosarcoma
   Malignant schwannoma
   Non-Hodgkin lymphoma*
   Squamous cell carcinoma from oropharynx (retromolar trigone)*
   Rhabdomyosarcoma (in the pediatric population)*
   Mandibular metastases

*These are more common lesions.

   c. Because during its early phases perineural tumor may be entirely microscopic, initial radiographic manifestations may be nonexistent. As the process progresses macroscopic perineural tumor may be contiguous or discontinuous along the nerve. Perineural tumor may pass through the skull-base foramen without causing bone changes on high-resolution CT images.
   d. Imaging of the MS must therefore include the entire course of cranial nerve V_3 from the mental foramen of the mandible to the root entry zone in the lateral pons, including the mandibular foramen, foramen ovale, and Meckel's cave.
   e. Failure to image and inspect cranial nerve V_3 in its entirety will result in missed perineural tumor spread and therapeutic mistakes (radiation-therapy port misses or inadequate surgical margins), leading to "early recurrence" along the proximal V_3. In this circumstance tumor

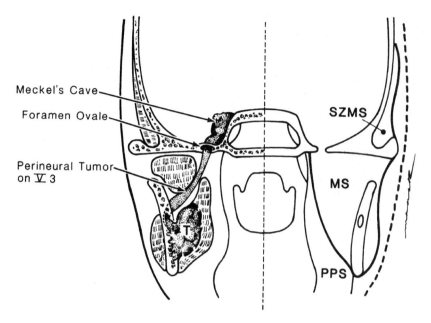

Meckel's Cave

Foramen Ovale

Perineural Tumor
on Ⅴ 3

SZMS

MS

PPS

Fig. 3-3   Coronal view showing the craniocaudad relationships of the masticator space depicting a malignant tumor (*T*) originating in the masticator space. The invasive malignancy has invaded the adjacent mandible, accessed the inferior alveolar nerve, and is tracking cephalad on this nerve to the skull base and beyond. Perineural tumor spread on the mandibular division of the trigeminal nerve has been seen to traverse the skull base through the foramen ovale, spread intracranial through Meckel's cavity and the preganglionic segment of the trigeminal nerve, and finally reach the pons at the root entry zone. In this case the perineural tumor can be seen spreading centrally as far as Meckel's cave. *MS*, Masticator space; *PPS*, parapharyngeal space; *SZMS*, suprazygomatic masticator space.

will be found during follow-up examination at the skull base near the foramen ovale and intracranially in Meckel's cave.
   f. Because MRI is more sensitive to perineural tumor spread, especially at the skull base and intracranial level, it is recommended over CT when noninfectious MS mass is under radiologic evaluation.
3. What is the status of the skull base and the suprazygomatic MS?
   a. Because the muscles of mastication attach to the skull base and the suprazygomatic MS, these areas must be imaged and inspected during MS examination.
   b. Infection spreads preferentially upward (the path of least resistance) in the MS. Osteomyelitis of the skull base with destruction of the pterygoid wing area requires significantly more antibiotic therapy.

Failure to recognize skull-base infection will lead to inadequate therapy and relapse.

c. Malignant tumor also preferentially spreads cephalad. Involvement of the skull base usually makes the tumor unresectable. Suprazygomatic MS tumor must be recognized so that radiation ports can be adjusted to this region.

4. What is the status of the mandible?
   a. Mandibular osteomyelitis requires subperiosteal surgical drainage and a longer course of antibiotic therapy.
   b. Malignancy invading the mandible is more likely to spread perineurally (following the inferior alveolar nerve distally along the inferior alveolar canal, or proximally along the main trunk of cranial nerve V_3).

5. Is the parotid duct involved?
   a. In the case of infection of the MS, calculus in the parotid duct may be causal. Draining an abscess of the MS without treating the ductal stone will not yield a lasting cure.
   b. Direct invasion of MS malignancy laterally will involve and obstruct the parotid duct. Surgical intervention must deal with the duct and the parotid gland if CT or MRI suggests that the duct is involved.
   c. CT is the examination of choice in evaluating patients with suspected infection of the MS. This is because of its ability to identify calculus disease and more readily define the presence or absence of mandibular osteomyelitis.

C. Pitfalls in imaging.

1. When a lesion is found within the MS, be sure that:
   a. The entire course of cranial nerve V_3 is imaged.
   b. The entire MS is imaged, including the suprazygomatic area.
   c. The lesion is not a MS pseudomass.

2. Masticator space pseudomasses.
   a. The three pseudomasses of the MS are:
      1) Asymmetric accessory parotid gland.
      2) Benign masseteric hypertrophy.
      3) Cranial nerve V_3 motor atrophy.
   b. Asymmetric accessory parotid glands.
      1) The accessory parotid glands are normally found on the surface of the masseter muscle just superficial to the MS.
      2) Anatomic studies reveal a 21% incidence of accessory parotid glands among the general population.
      3) When the patient clenches his or her teeth, the accessory parotid glands (when prominent or asymmetric) will feel like a lateral MS mass to the examining physician.

4) Imaging will reveal salivary-gland tissue resting on the surface of the masseter muscle. This tissue may appear quite prominent, but it should not be called a mass lesion if the density (on CT) or intensity (on MRI) parallels that of the adjacent parotid gland.

c. Benign masseteric hypertrophy.

1) This is a complex anomaly with multiple causes. The acquired form is most commonly secondary to bruxism (i.e., nocturnal molar grinding).

2) Masseter muscle enlargement may be either unilateral or bilateral.

3) CT or MRI will reveal homogeneous enlargement of one or both masseter muscles, with discrete outer margin to the muscle. When the lesion is bilateral, the findings are pathognomonic. If pterygoid and temporalis muscle hypertrophy accompanies the masseter muscle enlargement, the diagnosis can be made with confidence.

4) Comment. If unilateral masseter muscle mass is present without a definite history of bruxism, careful radiologic follow-up is important to exclude malignant tumor. Unilateral masseter mass with infiltrating margins should not be called benign masseteric hypertrophy.

d. Cranial nerve V_3 motor atrophy.

1) The motor root of the trigeminal nerve travels with the mandibular division (V_3), supplying innervation to the muscles of mastication as well as the anterior belly of the digastric, mylohyoid muscles and the tensor tympani and palatini muscles.

2) When injured by malignant tumor or retrogasserian rhizotomy, V_3 denervation atrophy occurs. This is seen as muscle fatty infiltration and volume loss from the ipsilateral MS.

3) CT or MRI will demonstrate increased fat and decreased muscle volume on the affected side within 6 weeks of the injury. Do not mistake the opposite normal side as a tumor.

D. Common lesions.

Q#3

1. Because there are limited normal-tissue types in the MS (muscle, mandible, V_3), only a few lesions are seen to originate in this location. These include sarcomas, non-Hodgkin lymphoma, and invasive squamous cell carcinoma. Of all disease types, odontogenic abscess is the most common lesion seen in the MS.

2. Inflammatory.

a. Odontogenic abscess.

1) Clinical presentation. Patient has bad dentition or a history of dental manipulation. Initial symptom is trismus. Physical examination is severely limited by the patient's unwillingness to be touched and inability to open the mouth. When the referring clinician describes the jaw as "lumpy," consider actinomycosis in the differential diagnosis.

Q#4

    a) The most common cause of MS abscess is secondary to seeding from infected teeth or following dental manipulation.

2) Imaging features. Fluid density (on CT) or intensity (on MRI) is seen within the MS surrounded by swollen, cellulitic tissue. If osteomyelitis of either the mandible or skull base is present, bone destruction is best visualized by CT (Fig. 3-4).

    a) In the special clinical setting of facial swelling following the removal of wires around the zygomatic arch used during treatment of facial fractures, carefully evaluate the suprazygomatic MS, because the risk is high for abscess formation in this area.

3) Comment. Because of the inability of the clinician to examine the patient, radiology is the best key to directing therapy. CT is the modality of choice because of its sensitivity to osteomyelitis and calculus disease compared with the less-sensitive MRI. Consider the following questions as the scans are reviewed:

    a) Is skull-base or mandibular osteomyelitis present? If so, surgical and antibiotic therapy are more extensive.

    b) Is there evidence for parotid calculus disease? Infection from the more superficial parotid duct area can spread into the adjacent MS.

    c) Are any other spaces involved in the deep face? In general, one drain is necessary for each space involved.

    d) Is the suprazygomatic MS involved? Because of the firm attachment of the superficial layer of deep surgical fascia to the periosteum of the inferior mandible, infection tends to spread upward to the skull base and the suprazygomatic MS.

3. Malignant tumor.

  a. Sarcoma

    1) Because the principal structures of the MS are the muscles of mastication and the mandible, primary malignant tumors are often sarcomas (soft-tissue sarcoma, chondrosarcoma, osteosarcoma).

    2) Chondrosarcoma arises from the region of the temporomandibular joint. Osteosarcoma can arise from any part of the mandible.

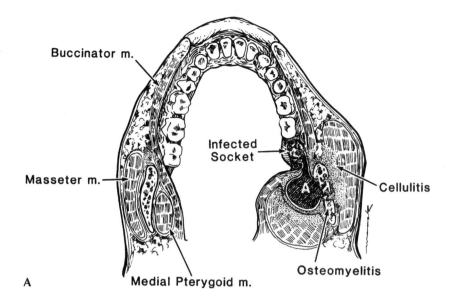

A

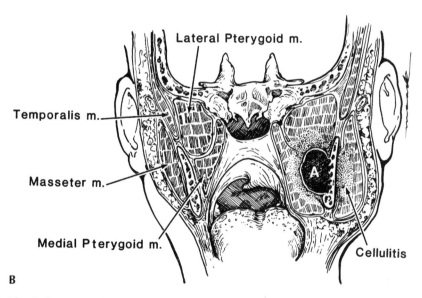

B

Fig. 3-4 **A**, Axial view at the level of the midoropharynx showing a masticator space abscess (*A*) secondary to an infected molar. The infected socket has fistulized the masticator space, causing both cellulitis and abscess. Note the mandibular osteomyelitis with resulting bony destructive changes. **B**, Coronal view through the oropharynx showing the same masticator space abscess as in **A**. The abscess and associated cellulitis cause bowing of the soft palate and uvula medially and of the masseter muscle and cheek laterally. Because the actual abscess pocket is in the medial portion of the masticator space, it can be drained via a peroral surgical approach.

3) Imaging features. When matrix forming, osteosarcoma may demonstrate tumorous new bone formation on CT, whereas chondrosarcoma may show chondroid calcifications within its mass. Otherwise CT or MRI will demonstrate infiltrating mass in the MS (usually with some element of mandibular destruction) indistinguishable from any other malignancy of this space.

b. Malignant schwannoma

1) Clinical presentation. Pain and numbness along the distribution of the inferior alveolar nerve (chin and jaw).

2) Pathologic findings. Also referred to as *neurogenous sarcoma*. "Fibrosarcoma" that originates from a nerve trunk. In the MS this lesion arises from the inferior alveolar nerve or masticator nerve.

3) Imaging features. CT or MRI will demonstrate a tubular mass along the course of cranial nerve V_3, mandibular foramen, usually involving the inferior alveolar nerve in the inferior alveolar canal. The main trunk of V_3 may be involved up to and through the foramen ovale of the skull base. The tumor may have already spread perineurally to the gasserian ganglion in Meckel's cave (Fig. 3-3).

c. Non-Hodgkin lymphoma.

1) Clinical presentation. The patient may have cranial nerve V_3 symptoms and MS mass as part of systemic non-Hodgkin lymphoma or as the first manifestation of limited head and neck disease. When the disease is already systemic, CT or MRI provides three-dimensional information for "involved field" radiation therapy planning.

2) Imaging features. Non-Hodgkin lymphoma of the MS cannot be radiographically distinguished from any other malignancy of the MS unless associated nodal disease, extranodal lymphatic disease (Waldeyer's ring), or multiple other extranodal extralymphatic sites (e.g., sinus, nose, orbit) are involved simultaneously. As a single focus, non-Hodgkin lymphoma in the MS looks like any other infiltrating malignant lesion.

d. Infiltrating squamous cell carcinoma.

1) Clinical presentation. Previous history of treated oropharyngeal or oral cavity squamous cell carcinoma is usually present. Patient returns with trismus and cranial nerve V_3 numbness.

2) Pathologic finding. Squamous cell carcinoma enters the MS either by direct extension from the faucial tonsil or retromolar trigone, or via perineural tumor spread along the inferior alveolar nerve usually involved during mandibular invasion from the oral cavity.

3) Imaging features. CT or MRI will show an infiltrating mass of the MS with or without perineural tumor along cranial nerve V_3.

If the primary tumor site was successfully treated, no mass may be present in the pharyngeal mucosal space.

SUGGESTED READING

Aspestrand F, Boysen M: CT and MR imaging of primary tumors of the masticator space. *Acta Radiologica* 33:518–522, 1992.

Braun IF, Hoffman JC: Computed tomography of the buccomasseteric region. I: anatomy. II: pathology. *AJNR* 5:605–616, 1984.

Braun IF, Torres WE, Landman JA, et al: Computed tomography of benign masseteric hypertrophy. *J Comput Assist Tomogr* 9:167–170, 1985.

Curtin HD: Separation of the masticator space from the parapharyngeal space. *Radiology* 163:195–204, 1987.

Hardin CW, Harnsberger HR, Osborn AG, et al: CT in the evaluation of the normal and diseased oral cavity and oropharynx. *Semin Ultrasound CT MR* 7:131–153, 1986.

Hardin CW, Harnsberger HR, Osborn AG, et al: Infection and tumor of the masticator space: CT evaluation. *Radiology* 157:413–417, 1985.

Harnsberger HR: CT and MRI of masses of the deep face. *Curr Probl Diagn Radiol* 16:143–173, 1967.

Hutchins LG, Harnsberger HR, Hardin CW, et al: The radiologic assessment of trigeminal neuropathy. *AJNR* 10:1031–1038, 1989.

Laine FJ, Braun IF, Jensen ME, et al: Perineural tumor extension through the foramen ovale: evaluation with MR imaging. *Radiology* 174:65–71, 1990.

Schellhas KP: MR imaging of muscles of mastication. *AJNR* 10:829–837, 1989.

4

The Parotid Space

CRITICAL IMAGING QUESTIONS: PAROTID SPACE

1. Is the lesion intraparotid or extraparotid?
2. Are the margins of the lesion discrete or indistinct? Does the lesion invade adjacent structures? Are there associated lymph nodes that are affected?
3. Is the lesion in the superficial or the deep lobe of the parotid gland? What is the relationship of the mass of the facial nerve?
4. Is the lesion single or multiple?

Answers to these questions are found in the text beside the question number (Q#) in the margin.

PAROTID SPACE (PS)

A. Normal anatomy.

1. Fascia. The superficial layer of the deep cervical fascia splits to encompass the parotid space (PS).
2. Contents (Fig. 4-1).
    Parotid gland.
    Facial nerve (cranial nerve VII).
    Retromandibular vein.
    External carotid artery.
    Intraparotid lymph nodes.
    a. Facial nerve. The intraparotid facial nerve creates a surgical plane that divides the gland into superficial and deep lobes.
        1) The intraparotid facial nerve is *not* routinely identified on either CT or MRI, even with high-resolution imaging. The linear, low

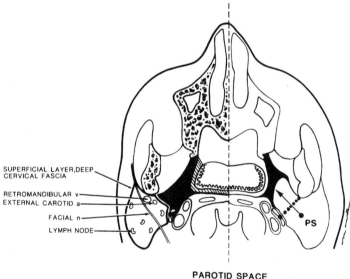

PAROTID SPACE

Fig. 4-1 *Left,* Superficial layer of the deep cervical fascia (*dark line*) completely encloses the parotid space (*PS*). The facial nerve divides the gland into superficial and deep lobes. Multiple intraglandular nodes as well as the retromandibular vein and external carotid artery make up the remainder of the contents of the parotid space. *Right,* Appearance of a PS mass. Note that the mass lesion involves the deep lobe of the parotid gland, with its center (*black dot*) lateral to the parapharyngeal space (*blackened area*) and its displacement pattern bowing the parapharyngeal space from lateral to medial. Widening of the stylomandibular notch (*dotted line*) also occurs in PS masses.

intensity seen on axial T1-weighted MRI is most likely the intra-parotid ductal ramifications and not the facial nerve.

2) The deep lobe of the parotid gland is sometimes referred to as the *parapharyngeal lobe*, because it projects to the lateral margin of the parapharyngeal space. This terminology is avoided here so as to not confuse deep-lobe lesions as parapharyngeal in origin.

3) Injury to the proximal intraparotid facial nerve results in loss of motor function in the muscles of facial expression for the entire ipsilateral face (peripheral facial nerve paralysis). The special functions of the facial nerve that result from branches in the temporal bone (lacrimation, stapedial reflex, taste in the anterior two thirds of the tongue) are spared by extracranial nerve VII injury.

4) See Chapter 19 for further discussion of the imaging issues involved in facial nerve dysfunction.

b. Vessels. Two vessels are usually seen in the PS. The retromandibular vein is the lateral of the two, and the external carotid artery is just medial to it. The facial nerve courses immediately lateral to the retromandibular vein (Fig. 4-1).

c. Lymph nodes. Because of late encapsulation of the parotid gland in embryogenesis, the PS has lymph nodes within the glandular parenchyma. As a result, the PS functions as a first-order drainage site for malignancies of the adjacent scalp, external auditory canal, and deep face.

1) The normal parotid gland contains 20 to 30 nodes.

2) This contrasts with the submandibular gland, which undergoes early encapsulation. None of the nodes of the submandibular gland are intraglandular.

d. Parotid duct (Stenson's duct). The parotid duct emerges from the anterior PS, runs anteriorly over the surface of the masseter muscle, then arches medially through the buccal space to pierce the buccinator muscle at the level of the upper (maxillary) second molar.

1) The parotid duct is routinely seen on thin-section (3-mm contiguous) axial CT. The best plane to ensure the visualization of the duct is parallel to the hard palate.

2) Thibault and co-workers (1993) showed that the linear, low-signal structure seen on T1-weighted MRI, previously thought to represent the intraparotid facial nerve, is actually the excretory ducts traversing the gland.

3. Extent and boundaries.

a. The PS is the most lateral space in the nasopharyngeal and oropharyngeal area, extending from the external auditory canal above to the level of the mandibular angle below.

    b. At times the parotid tail can dip inferiorly below the angle of the mandible. In this circumstance the parotid tail masses can present as angle of mandible masses.

        1) Excisional biopsy of such low-lying mass, unrecognized as being within the PS, often results in facial nerve injury.

    c. The posteromedial boundary of the PS is made up of the posterior belly of the digastric muscle and its fascia, which separates the PS from the carotid space.

    d. Directly medial to the PS is the parapharyngeal space (Fig. 4-1).

B. Imaging issues.

1. When first examining the CT or MRI scans of a mass lesion in the region of the PS, begin by determining whether the mass lesion is intraparotid or extraparotid.

Q#1

    a. Lesions of the adjacent deep face displace the parotid gland laterally. As a result, masses in this area are often thought to be parotid masses when in fact they may arise from the adjacent masticator, parapharyngeal, or carotid spaces. Do not be surprised if the clinician insists the lesion is in the PS but the imaging study shows differently.

        1) The designation of intraparotid vs. extraparotid mass is extremely important to the surgeon. It means the difference between a transparotid surgical approach, with control of the facial nerve (intraparotid mass), or some type of peroral or submandibular approach, where no attempt at facial nerve localization or control is made (extraparotid mass).

    b. With smaller lesions it is often easy to identify the mass as primary to the PS by noting that it is well within the parotid gland and has glandular tissue surrounding it. When the lesion is in the deep lobe of the parotid gland, however, it may be difficult to make this identification. Because the common diseases of the PS are quite different from the surrounding deep facial spaces, the designation of a mass as primary to the PS has great significance.

    c. A mass is primary to the PS when:

        1) The center of the mass is lateral to the parapharyngeal space (Fig. 4-1).

        2) The mass invades the parapharyngeal space laterally to medially, displacing the fat of the space medially (Fig. 4-1).

        3) The mass widens the distance between the angle of the mandible and the styloid process (stylomandibular notch or tunnel)

Q#2

   d. Once the mass has been identified as originating in the PS, the differential diagnosis (Table 4-1) should be reviewed.

     1) In most cases the patient will appear septic when an inflammatory lesion is present.

     2) In the case of a tumor the margins of the mass often can serve as a clue to whether it is benign or malignant. When benign, the tumor edges are usually discrete; when malignant, the margins are indistinct and seem to fade into the surrounding parotid gland.

     3) Comment. These guidelines should be viewed with great care. In reality the radiologic characterization of benign vs. malignant tumor is an imprecise science. Only when the lesion invades

Table 4-1   Parotid Space Mass: Differential Diagnosis

Congenital
First branchial cleft cyst
Hemangioma (in the pediatric population)
Lymphangioma (in the pediatric population)

Inflammatory
Abscess or cellulitis
Benign lymphoepithelial lesions (AIDS)
Reactive adenopathy

Benign tumor
Pleomorphic adenoma (benign mixed tumor)*
Warthin's tumor (papillary cystadenoma lymphomatosum)*
Oncocytoma
Lipoma
Facial nerve schwannoma or neurofibroma

Malignant tumor, primary
Mucoepidermoid carcinoma*
Adenoid cystic carcinoma*
Non-Hodgkin lymphoma
Acinic cell carcinoma
Malignant mixed tumor
Squamous cell carcinoma

Malignant tumor, metastatic (within parotid nodes)
Skin squamous cell carcinoma*
Melanoma*
Non-Hodgkin lymphoma

*These are more common lesions

adjacent structures or nodal seeding is identified can the radiologist come down hard on the side of malignancy.

2. What is the relationship of the mass to the facial nerve?

Q#3

    a. If the location of the facial nerve plane is known, it is possible to estimate the position of the facial nerve as superficial, deep, or in the same plane as the mass.

    b. A superficial-lobe PS mass is removed by superficial parotidectomy. A deep-lobe mass requires total parotidectomy, with significantly greater risk for injury to the facial nerve.

    c. With CT the facial nerve plane is extrapolated as a line connecting the stylomastoid foramen to a point just lateral to the retromandibular vein. MRI often allows direct visualization of the facial nerve plane.

    d. When parotid malignancy is suspected on either clinical or radiologic grounds, a search for perineural tumor spread along the course of the facial nerve must be conducted.

        1) Comment. Remember that the tumor may run either antegrade (to the motor endplates of cranial nerve VII) or retrograde (along the mastoid segment of VII in the temporal bone) along the facial nerve (Fig. 4-2).

3. Is the lesion single or multiple?

Q #4

    a. With a single lesion of the parotid gland, all of the possible differential diagnosis (Table 4-1) must be considered.

    b. Multiple masses in the parotid gland limit the diagnostic possibilities to Warthin's tumor, acinic cell carcinoma, nodal diseases such as skin cancer metastases (squamous cell carcinoma, melanoma) and non-Hodgkin lymphoma, and benign lymphoepithelial cysts (AIDS) (Table 4-2).

4. Which lesions need to be imaged?

    a. Lesions of the PS that are superficial (i.e., the clinician can "get his fingers around it") first can be needle aspirated. If cytopathology reveals benign mixed tumor, superficial parotidectomy is usually curative and no imaging is required.

    b. Lesions can be extraparotid or intraparotid in the deep lobe, or they can involve multiple deep facial spaces. Whenever clinical doubt exists as to its location, the lesion should be imaged with CT (when infection is suspected) or MR (when tumor is suspected).

5. Which imaging method should be used?

    a. If the clinical setting suggests parotid ductal disease (recurrent, diffuse parotid swelling associated with eating), thin-section ($\leq$ 3mm)

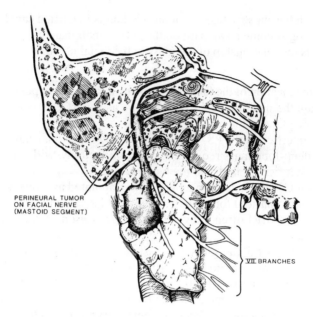

Fig. 4-2 Drawing depicting malignant parotid tumor (*T*) spreading in a perineural fashion along the course of the facial nerve into the temporal bone through the stylomastoid foramen. The mastoid segment of the facial nerve is involved within the temporal bone.

Table 4-2   Multiple Lesions of the Parotid Space: Differential Diagnosis

Inflammatory or Infectious
  Reactive lymphadenopathy
  Benign lymphoepithelial lesions (AIDS)
  Sarcoid

Primary tumor
  Warthin's tumor
  Acinic cell carcinoma
  Non-Hodgkin lymphoma (within parenchyma)

Nodal tumor
  Metastatic tumor
  Non-Hodgkin lymphoma (within parotid nodes)
  Skin malignancy
  Squamous cell carcinoma
  Melanoma

CT is probably the best initial imaging modality. Tailored CT may reveal a dilated parotid duct with or without obstructing calculus. Alternatively, CT may show a picture suggesting Sjögren's syndrome or AIDS. Sialography is still used when the CT picture does not fully explain the problem if ductal stenosis or calculus remains a clinical concern.

b. When parotid abscess is suspected, CT with contrast allows identification of abscess vs. cellulitis, and it will often demonstrate a ductal calculus when present. In 60% of cases parotid ductal calculi are visible on CT. MRI may not show calculus disease.

c. For suspected tumor in the PS (painful mass with or without facial nerve paralysis), MRI is the superior method for demonstrating tumor extent, relationship of the tumor to the facial nerve, and perineural tumor spread along the facial nerve into the temporal bone.

C. Pitfalls in imaging the PS.

1. The parotid gland becomes progressively more fatty with age.

a. A child's gland may appear as tissue or muscle density on CT. Avoid overdiagnosing "infiltrating tumor" in the young parotid gland.

b. MRI shows the young parotid gland as intermediate signal on T1-weighted imaging. Contrast enhancement with MRI in this setting requires fat-suppression techniques to be of use.

2. The general rule that benign tumors are well circumscribed will at times break down in the case of low-grade mucoepidermoid carcinoma. These lesions are rare, but they can mimic benign mixed tumors both clinically and radiographically. Most likely these lesions originally provoked the surgeon's adage that "all parotid masses must come out."

3. Chronic inflammatory disease of the PS may mimic malignant tumor radiologically because of the indistinct margins. Conversely, tumor obstruction of the parotid ductal system may create the clinical appearance of parotid infection.

4. When prominent, the accessory parotid glands will appear as asymmetric masses over the masseter muscle. Inasmuch as accessory parotid glands are present in 21% of normal anatomic dissections, this problem is not infrequent. On CT or MRI "normal" parotid tissue will be seen in this location. This is a clinical pseudomass and need not be removed.

D. Common lesions.

1. Congenital.

a. First branchial cleft cyst.

1) Clinical presentation. The typical patient with a first branchial cleft cyst is a middle-aged woman with a history of multiple parotid abscesses unresponsive to drainage and antibiotics. Otor-

rhea is present when the cyst connects to the bony-cartilaginous junction of the external auditory canal. If an external sinus is present, it is found in the skin at the angle of the mandible.

2) Pathogenesis. Abnormal embryogenesis of the first branchial apparatus. This accounts for 8% of all branchial complex anomalies. The spectrum of developmental abnormalities includes cysts, sinuses, fistulas, and various combinations of these entities.

3) Imaging features. CT or MRI will show a cystic mass superficial to, within, or deep to the parotid gland. Wall thickness varies with the degree of inflammation. CT is the preferred imaging tool when this entity is suspected because of its superior ability in defining the cystic nature of the lesion and associated bony changes (tract through external auditory canal or adjacent temporal bone).

4) Comment. Pathologists have trouble with this diagnosis, because it is rare. They may mistakenly label it an "ectatic duct" or a "parotid cyst."

b. Hemangioma.

1) Clinical presentation. Unilateral parotid swelling seen shortly after birth. The mass is usually soft and compressible. Bluish discoloration is usually visible over the skin, especially with crying.

2) Imaging features. CT is characteristic with holoparotid, intense, uniform enhancement.

3) Comment. This lesion ordinarily involves the entire parotid gland. The facial nerve therefore passes directly through it. Because many of these lesions spontaneously involute, surgery should be postponed if possible to avoid injury to the facial nerve.

2. Infectious or inflammatory diseases.

a. Parotid abscess.

1) Clinical presentation. Unilateral cheek swelling associated with fever, chills, and elevated white-blood-cell count. Usually not a subtle clinical diagnosis.

2) Imaging features. Swollen, enhancing parotid (cellulitis) with focal area(s) of rim-enhancing cyst(s). The parotid duct may be dilated with or without calculus.

3) Comment. CT is the preferred modality in the setting of suspected abscess, because MRI may miss the causal calculus.

b. Sjögren's syndrome.

1) Clinical presentation. Triad of enlarged salivary glands with xerostomia (i.e., dry mouth), enlarged lacrimal glands with ker-

atoconjunctivitis sicca, and connective tissue disease (most commonly rheumatoid arthritis).
  2) Imaging features.
      a) Sialography reveals four progressive patterns: punctate type, globular type, cavitary type, and destructive type.
      b) CT and MRI in more advanced cases will most commonly reveal bilateral parotid enlargement with a honeycombed appearance. Pseudotumors indistinguishable from glandular non-Hodgin lymphoma also may be seen.
  3) Comment. Patients with Sjögren's syndrome have an increased risk of developing a lymphoma, which often has an aggressive biologic course.
  c. Benign lymphoepithelial lesions of AIDS.
      1) Clinical presentation. Bilateral parotid swelling associated with cervical adenopathy in a seropositive for human immunodeficiency virus.
      2) Imaging features. CT or MRI will show bilateral parotid enlargement with intraglandular cystic and cystic–solid lesions. Cervical reactive adenopathy is associated.
      3) Comment. The term *benign lymphoepithelial cysts* has been replaced with *benign lymphoepithelial lesions*, because it is now recognized that both cystic and solid lesions may be present within the parotid gland.
3. Benign tumor.
  a. Benign mixed tumor (pleomorphic adenoma).
      1) Clinical presentation. The patient is usually older than 50 years and has a slow-growing lump in the cheek.
      2) Pathologic findings. Most common (80%) benign parotid tumor. Histologic studies reveal a mixture of epithelial and myoepithelial cells.
      3) Imaging features. CT or MRI will show a sharply marginated mass, which may be round, oval, or lobulated.
          a) Other CT features. Variable enhancement, infrequent dystrophic calcification, and internal pockets of low density when large secondary to "mucoid matrix."
          b) Other MRI features. Very hyperintense on T2-weighted images, and internal pockets of hyperintensity when the tumor is large secondary to "mucoid matrix."
  b. Warthin's tumor (papillary cystadenoma lymphomatosum).
      1) Clinical presentation. Of these patients, 80% are male, older than 50 years, and have a slow-growing mass in the parotid tail region.
      2) Pathologic findings. Second most common benign tumor of the PS. Tumor arises from heterotopic salivary-gland tissue within

parotid lymph nodes. Found in the parotid gland only. Bilateral in 10% to 15% of cases.

3) Imaging features. Well circumscribed and usually 3 to 4 cm in diameter. Internal architecture that is a complex mixture of solid and cystic components on CT or MRI suggests this diagnosis. May be multiple or bilateral.

  c. Oncocytoma.

1) Clinical presentation: Occurs exclusively in adults older than 50 years.

2) Pathologic findings. Oncocytes are large cells with granular eosinophilic cytoplasm that may be found in groups, normally in the parotid gland. An *oncocytoma* describes a solid tumor composed entirely of oncocytes.

3) Imaging features. Nonspecific compared with benign mixed tumor.

4. Malignant tumor, primary.

  a. The smaller the salivary gland, the greater the chance that a mass is malignant. Sublingual gland masses are malignant approximately 70% of the time, submandibular gland masses 60%, and parotid gland masses 20%.

  b. Mucoepidermoid carcinoma.

1) Clinical presentation. Rock-hard mass with associated pain or itching over the course of the facial nerve signals a malignant parotid tumor. Facial nerve paralysis is an ominous sign. Most common malignant parotid tumor in children.

2) Pathologic findings. Most common malignant lesion of the parotid gland. Arises from glandular ductal epithelium. Histologic grade of tumor relates to clinical and radiographic presentation. Low-grade lesion may feel and look like benign mixed tumor.

3) Imaging features. Related to histologic grade. Low-grade lesions are well circumscribed; high-grade lesions are poorly marginated and infiltrating. Remember to search for perineural tumor spread along the course of the facial nerve into the mastoid segment within the temporal bone.

  c. Adenoid cystic carcinoma (cylindroma).

1) Clinical presentation. Same as described for mucoepidermoid carcinoma. In addition, the combination of cranial nerve VII and V_3 neuropathy suggests the diagnosis of adenoid cystic carcinoma of the deep lobe of the parotid gland.

2) Pathologic findings. Tumor arises from peripheral ducts of the parotid gland. Tends to be infiltrating, with a propensity to spread in a perineural fashion along the facial nerve into the temporal bone.

3) Imaging features. CT or MRI will demonstrate an infiltrating mass within the parotid gland. The mastoid or descending portion of the facial nerve must be included in the examination.

   d. Acinic cell carcinoma.
   1) Clinical presentation. Same as described for adenoid cystic carcinoma.
   2) Pathologic findings. Second most common multiple or bilateral tumor (behind Warthin's tumor). Probably arises in the terminal portion of the ductal system. Accounts for 2% to 4% of all major salivary gland malignancy.
   3) Imaging features. Nonspecific.
   e. Malignant tumor, metastatic.
   1) Because the parotid gland undergoes late encapsulation, incorporating lymph nodes within its capsule, it functions as a site for nodal tumor.
   2) Both squamous cell carcinoma and melanoma primary to the skin of the lateral head and external auditory canal can metastasize to the node of the parotid gland. If needle biopsy of a parotid mass reveals either of these lesions, careful physical examination of the scalp and external auditory canal is essential to discover the primary site.
   3) Non-Hodgkin lymphoma can occur either in the nodes or the parenchyma of the parotid gland. In most cases the disease probably begins in the parotid nodes, with "parenchymal disease" resulting when non-Hodgkin lymphoma becomes extranodal.

E. Imaging techniques and protocols.

1. Computed tomography.
   a. Use a lateral scout to assign the angle that maximally avoids dental-filling artifact. Angling parallel to the hard palate above the fillings and parallel to the inferior mandible inferior to the fillings often minimizes the loss of information that results from scanning through fillings.
   b. Contiguous, 3-mm sections with high mAs and moderate magnification are used routinely.
   c. Scan from the lower temporal bone (descending facial nerve canal) until the parotid tail is imaged completely. The hyoid bone represents a useful distal endpoint, because the scan encompasses both the parotid tail and the first-order drainage nodes (high-deep cervical nodes/jugulodigastric node).
   d. Contrast strategy. Bolus (50-mL, 240-contrast medium) followed by rapid drip of 150-ml, 240–iodinated contrast medium. This strategy creates maximal intravascular contrast, which allows the differentia-

tion of vessels from nodal tumor. When spiral technology is available, a significant decrease in the amount of contrast used can be anticipated.

2. Magnetic resonance imaging.
   a. MRI is not used if any suspicion of infection exists, because it will not visualize ductal calculus. When evaluation of tumor is the main imaging issue, MRI delineates the margins and relationship of a mass to the facial nerve better than CT.
   b. Axial and coronal T1-weighted MRI (TR/TE, 500–600/15–30) obtained with 5 mm or less closely spaced (maximum skip, 1 mm) sections are used.
   c. Axial and coronal T2-weighted MRI (TR, 2000) from the midtemporal bone to the hyoid bone further characterize any lesion discovered on T1-weighted imaging.
   d. Contrast usually does not add to the diagnostic information provided by MRI unless deeper and cephalad infiltration is present on the non-contrast images.

3. The clinicoradiographic protocol for the evaluation of a parotid abnormality has multiple permutations. The protocol is constructed on the following major principles:
   a. If a mass is palpable, needle aspiration is completed. For benign tumors clearly in the superficial lobe of the parotid gland, superficial parotidectomy is performed without imaging.
   b. For malignant tumors and benign lesions with margins unclear by palpation, CT or MRI is performed to answer the imaging questions enumerated earlier.
   c. For diffuse swelling (especially when bilateral) CT or MR is initially used, but sialography is kept in reserve if the initial imaging study is inconclusive.
   d. If CT or MRI suggests parotid ductal disease (calculi or stenosis), sialography is done if clinical questions are left unanswered by the initial study.
   e. If a sialogram has been done that suggests a mass, MRI is used if deep-tissue margins are still in question.

SUGGESTED READING

Batsakis JG: *Tumors of the head and neck: clinical and pathological considerations*, ed 2. Baltimore, 1979, Williams & Wilkins.

Bryan RN, Mawad ME, Sandlin ME, et al: CT imaging of the salivary glands. *Semin Ultrasound CT MR* 7:154–165, 1986.

Bryne MN, Spector JG: Parotid masses: evaluation, analysis, and current management. *Laryngoscope* 98:99–105, 1988.

Bryne MN, Spector G, Garvin CF, et al: Preoperative assessment of parotid masses: a comparative evaluation of radiologic techniques to histopathologic diagnosis. *Laryngoscope* 99:284–292, 1989.

Casselman JW, Mancuso AA: Major salivary gland masses: comparison of MR imaging and CT. *Radiology* 165:183–189, 1987.

Eneroth EM: Incidence and prognosis of salivary gland tumours at different sites: a study of parotid, submandibular and palatal tumours in 2632 patients. *Acta Otolaryngol* 273:174–178, 1970.

Freling NJM, Molenaar WM, Vermey A, et al: Malignant parotid tumors: clinical use of MR imaging and histologic correlation. *Radiology* 185:691–696, 1992.

Holiday RA, Cohen WA, Schinella RA, et al: Benign lymphoepithelial parotid cysts and hyperplastic cervical adenopathy: a new CT appearance. *Radiology* 168:439–441, 1988.

Kane WJ, McCaffrey TV, Olsen KD, et al: Primary parotid malignancies: a clinical and pathologic review. *Arch Otolaryngol Head Neck Surg* 117:307–315, 1991.

Kirshenbaum KJ, Nadimpalli SR, Friedman M, et al: Benign lymphoepithelial parotid tumors in AIDS patients: CT and MR findings in nine cases. *AJNR* 12:271–274, 1991.

McGahan JP, Walter JP, Bernstein L: Evaluation of the parotid gland. *Radiology* 152:453–458, 1984.

Mandelblatt SM, Braun IF, Davis PC, et al: Parotid masses: MR imaging. *Radiology* 163:411–414, 1987.

Minami M, Tanioka H, Oyama K, et al: Warthin tumor of the parotid gland: MR-pathologic correlation. *AJNR* 14:209–214, 1993.

Mirich DR, McArdle CB, Kulkarni MV: Benign pleomorphic adenomas of the salivary glands: surface coil MR imaging versus CT. *J Comput Assist Tomogr* 1:65–69, 1988.

Mukherji SK, Tart RP, Slattery WH, et al: Evaluation of first branchial anomalies by CT and MR. *J Comput Assist Tomogr* 17:576–581, 1993.

Pollei SR, Harnsberger HR: The radiologic evaluation of the parotid space. *Semin Ultrasound CT MR* 11:486–503, 1990.

Som PM, Shugar JMA, Stollman AL, et al: Benign and malignant parotid pleomorphic adenomas: CT and MR studies. *J Comput Assist Tomogr* 12:65–69, 1988.

Sone S, Higashihara T, Morimoto S, et al: CT of parotid tumors. *AJNR* 3:143–147, 1982.

Swartz JD, Rothman MI, Marlowe FI, et al: MR imaging of parotid mass lesions: attempts at histopathologic differentiation. *J Comput Assist Tomogr* 13:789–796.

Tabor EK, Curtin HD: MR of the salivary glands. *Radiol Clin North Am* 27:379–392, 1989.

Takashima S, Nagareda T, Noguchi Y, et al: CT and MR appearance of parotid pseudotumors in Sjögren's syndrome. *J Comput Assist Tomog* 16:376–383, 1992.

Takashima S, Takeuchi N, Morimoto S, et al: MR imaging of Sjörgren's syndrome: correlation with sialography and pathology. *J Comput Assist Tomog* 15:393–400, 1991.

Teresi LM, Lufkin RB, Wortham DG, et al: Parotid masses: MR imaging. *Radiology* 163:405–409, 1987.

Thibault F, Halimi P, Bely H, et al: Internal architecture of the parotid gland at MR imaging: facial nerve or ductal system? *Radiology* 188:701–704, 1993.

Vogl TJ, Dresel SHJ, Spath M, et al: Parotid gland: plain and gadolinium-enhanced MR imaging. *Radiology* 177:667–674, 1990.

5

The Carotid Space

CRITICAL IMAGING QUESTIONS: CAROTID SPACE

1. What radiologic features characterize a lesion as primary to the carotid space (CS)?
2. What statistically common lesions are unique to the CS?
3. Does the CS lesion appear vascular (i.e., marked enhancement on CT or "channel voids" on MRI) or avascular? Why is it important to differentiate these specific radiologic features?
4. Is the CS lesion adjacent or intrinsic to the carotid artery or jugular vein?
5. Does the CS lesion involve the jugular foramen or the basal cistern? What tumors are in this limited differential diagnosis?

Answers to these questions are found in the text beside the question number (Q#) in the margin.

CAROTID SPACE (CS)

A. Normal anatomy.

1. Fascia. All three layers of deep cervical fascia condense to form the tenacious fascia surrounding the carotid space (CS), which is known as the *carotid sheath*.
2. Contents. (Fig. 5-1, *left*).
   Common or internal carotid artery (level dependent).
   Internal jugular vein.
   Cranial nerves IX, X, XI, XII: nasopharyngeal CS.
   Cranial nerve X only: oropharyngeal and infrahyoid CS.
   Sympathetic plexus.
   Lymph nodes.
   a. Carotid sheath.
       1) The carotid sheath comprises all three layers of the deep cervical fascia.

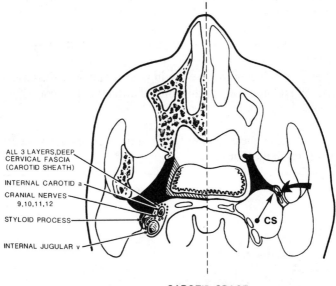

CAROTID SPACE

Fig. 5-1 *Left,* Three layers of the deep cervical fascia constitute the carotid sheath (*dotted-dashed-solid line*). The internal carotid artery, internal jugular vein, and cranial nerves IX through XII are the principal occupants of the CS at this level. *Right,* Axial drawing through the low nasopharynx illustrates a carotid space (*CS*) mass. Its center (*black dot*) is posterior to the parapharyngeal space fat (*black area*). The displacement pattern of the mass is from posterior to anterior, bowing the parapharyngeal space anteriorly and displacing the styloid process (*curved arrow*) anterolaterally.

2) It is a more substantive fascia in the extracranial head and neck that prevents disease outside the CS from entering and disease within the CS from spreading into the surrounding deep spaces.

3) The carotid sheath is a well-defined structure below the carotid bifurcation, but it is often incomplete or absent in the area of the oropharynx and nasopharynx.

  b. CS vessels.

1) The internal carotid artery (ICA) arises from the common carotid artery at approximately the level of the hyoid bone. Ectasia, aneurysm, or pseudoaneurysm of the ICA can mimic vascular tumor of the CS.

2) The internal jugular vein usually runs posterolaterally with the ICA (Fig. 5-1) throughout the deep face and neck. Jugular vein thrombosis can mimic necrotic tumor of the CS.

  c. CS nerves.

1) The vagus nerve is the single most important nerve within the CS. It is located in the posterior notch formed by the common and internal carotid arteries and the internal jugular vein throughout the entire extracranial CS.

    a) Comment. Because the vagus nerve is the only cranial nerve traversing the entire CS, the discussion of vagus nerve imaging found in the chapter on lower cranial nerves is particularly important. The issues of radiologic evaluation of vagal neuropathy and CS lesions are inextricably linked.

2) The glossopharyngeal, spinal accessory, and hypoglossal cranial nerves (IX, XI, and XII, respectively) are also seen in the nasopharyngeal CS, but all three soon leave the CS at approximately the level of the soft palate.

3) The sympathetic plexus is most easily remembered for imaging purposes as an occupant of the CS. Careful dissection, however, will find this nerve plexus to be in the medial fascial wall of the CS (i.e., in the common wall between the CS and the retropharyngeal space).

  d. CS lymph nodes.

1) The highest nodes of the deep cervical chain are found with the carotid sheath at the level of the oropharynx and known as *jugulodigastric nodes.*

2) In any discussion of the infrahyoid neck, the CS is important because of its close association with the deep cervical nodal chain.

3. Extent and boundaries.

  a. The CS extends from the skull base to the aortic arch. In describing an abnormality, subdividing the CS into nasopharyngeal, oropharyngeal, cervical, and mediastinal segments helps one to communicate effectively with the referring physician.

1) It is important to recognize that the cephalad margin of the CS feeds directly into the jugular foramen. This critical anatomic relationship creates the potential for extracranial spread of cisternal and skull base lesions (e.g., meningioma, glomus jugulare paraganglioma) and intracranial spread of nasopharyngeal CS lesions (e.g., vagal schwannoma).

2) Only the suprahyoid CS is discussed here. The infrahyoid CS is discussed in the chapter covering the infrahyoid neck.

b. The nasopharyngeal carotid space is also referred to in the literature as the *retrostyloid parapharyngeal space*.

1) This latter terminology is not used here, because it may confuse the discussion of differential diagnosis. Tissues of the carotid space are unique compared with the fatty triangle of the parapharyngeal space, allowing a unique, space-specific differential diagnosis to be described for lesions of this space.

c. Bordering spaces (see Figs. 1-4 and 1-5).

1) Lateral to the CS is the parotid space. The posterior belly of the digastric muscle and its associated superficial layer of deep cervical fascia separate the CS from the parotid space.

2) Anterior to the CS is the parapharyngeal space fat.

3) Medial to the CS is the lateral margin of the retropharyngeal space. Diseases involving the lateral retropharyngeal nodes can be confused with CS lesions if one is not mindful of their close proximity (see Chapter 6).

B. Imaging issues.

1. How can a lesion be identified with certainty as arising in the CS?

Q#1

a. A mass is primary to the carotid space if:

1) The center of the mass is within the area of the ICA and internal jugular vein and posterior to the parapharyngeal space (Fig. 5-1, *right*).

2) The mass invades or encroaches on the parapharyngeal space from posterior to anterior, displacing the PPS fat anteriorly.

   a) When the mass is in the nasopharyngeal CS, displacement of the parapharyngeal space fat is accompanied by anterolateral displacement of the styloid process.

   b) When the mass begins in the posterior portion of the CS (e.g., vagal schwannoma or neurofibroma, or paraganglioma), the

          ICA will be seen draped over the anterior margin of the CS mass.

   b. Once the mass has been localized to the CS, the differential diagnosis (Table 5-1) should be consulted. Matching the characteristic radiologic features of the lesion to common entities of the CS often will yield a short list of possible diagnoses.

   c. Unlike those of some other deep facial spaces, CS lesions are quite characteristic in their radiologic appearance, making the process of discovery and spatial localization blissfully histopathologic.

2. What other questions must be answered to help sort out what these lesions might be?

Q#2

   a. What are the statistically common lesions of the CS?

     1) The three most common lesions of the CS are:

Table 5-1   Differential Diagnosis of Carotid Space Mass

Pseudomass
   Ectatic common or internal carotid artery*
   Asymmetric internal jugular vein*

Inflammatory
   Carotid space cellulitis or abscess

Vascular lesions
   Jugular vein thrombosis or thrombophlebitis*
   Internal carotid artery thrombosis, mural thrombus, aneurysm, or
     pseudoaneurysm*
   Internal carotid artery dissection

Benign tumor
   Paraganglioma*
     Glomus jugulare
     Glomus vagale
     Carotid body tumor
   Neural sheath tumor
     Schwannoma*
     Neurofibroma
   Meningioma (from jugular foramen)

Malignant tumor
   Squamous cell carcinoma nodal metastasis*
   Direct invasion by primary squamous cell carcinoma
   Non-Hodgkin lymphoma

*These are more common lesions

a) Paraganglioma (glomus jugulare, vagale or carotid body tumor).
b) Schwannoma, usually vagal.
c) Squamous cell carcinoma nodal metastasis.

Q#3

b. Does the lesion appear vascular?

1) On enhanced CT scans, the mass should have approximately the same density as the adjacent vessels for the radiologist to suggest it is vascular. CT with the bolus-drip technique is assumed.
2) On MRI, observation of serpiginous flow or channel voids suggests a vascular mass.
3) Bright enhancement on CT or flow voids on MRI suggest the diagnosis of paraganglioma. At times "vascular neural sheath lesions," especially schwannoma, cannot be differentiated from paraganglioma. This differentiation is not critical, however, because preoperative embolization and the same surgical approach is used for both.

Q#4

c. What is the relationship of the CS mass to the ICA and internal jugular vein?

1) Careful consideration as to whether the lesion is a vascular pseudomass (e.g., ectatic ICA) or a nonsurgical vascular lesion (e.g., a thrombosed ICA or internal jugular vein) will obviate resection of these nonsurgical abnormalities.
2) The important feature to observe in this setting is the relationship between the lesion and the vessels of the CS (i.e., is the lesion extrinsic to the CS vessels?).

Q#5

d. Does the CS lesion extend into the jugular foramen or basal cisterns?

1) Lesions of the nasopharyngeal CS may project cephalad to involve the jugular foramen and the basal cisterns. Because head and neck surgeons usually view the skull base as the end of their surgical field, a neurosurgeon or head and neck surgeon trained in the skull base must be involved if the lesion penetrates the skull base and basal cisterns.
2) Conversely, if the lesion begins in the jugular foramen, it may spread inferiorly into the nasopharyngeal CS. In this manner lesions such as glomus jugulare paraganglioma and jugular foramen meningioma may access the extracranial head and neck. Because neurosurgeons generally see the lower margins of the

jugular foramen as the end of their surgical dissection, a head and neck surgeon must be on the surgical team for these dumb-bell lesions.

3) Lesions involving the basal cistern, jugular foramen, and nasopharyngeal carotid space are limited in number and include:
   a) Jugular foramen paraganglioma.
   b) Cranial nerves IX through XI schwannoma.
   c) Cranial nerves IX through XI neurofibroma.
   d) Jugular foramen meningioma.

C. Common lesions (Table 5-1).

1. Pseudomasses.
   a. Ectatic common or internal carotid artery.
   1) Clinical presentation. A pulsatile mass is seen or felt in the anterolateral neck or posterolateral pharyngeal wall. The diagnosis of paraganglioma is questioned by the referring physician.
   2) Imaging features. A tubular, tortuous, sometimes dilated common carotid artery or internal carotid artery is seen on CT (enhancing) scans or MRI (flow void) in the location of the normal carotid artery. At times when the vessel folds sharply on itself, the appearance of an enhancing CS mass is suggested on CT scans.
   3) Comment. Do not mistake this nonsurgical pseudomass for a "vascular tumor." If questions still exist after CT scans, MRI with magnetic resonance angiography will settle the issue. In most cases the diagnosis can be made from CT or standard MRI alone.
   b. Asymmetric internal jugular vein.
   1) Clinical presentation. Incidental finding on CT scans, or MRI, or vague fullness in the neck noted by referring physician.
   2) Imaging features. Large, tubular, enhancing structure (on CT) or flow void (on MRI) in the normal location of the internal jugular vein.
   3) Comment. A wide range of normal variation exists in symmetry of the internal jugular veins of the deep face and neck, from complete absence of one vein to perfect bilateral symmetry.

2. Inflammatory.
   a. Cellulitis or abscess.
   1) Clinical presentation. Patients with infection of the extracranial head and neck are generally quite sick, with fever, elevated white blood cell count, and tenderness in the infected area. The CS is usually involved secondarily with infection, similar to the parapharyngeal space. When the CS is infected, hoarseness (i.e., vagus nerve malfunction) is also noted.

    2) Imaging appearance. Cellulitis is seen as a loss of soft-tissue planes within the CS without focal fluid collection. Abscess is diagnosed by identification of a focal area of fluid (i.e., pus). CS infection is usually very localized by the tenacious carotid sheath.

    3) Comment. CS abscess is a surgical emergency! The clinician must be notified immediately in suspected cases. Delay in surgical intervention can result in perforation of the carotid artery and exsanguination.

3. Vascular lesions.

  a. Jugular vein thrombosis or thrombophlebitis.

    1) Clinical presentation. Patients often have a history of previous central venous catheterization, drug abuse, or malignancy. The acute thrombophlebitic phase of this process clinically mimics infection (i.e., tender red mass and fever); the chronic thrombotic phase can appear like a tumor (i.e., hard, nontender mass).

    2) Imaging features.

      a) CT. Findings depend on the stage of the disease. The acute thrombophlebitic phase shows loss of soft-tissue planes surrounding the enlarged, thrombus-filled, internal jugular vein. The vasa vasorum of the venous wall may enhance as a thin white rim. The more chronic thrombotic phase appears as a well-marginated tubular mass without loss of surrounding soft-tissue planes.

      b) MRI. In the subacute phase of jugular vein thrombosis, MRI demonstrates a tubular mass with high signal on T1-weighted images secondary to T1 shortening from the paramagnetic effect of methemoglobin.

  b. Common carotid artery or ICA thrombosis, mural thrombus, aneurysm, or pseudoaneurysm.

    1) Clinical presentation. Carotid artery thrombosis and mural thrombus with stenosis may present with transient ischemic attack or cerebrovascular accident (i.e., stroke). Pseudoaneurysm usually follows penetrating trauma with injury to the vessel or deceleration injury with carotid artery dissection and associated pseudoaneurysm formation.

    2) Imaging features. Enhanced CT shows complete carotid artery luminal obliteration (i.e., thrombosis) or partial obliteration (e.g., mural thrombus). Pseudoaneurysm is seen as a CS mass with at least partial filling of its lumen. MRI shows partial or complete loss of the carotid artery flow void. The clot associated with the thrombosis, mural thrombus, or pseudoaneurysm often will show a complex mixture of signal intensities on T1-weighted

images secondary to the multiple ages of the blood within the clot.

3) Comment. Jugular vein or carotid artery thrombosis associated with primary or recurrent squamous cell carcinoma of the extracranial head and neck, as is often the case, can be misdiagnosed by an unwary radiologist as "necrotic adenopathy." Avoid this pitfall by observing their tubular nature (i.e., the abnormality is present on multiple sequential axial images).

4. Benign tumor.

   a. Paraganglioma (Table 5-2).

   1) Clinical presentation. Slowly enlarging (over years) mass of the CS. When the tumor involves the jugular foramen of the skull base, cranial nerve compressive ischemia results in variable neuropathy of cranial nerves IX through XII. Skull base involvement also may present as pulsatile tinnitus.

   2) Pathologic findings.

   a) Benign tumor arising from neural crest paraganglion cells of the extracranial head and neck.

   b) Multiple tumors seen in 3% to 5% of patients overall and 20% to 30% with a family history.

   3) Imaging features.

   a) CT. *Intensely* enhancing mass of the CS. The only other common diagnosis for this CT appearance is vascular schwannoma. Metastatic hypernephroma may have this appearance but is extremely rare in this location. When the bone of the jugular foramen is involved, the jugular spine is eroded and the bony changes are irregular and *permeative* (compare bone findings in schwannoma and neurofibroma).

   b) MRI. When the lesion is larger than 2 cm, the MRI appearance is distinctive. Tubular mass within the CS is nicely delineated by sagittal or coronal imaging planes. Serpiginous flow

Table 5-2   Types of Paraganglioma

Name	Location	Associated structure
Glomus tympanicum	Cochlear promontory on medial wall of the middle ear cavity	Jacobsen's nerve
Glomus jugulare	Jugular foramen	Jugular ganglion
Glomus vagale	Naso- and oropharyngeal carotid space	Nodose ganglion of the vagus nerve
Carotid body tumor	Carotid bifurcation	Carotid body

voids within the mass look like "pepper" (i.e., focal hypo-intensity) and are usually obvious, whereas small areas of sub-acute hemorrhage within the tumor look like "salt" (i.e., focal hyperintensity on T1-weighted images) and are seen less frequently. When seen together, this heterogeneous "salt-and-pepper" appearance is characteristic of paraganglioma.

4) The lesion is named by its anatomic location. Paraganglioma at the common carotid bifurcation is termed a *carotid body tumor*. When seen above the bifurcation to the skull base, *glomus vagale paraganglioma* is used. When originating in the jugular foramen and involving the carotid space from above, the term *glomus jugulare paraganglioma* is used (Fig. 5-2).

5) Comment. When a CS mass is identified as probable paraganglioma, a careful search for a second, synchronous lesion is

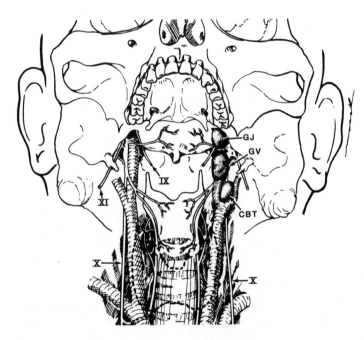

Fig. 5-2   Anterior view of the carotid space showing the three major areas where paragangliomas are found. Paragangliomas are named by their anatomic location. When they occur in the bifurcation notch, they are referred to as *carotid body tumor* (*CBT*). In the area between the carotid bifurcation and the skull base, the term *glomus vagale* (*GV*) is used. *Glomus jugulare paraganglioma* (*GJ*) occur in the jugular foramen and may extend inferiorly into the nasopharyngeal carotid space or superiorly into the basal cistern.

important, especially when a family history of paraganglioma exists.
- b. Schwannoma.
    1) Clinical presentation. Painless, slow-growing mass in the antero-lateral neck or the posterolateral oropharynx or nasopharynx. They may become painful, with associated cranial neuropathy (cranial nerves IX to XII) when involving the jugular foramen of the skull base. When present in a patient with neurofibromatosis, schwannoma may be multiple.
    2) Pathologic findings.
        a) This tumor arises from Schwann cells, which surround the peripheral nerves, providing mechanical protection, producing the myelin sheath, and serving as a tract for nerve regeneration.
        b) Schwannoma is an encapsulated tumor with two components: a cellular component (i.e., Antoni type A tissue); and a loose, myxoid component (i.e., Antoni type B tissue). The presence of these two components allows the pathologist to differentiate schwannoma from neurofibroma.
        c) The most commonly involved peripheral nerves are the cervical spinal roots, the vagus nerve, and the sympathetic plexus.
    3) Imaging features.
        a) CT shows a fusiform, well-encapsulated, tissue-density mass in the CS, with displacement of the ICA anteriorly (i.e., vagal schwannoma). When the schwannoma extends into the jugular foramen of the skull base, the bone is smoothly scalloped, a feature that clearly differentiates it from the permeative bony changes of paraganglioma.
        b) MRI demonstrates the fusiform shape better than CT in the sagittal and coronal plane. Conspicuous absence of flow voids in the tumor helps to differentiate schwannoma from paraganglioma, and MRI with contrast reveals a uniformly enhancing, well-circumscribed, fusiform mass on T1-weighted images.
    4) Comment. The more vascular schwannoma may not be radiologically separable from paraganglioma. Bone changes may help the differentiation; however, a transcervical surgical approach and preoperative embolization are used in the treatment of both lesions.
- c. Neurofibroma.
    1) Clinical presentation. Symptoms depend on the nerve involved. Only 10% of patients with neurofibromas have von Reckling-

hausen syndrome. Younger patients (i.e., those 20 to 30 years of age) have solitary neurofibromas.

    2) Pathologic findings.

       a) Benign, nonencapsulated, well-circumscribed tumor of the peripheral nerves.

       b) Histologic studies demonstrate swirls of neuronal elements.

       c) Some neurofibromas undergo considerable fatty degeneration.

    3) Imaging features.

       a) CT shows a well-circumscribed, low-density, fusiform mass. Density may vary, but a low, almost water density is characteristic of neurofibroma.

       b) MRI features of neurofibroma are indistinguishable from those of schwannoma, except in the case of a plexiform lesion, where central low intensity from the central fibrous core is seen.

  d. Meningioma.

    1) Clinical presentation. Symptoms depend on nerve compression (cranial nerves IX through XI) within the jugular foramen.

    2) Pathologic findings. Same as any dural-based, intracranial meningioma.

    3) Imaging features.

       a) Both CT and MRI reveal a well-circumscribed mass/lesion hanging out the bottom of the jugular foramen into the nasopharyngeal carotid space. The lesion also may project cephalad into the basal cistern, creating a dumb-bell appearance on coronal images.

       b) CT may show calcification as well as hypertrophic bony changes in the adjacent skull base bones. Intense enhancement is visible when contrast is administered.

       c) MRI will show intense contrast enhancement on T1-weighted images. A dural tail also may be associated. Conventional T2-weighted, spin echo images often will show susceptibility changes (i.e., blotchy low intensity) when calcification is present within the lesion.

5. Malignant tumor.

  a. Squamous cell carcinoma nodal metastasis.

    1) Clinical presentation. In most cases the patient has a previously diagnosed primary squamous cell carcinoma of the mucosa of the upper aerodigestive tract mucosa. In cases where the primary tumor is clinically or radiologically occult, nodal mass may be the only manifestation of the malignancy.

    2) Imaging features. CT or MRI will show single or multiple, oval to round masses immediately adjacent to the CS from the level of

the oropharynx to that of the clavicle. Enhanced CT or gadolinium-enhanced MRI may delineate inhomogeneity to the internal architecture of the nodal mass as a marker of malignancy.

3) Comment. A nodal mass in or adjacent to the CS at the level of the oropharynx is a jugulodigastric or a high, deep cervical chain node. A nodal mass above the level of the hard palate, however, is in the lateral retropharyngeal nodal chain, not the CS. For further discussion of this concept, see Chapter 13.

b. Non-Hodgkin lymphoma.

1) Clinical presentation. Early non-Hodgkin lymphoma may present as nodal neck disease in the CS. More advanced disease usually involves thoracic and abdominal nodes along with CS adenopathy.

2) Imaging features. Enhanced CT or MRI will show homogeneous, oval to round, single or multiple CS masses. In the absence of treatment the nodes are rarely "necrotic," unless the lymphoma is particularly undifferentiated.

6. Summary.

a. The carotid space contains vessels, nerves, and nodes. As expected, the main lesions of this space include vascular pseudomasses and diseases, nerve-related tumors, and nodal tumor. Many CS lesions have characteristic radiologic features that allow the radiologist to make near-histopathologic diagnoses from images of the lesion.

SUGGESTED READING

Albertyn LE, Alcock MK: Diagnosis of internal jugular vein thrombosis. *Radiology* 162:505–508, 1987.

Braun IF, Hoffman JC, Malko JA, et al: Jugular vein thrombosis: MR imaging. *Radiology* 157:357–360, 1985.

Cohen LM, Schwartz AM, Rock SD: Benign schwannomas: pathologic basis for CT inhomogeneities. *Am J Roentgenol* 147:141–143, 1986.

Duvall ER, Gupta KL, Vitek JJ, et al: CT demonstration of extra-cranial carotid artery aneurysm. *J Comput Assist Tomogr* 10:404–408, 1986.

Eriksen C, Girdhar-Gopal H, Lowry LD: Vagal paragangliomas: a report of nine cases. *Am J Otolaryngol* 12:278–287, 1991.

Fishman EK, Pakter RL, Gayler BW, et al: Jugular venous thrombosis: diagnosis by computed tomography. *J Comput Assist Tomogr* 8:963–968, 1984.

Fruin ME, Smoker WRK, Harnsberger HR: The carotid space of the infrahyoid neck. *Semin Ultrasound CT MR* 12:224–240, 1991.

Fruin ME, Smoker WRK, Harnsberger, HR: The carotid space in the suprahyoid neck. *Semin Ultrasound CT MR* 11:504–519, 1990.

Goldberg HI, Grossman RI, Gomori JM, et al: Cervical internal carotid artery dissection hemorrhage: diagnosis using MR. *Radiology* 158:157–161, 1986.

Harnsberger HR: CT and MRI of masses of the deep face. *Curr Probl Diagn Radiol* 16:143–173, 1987.

Haynes DS, Schwaber MK, Netterville JL: Internal carotid artery aneurysms presenting as neck masses. *Otolaryngol Head Neck Surg* 107:787–791, 1992.

Hodge KM, Byers RM, Peters LJ: Paragangliomas of the head and neck. *Arch Otolaryngol Head Neck Surg* 114:872–877, 1988.

Jacobs JM, Harnsberger HR, Lufkin RB, et al: Vagal neuropathy: evaluation with CT and MR imaging. *Radiology* 164:97–102, 1987.

Kumar AJ, Kuhajda FP, Martinez CR, et al: Computed tomography of extracranial nerve sheath tumors with pathological correlation. *J Comput Assist Tomogr* 7:857–865, 1983.

Lloyd GAS, Cheesman AD, Phelps PD, King CMP: The demonstration of glomus tumours by subtraction MRI. *Neuroradiology* 34:470–474, 1992.

Olsen WL, Dillon WP, Kelly WM, et al: MR imaging of paragangliomas. *Am J Roentgenol* 148:201–204, 1987.

Silver AJ, Mawad ME, Hilal SK, et al: Computed tomography of the carotid space and related cervical spaces. I: anatomy. II: neurogenic tumors. *Radiology* 150:723–735, 1984.

Som PM, Biller HF, Lawson W, et al: Parapharyngeal space masses. An updated protocol based upon 104 cases. *Radiology* 153:149–156, 1984.

Som PM, Lanzieri CF, Sacher M, et al: Extracranial tumor vascularity: determination by dynamic CT scanning. I: concepts and signature curves. II: the unit approach. *Radiology* 154:401–412, 1985.

Suh JS, Abenoza P, Galloway HR, et al: Peripheral (extracranial) nerve tumors: correlation of MR imaging and histologic findings. *Radiology* 183:341–346, 1992.

Vogl T, Bruning R, Schedel H, et al: Paragangliomas of the jugular bulb and carotid body: MR imaging with short sequences and Gd-DTPA enhancement. *AJNR* 10:823–827, 1989.

6

The Retropharyngeal Space

CRITICAL IMAGING QUESTIONS: RETROPHARYNGEAL SPACE

1. Why is a mass in the retropharyngeal space (RPS) asymmetric (involving only one side) in the nasopharynx and oropharynx but symmetric (involving both sides) in the infrahyoid neck?
2. What radiologic features define a mass as primary to the RPS?
3. What key CT or MRI observation allows differentiation of a mass in the RPS vs. the perivertebral space?
4. Under what circumstances can a lesion that looks like an abscess of the RPS on CT or MRI scans not be an abscess of that space?

Answers to these questions are found in the text beside the question number (Q#) in the margin.

RETROPHARYNGEAL SPACE (RPS)

A. Normal anatomy.

1. Fascia. The retropharyngeal space (RPS) is the potential space formed between the middle layer and the deep layer of deep cervical fascia (Figs. 6-1 and 6-2). Practically speaking, this space will be seen on cross-sectional imaging between the pharyngeal constrictor muscles anteriorly and the prevertebral muscles posteriorly. In its undiseased state the RPS is seen as a thin line of fat, which may be more prominent in patients with obesity.

   a. The lateral walls of the RPS are comprised of a slip of deep cervical fascia called the *alar fascia*.

   b. A second slip of deep cervical fascia can be seen separating the RPS from the danger space (DS) (Fig. 6-1). The importance of the DS is that it serves as a conduit for RPS infection and tumor to reach the mediastinum inferiorly. Otherwise, lesions of the RPS and DS are radiologically indistinguishable from one another and are therefore discussed under the general heading of RPS pathology.

   c. A median raphe divides the RPS into two halves. The median raphe is often difficult to identify with imaging when the RPS is normal.

2. Contents (Figs. 6-1 through 6-3). The RPS has few important structures within its boundaries:

   Fat.

   Lymph nodes.

      Lateral nodes (nodes of the Rouviere).

      Medial nodes.

   a. Lymph nodes.

      1) The lateral retropharyngeal nodal group (the nodes of Rouviere) is found in the high oropharynx and nasopharynx. The nodes are considered normal if they are less than 1 cm in diameter. The younger the person being imaged, the more likely these nodes will be seen and be normal.

         a) These nodes can be seen routinely on MRI scans. They are far less well seen on CT scans. Therefore if retropharyngeal nodal tumor is being sought radiologically, MRI is the superior imaging modality.

      2) The medial retropharyngeal nodal group is found only from the level of the nasopharynx to the upper hypopharynx. These nodes are not normally seen on CT or MRI scans.

Q #1

      3) There are no lymph nodes in the RPS below the level of the hyoid bone. Consequently, when infection or tumor involves the

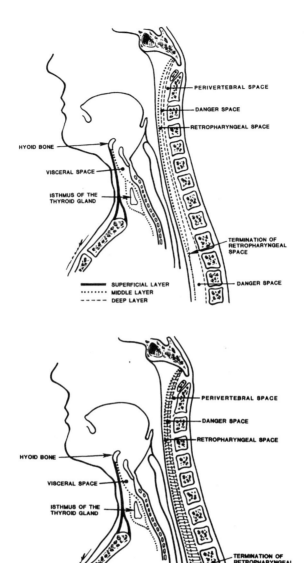

Fig. 6-1 **A**, Sagittal drawing of the extracranial head and neck depicting the complete craniocaudal extent of the retropharyngeal, danger, and perivertebral spaces. All three spaces traverse the distance from the skull base to approximately the level of the T3 vertebral body. **B**, The danger space provides an inferior route for disease of the retropharyngeal space to access the mediastinum. From an imaging standpoint, the retropharyngeal space cannot be distinguished from the danger space in either the normal or diseased state. These two spaces are crosshatched to emphasize this point.

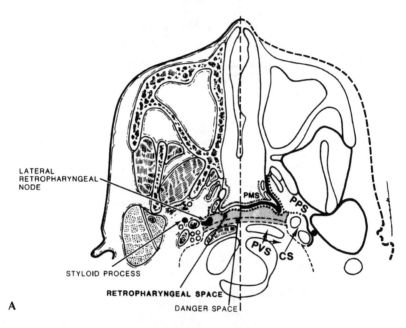

LATERAL
RETROPHARYNGEAL
NODE

STYLOID PROCESS

RETROPHARYNGEAL SPACE

A

DANGER SPACE

Fig. 6-2 Transaxial drawings through nasopharynx (A), low oropharynx (B), and infrahyoid neck (C) illustrate the fascia and contents of the retropharyngeal (*RPS*), danger (*DS*), and perivertebral spaces (*PVS*). **A**, The nasopharyngeal RPS has the middle layer of deep cervical fascia (*dotted line*) as its anterior border. Its posterior border is supplied by a slip of the deep layer of deep cervical fascia (*dashed line*), and the lateral margin comes from an anterior slip of this same fascia. At the nasopharyngeal level the RPS contains fat and both medial and lateral retropharyngeal nodes. Just posterior to the RPS is the danger space, which contains only fat. The nasopharyngeal PVS is circumscribed by the deep layer of deep cervical fascia (*dashed line*). **B**, The oropharyngeal RPS has the middle layer of deep cervical fascia (*dotted line*) as its anterior border. Its posterior border is supplied by a slip of the deep layer of deep cervical fascia (*dashed line*), and the lateral margin comes from an anterior slip of this same fascia. At the oropharyngeal level the RPS contains fat and medial retropharyngeal nodes. **C**, The infrahyoid RPS has the

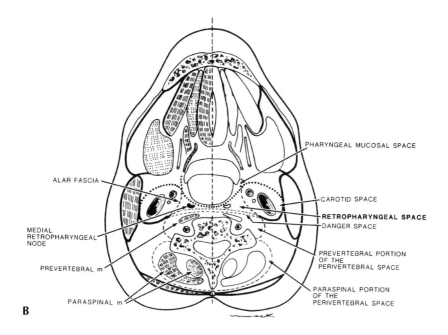

PHARYNGEAL MUCOSAL SPACE

ALAR FASCIA

CAROTID SPACE

RETROPHARYNGEAL SPACE
DANGER SPACE

MEDIAL
RETROPHARYNGEAL
NODE

PREVERTEBRAL PORTION
OF THE
PERIVERTEBRAL SPACE

PREVERTEBRAL m

PARASPINAL PORTION
OF THE
PERIVERTEBRAL SPACE

PARASPINAL m

B

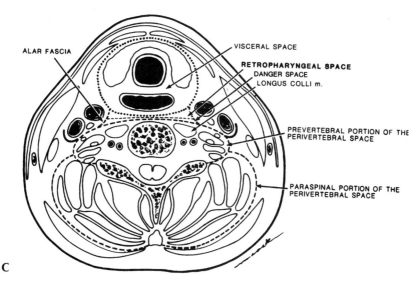

ALAR FASCIA

VISCERAL SPACE

RETROPHARYNGEAL SPACE
DANGER SPACE
LONGUS COLLI m.

PREVERTEBRAL PORTION OF THE
PERIVERTEBRAL SPACE

PARASPINAL PORTION OF THE
PERIVERTEBRAL SPACE

C

middle layer of deep cervical fascia (*dotted line*) as its anterior border. Its posterior border is supplied by a slip of the deep layer of deep cervical fascia (*dashed line*), and the lateral margin comes from an anterior slip of this same fascia. At the infrahyoid level the RPS contains only fat.

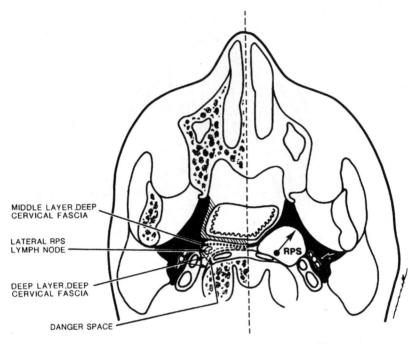

MIDDLE LAYER ,DEEP
CERVICAL FASCIA

LATERAL RPS
LYMPH NODE

DEEP LAYER ,DEEP
CERVICAL FASCIA

DANGER SPACE

A   **RETROPHARYNGEAL SPACE**

Fig. 6-3   The types of retropharyngeal masses in the nasopharynx (A), oropharynx (B), and the infrahyoid neck (C). **A,** *Left,* The middle layer of deep cervical fascia (*dotted line*) forms the anterior wall of the normal RPS, and a slip of the deep layer of deep cervical fascia (*dashed line*) forms the lateral and posterior walls. Fat and the medial and lateral retropharyngeal nodal chain are the only contents of the RPS. Note the danger space between the RPS and prevertebral portion of the perivertebral space. *Right,* Axial drawing through the low nasopharynx shows the appearance of a nodal retropharyngeal space mass (*RPS*). The mass is depicted as unilateral, beginning in the lateral retropharyngeal nodal chain, with its center (*black dot*) posteromedial to the parapharyngeal space (*black area*). The displacement pattern of this RPS mass is from posteromedial to anterolateral, with bowing of the parapharyngeal space anteromedially. Note the lack of displacement of the styloid process (*outlined arrow*). **B,** Axial drawing at the level of the oropharynx showing a "bow tie"–shaped RPS mass/lesion displacing the pharyngeal mucosal space (*PMS*) anteriorly and the danger space (*DS*)/perivertebral space (*PVS*) posteriorly. Note the flattening of the prevertebral muscles (*arrows*) posteriorly. **C,** RPS mass at the level of the infrahyoid neck. Axial drawing through the thyroid shows a "bow tie"–shaped mass in the infrahyoid RPS. At this level the RPS mass displaces the visceral space (*VS*) anteriorly while flattening the danger space and prevertebral space muscles posteriorly. *CS,* Carotid space; *MS,* masticator space; *PPS,* parapharyngeal space; *PS,* parotid space.

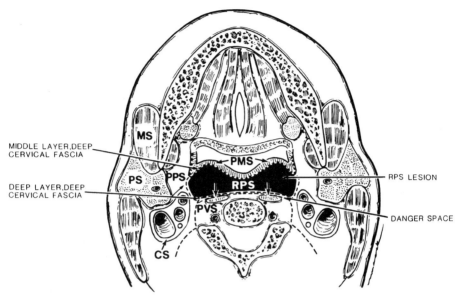

MIDDLE LAYER,DEEP
CERVICAL FASCIA

DEEP LAYER,DEEP
CERVICAL FASCIA

RPS LESION

DANGER SPACE

B   **RETROPHARYNGEAL SPACE**

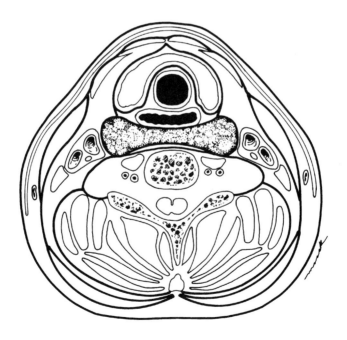

C   **RETROPHARYNGEAL SPACE**

suprahyoid RPS, the disease is usually asymmetric and on the side of the initial diseased node.

  a) When the infrahyoid RPS is diseased, the process is seen throughout the space and on both sides, because tumor or infection spreads freely through the fatty RPS without being confined initially within a nodal capsule.

3. Extent and boundaries.

 a. The RPS extends as a potential space from the skull base above to approximately the level of the T4 vertebral body (Fig. 6-1).

 b. The RPS serves as a conduit through which infection spreads from the neck to the mediastinum. Although this potentially lethal complication of deep neck infections is not frequently seen in this era of antibiotics, the potential for abscess to spread into the mediastinum via the RPS must be recognized and the scan extended sufficiently so that the condition can be diagnosed if present.

  1) Reviewing Fig. 6-1, you will see that the danger space serves as the caudal conduit for retropharyngeal disease to access the mediastinum. If it were not for this strategic anatomic relationship, it would be quite easy to ignore the DS altogether.

 c. Bordering spaces. The RPS maintains constant relationships with the surrounding deep neck spaces throughout the suprahyoid and infrahyoid neck. Anterior to the RPS is the pharyngeal mucosal space; lateral to the RPS is the carotid space; and posterior to the RPS are the DS and the perivertebral space (PVS).

 d. In the surgical and anatomic literature the term danger space is used to describe a midline posterior space, which is found between the RPS and the PVS. The danger space is found between two leaves of the deep layer of deep cervical fascia. Although the danger space exists as a potential space of the extracranial head and neck, for all practical purposes it can be grouped with the RPS. Both spaces traverse the neck into the mediastinum, and both are posterior, in the midline, and anterior to the PVS. An inflammatory or neoplastic mass in either the danger space or RPS cannot be differentiated by CT or MRI. Therefore, for our purposes, these spaces are treated as one and discussed together under the subject of the RPS.

B. Imaging issues.

1. What radiologic features define a lesion as primary to the RPS?

Q#2

 a. A mass is considered primary to the RPS in the suprahyoid neck when:

1) The center of the mass is posteromedial to the parapharyngeal space and directly medial to the carotid space (Fig. 6-3*A*).
2) The mass encroaches on the parapharyngeal space posteromedially to anterolaterally. (Compare this with the discussion of features that define a mass as primary to the carotid space in Chapter 5).
3) The mass is anterior to the prevertebral muscles regardless of its size.
4) Unless the RPS mass is very large, the styloid process is not displaced anteriorly.

  b. A mass is considered primary to the RPS in the lower oropharynx or infrahyoid neck when:

1) The mass is "bow-tie" shaped or oval in the posterior midline (Fig. 6-3*B*,*C*).

Q#3

2) The mass flattens and remains anterior to the prevertebral muscles. This second observation permits definite distinction between a mass in the RPS and one in the PVS.

  c. Once the mass is determined to be primary to the RPS, the space-specific differential diagnosis (Table 6-1) should be reviewed. Matching the radiologic features of the lesion in question with those of the statistically common RPS lesions will yield a short list of diagnostic possibilities.

2. When an abscess is identified as centered in the RPS, does any evidence exist on CT or MRI scans for spread into the mediastinum?

  a. Extension of an RPS abscess into the mediastinum usually is not a subtle finding. The critical mistake in this setting is to terminate the imaging study before the complete extent of the abscess is seen.

C. Pitfalls in imaging.

1. When a lesion is found within the RPS, be sure that:

  a. The nasopharynx is imaged when the lesion appears nodal. The nasopharynx is the most common primary site of squamous cell carcinoma (SCCa) that spreads into the nodes of the RPS.

1) The nasopharyngeal mucosal space is also the most common site to harbor a clinically occult primary SCCa.

  b. The entire lower extent of the lesion is imaged to exclude the possibility of mediastinal spread.

2. RPS pseudomasses.

  a. The three pseudomasses of the RPS are:

1) Tortuous carotid artery.

Table 6-1   Differential Diagnosis of Retropharyngeal Space Mass

Pseudomass

   Tortuous carotid artery

   Edema fluid or lymph spilling into the retropharyngeal space secondary to deep
      venous or lymphatic obstruction

Congenital

   Hemangioma

   Lymphangioma

Inflammatory

   Reactive adenopathy*

   Cellulitis*

   Suppurative adenopathy (intranodal abscess)*

   Abscess*

Benign tumor

   Lipoma

Malignant tumor

   Nodal metastases

      Squamous cell carcinoma of head and neck origin (especially from the
         nasopharynx)*

      Melanoma

      Thyroid carcinoma

   Nodal non-Hodgkin lymphoma*

   Direct invasion from primary squamous cell carcinoma (especially posterior
      wall primary lesions)*

*These are common lesions of the retropharyngeal space.

   2)   Edema fluid from deep venous obstruction.
   3)   Lymph fluid from tumor-induced lymphatic obstruction in the
        neck.
 b. Tortuous carotid artery.
   1)   Atherosclerotic ectasia of the carotid artery at times will project
        the carotid artery medially into the lateral aspect of the RPS.
        This artery is not actually in the RPS in this instance, but it does
        bow the lateral alar fascia so that it appears to be inside the RPS
        on CT or MRI scans.
   2)   Clinical presentation. "Pulsatile mass" in the lateral pharynx.
        The clinician suspects paraganglioma or other vascular tumor.
   3)   When the vascular loop is very angular, the carotid artery may
        look like a vascular mass or carotid artery aneurysm on CT scan.
        Careful scrutiny will reveal the true nature of this pseudomass.

4) When both carotid arteries are involved, this is referred to as the infamous "kissing carotids."

Q#4

c. Edema fluid from deep venous obstruction in the lower neck or mediastinum.

1) In patients with superior vena cava syndrome or internal jugular vein thrombosis, fluid is frequently seen collected within the RPS.

2) Although the mechanism of this phenomenon is not known, increased venous pressure may result in transudation of the fluid from the obstructed venous system to the RPS. In other words the RPS is serving as a reservoir.

3) Radiologically, edema fluid within the RPS can look identical to a RPS abscess. If fluid is seen within the RPS in association with venous or lymphatic (see below) obstruction and without clinical evidence for infection, conservative management may be indicated. In such cases the radiologist can be critical to correct patient management.

   a) In equivocal cases CT-guided or direct diagnostic needle aspiration can help to avoid unnecessary surgery.

d. Lymph fluid is collecting in the RPS from lymphatic obstruction secondary to lower neck or mediastinal tumor.

1) Patients with malignant tumor of the lower neck and mediastinum sometimes have fluid collected in the RPS.

2) Again, the mechanism of lymph accumulation is unknown but presumably related to the RPS taking up the excess lymphatic fluid (i.e., reservoir effect).

3) Lymphatic engorgement of the dermal and deeper tissue spaces is seen in conjunction with collection of fluid in the RPS.

D. Common lesions.

1. Inflammatory.

a. Clinical considerations.

1) In the pediatric population, infection usually begins in the lymphatic tissues of Waldeyer's ring. When the infection seeds the retropharyngeal nodes, the child will manifest swelling of the posterior wall of the pharynx, difficulty swallowing, and elevated temperature.

2) In adults, infection usually results from the spread from vertebral osteomyelitis (secondary to genitourinary infection) or following cervical spine surgery. Plain-film imaging of the cervical spine may set off the search for the extent of deep tissue infection.

   b. Reactive adenopathy.

     1) Clinical considerations. When the infection first spreads to the retropharyngeal nodes, the initial response is swelling of the node without suppuration.

     2) Imaging features. A reactive RPS node looks like an enlarged version of a normal lymph node in this area (Fig. 6-4*A*). The node maintains its normal oval or kidney-bean shape and shows no evidence for central cystic or necrotic change.

     3) Comment. Homogeneous, oval lymph nodes smaller than 1 cm in diameter normally can be found in the RPS on CT or MRI scans. The younger the patient, the more likely these nodes will be seen.

   c. Suppurative adenopathy.

     1) Clinical considerations. After "reacting" to the initial onslaught of infectious spread to the RPS nodes, a second phase of nodal metamorphosis occurs, where the inside of the node transforms into an intranodal abscess. The result is the formation of a suppurative node.

     2) Imaging features. Suppurative adenopathy has the appearance of a cystic mass in the location of known RPS nodes (Fig. 6-4*A*). Some amount of adjacent cellulitis or early abscess may be seen in the adjacent RPS.

   d. RPS cellulitis or abscess.

     1) Clinical presentation. The patient with cellulitis or abscess of the RPS is usually very sick, with high fever, sore throat, and elevated white blood cell count. The posterior wall of the pharynx bulges toward the examiner. In the pediatric population the RPS abscess forms because of rupture of the suppurative adenopathy into the adjacent RPS (Fig. 6-4*B,C*).

     2) Plain lateral radiographs taken during inspiration reveal prevertebral soft-tissue swelling. CT scans will show RPS abscess as fluid filling the RPS from side to side (Fig. 6-4*C*) If the abscess remains untreated, it may spread either inferiorly via the DS into the mediastinum or locally into adjacent spaces (i.e., transpatial abscess).

     3) Comment. The term *cellulitis* is used when infection occurs early and the tissues are swollen without focal fluid identified.

     4) Contemporary treatment. When infection is found the early stages (e.g., reactive or suppurative node, and/or cellulitis), antibiotic therapy and follow-up imaging are usually considered to be the treatment of choice. When the suppurative node has ruptured and the RPS has filled with pus (Fig. 6-3*B,C*), surgical intervention is warranted.

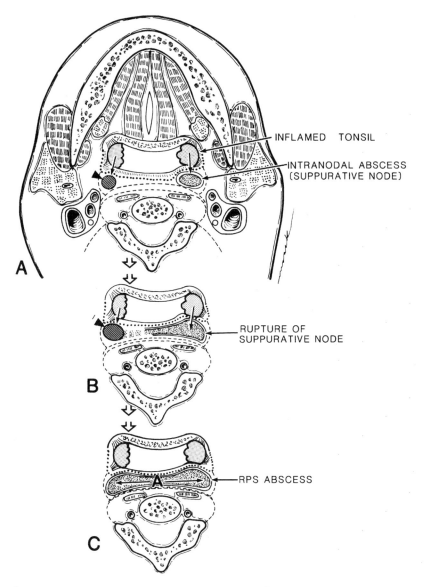

INFLAMED TONSIL

INTRANODAL ABSCESS (SUPPURATIVE NODE)

RUPTURE OF SUPPURATIVE NODE

RPS ABSCESS

Fig. 6-4 Temporal progression of retropharyngeal space infection from suppu-rative adenopathy to abscess. **A,** In the child the infected lymphatic tissue of Waldeyer's ring seeds the nodes in the retropharyngeal space (*short arrows*). The nodes are initially reactive (i.e., enlarge without internal architectural disruption; *arrowhead*). If untreated, the nodes will eventually suppurate, forming an intra-nodal abscess (i.e., enlarged node with central fluid). **B,** Suppurative nodes will go on to rupture into the retropharyngeal space if no treatment ensues (*arrowhead*). **C,** Untended, the abscess (*A*) spreads to fill the retropharyngeal space. From there, spread occurs inferiorly via the danger space into the mediastinum or locally beyond the confines of the boundary fascia into adjacent deep tissue spaces.

2. Congenital.
   a. Hemangioma–lymphangioma spectrum.
      1) When the RPS is involved by a lesion in the hemangioma–lymphangioma spectrum, the lesion usually is transpatial (i.e., involving multiple contiguous spaces).
      2) CT scans reveal a hypervascular infiltrating mass (i.e., hemangioma) or a hypodense lobular mass (i.e., lymphangioma).
3. Benign tumor.
   a. Lipoma.
      1) Benign tumors of the RPS are rare. Because this space contains only fat, lipoma is the only benign tumor seen with any frequency.
      2) CT or MRI will show an enlarged RPS with some displacement of surrounding structures.
4. Malignant tumor.
   a. Nodal metastases from SCCa.
      1) Clinical presentation. In most cases the patient has a known primary tumor of the pharyngeal mucosal space of the nasopharynx or posterior wall of the oropharynx or hypopharynx. Uncommonly, the primary tumor site is clinically occult.
      2) Imaging features. On CT or MRI scans, nodes are seen in the nasopharynx or oropharynx in the RPS that are larger than 1 cm in diameter, at times with central inhomogeneity. SCCa nodal metastasis is the most common cause of retropharyngeal nodal tumor.
      3) Comment. In the more unusual case where a patient is not known to have a primary SCCa but has RPS malignant adenopathy on CT or MRI scans, careful inspection of the pharyngeal mucosal space of the nasopharynx and hypopharynx may reveal the clinically occult, submucosal primary lesion.
   b. Other nodal metastases to the RPS.
      1) Two other malignant tumors have a propensity for the lymph nodes of the RPS:
         a) Melanoma.
         b) Thyroid carcinoma.
      2) In either case the tumor may present as a submucosal mass in the back of the throat. That is, RPS lymph nodes may be the first evidence of systemic melanoma or nodal spread of thyroid carcinoma.
      3) Imaging features. If the melanoma is melanotic, paramagnetic effect may cause T1 shortening on T1-weighted images (i.e., high signal). In the case of thyroid nodal metastases, high signal within the node on T1-weighted images may result from high protein (thyroglobulin) content.

    c. Non-Hodgkin lymphoma.
        1) Just as non-Hodgkin lymphoma may be found in any of the other nodal sites in the extracranial head and neck, it can be found in the lymph nodes of the RPS.
        2) Imaging features. If nodal involvement of the RPS is seen in its earlier phase, the mass will be unilateral and homogeneous. As the disease progresses it may become extranodal, with the mass filling the RPS with tissue-density (CT) or tissue-intensity (MR) material from side to side.
        3) Comment. In most cases non-Hodgkin lymphoma is found simultaneously in multiple nodal chains, including the retropharyngeal nodes; however, retropharyngeal nodal involvement may be the initial finding.
    d. Direct invasion of the RPS by primary SCCa.
        1) Clinical features. Primary SCCa usually is already known to be present either in the nasopharynx or the posterior wall of the oropharynx or hypopharynx.
        2) Imaging features. CT or MRI scans show direct extension of the primary SCCa from its site of origin in the nasopharynx, oropharynx, or hypopharynx into the RPS. In most cases the primary tumor is on the posterior wall. Once inside the RPS, SCCa can move easily in a cephalocaudal direction through the RPS fat, because there are no fascial barriers to inhibit its progress.
          a) Retropharyngeal adenopathy is often associated with direct invasion.

SUGGESTED READING

Baker LL, Dillon WP, Hieshima GB, et al: Hemangiomas and vascular malformations of the head and neck: MR characterization. *AJNR* 14:307–314, 1993.

Barratt GE, Koopmann CF, Coulthard SW: Retropharyngeal abscess—a ten-year experience. *Laryngoscope* 94:455–463, 1984.

Davis WL, Harnsberger HR, Smoker WRK, et al: Retropharyngeal space: evaluation of normal anatomy and diseases with CT and MR imaging. *Radiology* 174:59–64, 1990.

Davis WL, Smoker WRK, Harnsberger HR: The normal and diseased infrahyoid retropharyngeal, danger and prevertebral spaces. *Semin Ultrasound CT MR* 12:241–256, 1991.

Davis WL, Smoker WRK, Harnsberger HR: The normal and diseased retropharyngeal and prevertebral spaces. *Semin Ultrasound CT MR* 11:520–533, 1990.

Glasier CM, Stark JE, Jacobs RF, et al: CT and ultrasound of retropharyngeal abscesses in children. *AJNR* 13:1191–1195, 1992.

Harnsberger HR: CT and MRI of masses of the deep face. *Curr Probl Diagn Radiol* 16:142–173, 1987.

Harnsberger HR, Bragg DG, Osborn AG, et al: Non-Hodgkin's lymphoma of the head and neck: CT evaluation of nodal and extranodal sites. *Am J. Roentgenol* 149:785–791, 1987.

Mancuso AA, Harnsberger HR, Muraki A, et al: CT of cervical and retropharyngeal lymph nodes: normal anatomy, variants of normal, and applications in staging head and neck cancer. I: normal anatomy. II: pathology. *Radiology* 148:709–723, 1983.

Nyberg DA, Jeffrey B, Brant-Zawadzki M, et al: CT of cervical neck infections. *J Comput Assist Tomogr* 9:788–796, 1985.

Paonessa DF, Goldstein JC: Anatomy and physiology of head and neck infections (with emphasis on the fascia of the face and neck). *Otolaryngol Clin North Am* 9:561–580, 1976.

Welsh LW, Welsh JJ, Gregor FA: Radiographic analysis of deep cervical abscesses. *Ann Otol Laryngol* 101:854–859, 1992.

Wong YK, Novotny GM: Retropharyngeal space: a review of anatomy, pathology, and clinical presentation. *J Otolaryngol* 7:528–536, 1978.

Yuh WTC, Buehner L, Kao SCS, et al: Magnetic resonance imaging of pediatric head and neck cystic hygroma. *Ann Otol Rhinol Laryngol* 100:737–742, 1991.

Zadvinskis DP, Benson MT, Kerr HH, et al: Congenital malformations of the cervicothoracic lymphatic system: embryology and pathogenesis. *RadioGraphics* 12:1175–1189, 1992.

7

The Perivertebral Space

CRITICAL IMAGING QUESTIONS:
PERIVERTEBRAL SPACE

1. Why is it more anatomically correct to call the space deep to the deep layer of deep cervical fascia the *peri*vertebral rather than the *pre*vertebral space?
2. Explain the tendency of perivertebral space lesions to end up in the epidural area instead of the more superficial spaces of the neck?
3. What radiologic features define a mass as primary to the perivertebral space?
4. What key CT or MRI observation allows differentiation of a perivertebral space mass and a retropharyngeal space mass?

Answers to these questions are found in the text beside the question number (Q#) in the margin.

PERIVERTEBRAL SPACE (PVS)

A. Terminology

Q#1

1. In the first edition of this book and much of the supporting radiologic literature, the perivertebral space has been referred to as the *prevertebral space* (Fig. 7-1 and 7-2). The name is changed here, because one quick look at the space beneath the deep layer of the deep cervical fascia reveals that only the anterior portion is indeed prevertebral (Latin for "in front of the vertebral body").

2. The paraspinal portion of this space is to the side and behind the vertebrae in the cervical neck (Fig. 7-2*A*,*B*). Calling this area the paraspinal portion of the *pre*vertebral space goes against most readers' rational sensibilities. Hence the change to *peri*vertebral space.

3. Renaming this space the *perivertebral* (Greek for "around") *space* is an

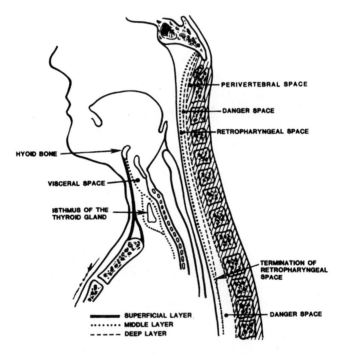

Fig. 7-1   Sagittal drawing of the extracranial head and neck depicting the craniocaudal extent of the perivertebral space (*crosshatched area*). Note that most anatomists recognize this space in some form from the clivus above to the coccyx below. If a lesion breaks out of the prevertebral portion of the perivertebral space anteriorly, it must traverse the danger space and then the retropharyngeal space on its way into the more anterior visceral space. More commonly it is forced into the epidural space by the tenacious deep layer of deep cervical fascia.

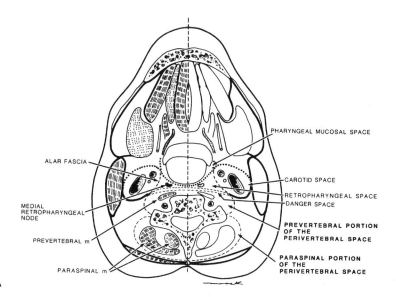

A

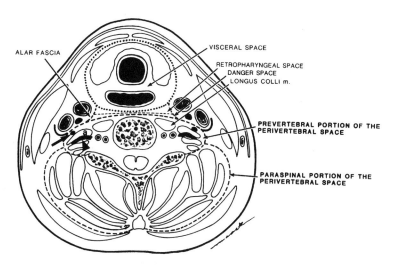

B

Fig. 7-2 Axial drawings of the normal perivertebral space (*PVS*) in the suprahyoid (A) and infrahyoid (B) neck. **A,** In the suprahyoid neck the deep layer of deep cervical fascia (*dashed line*) circumscribes both the prevertebral and paraspinal PVS, attaching to the transverse process laterally, making these two areas distinct. The prevertebral portion of the PVS contains the prevertebral muscles, vertebral artery and vein, and the vertebral body. The paraspinal portion of the PVS contains only the paraspinal muscles and fat. **B,** In the infrahyoid neck the PVS again can be seen as two relatively distinct areas enclosed by the deep layer of deep cervical fascia (*dashed line*). In the infrahyoid neck the prevertebral portion of the PVS has the phrenic nerve (*arrow*) and the brachial plexus roots (*arrowhead*) within it. Note that the brachial plexus roots pass just posterior to the anterior scalene muscle (*a*). As in the suprahyoid neck, the paraspinal portion of the PVS only contains the paraspinal muscles and fat.

attempt to regain the moral high ground in this discussion. Henceforth this book will refer to *prevertebral* and *paraspinal* portions of the *perivertebral space* (PVS) (Fig 7-2*A, B*).

4. This discussion is further confused by the fact that the anatomic literature freely refers to the deep layer of the deep cervical fascia as the *prevertebral fascia*. Again, only the anterior portion of this fascia is *pre*vertebral. The remainder encloses the paraspinal area posterolaterally. To keep the confusion to a minimum, this book will refer to the *deep layer of deep cervical fascia* only and dispense with the term *prevertebral fascia*.

B. Normal Anatomy.

1. Fascia. The deep layer of deep cervical fascia forms the PVS as it arches anteriorly from the cervical spine transverse process to the opposite transverse process (Figs. 7-1 and 7-2). This fascia continues posteriorly to completely enclose the paraspinal muscles and attach to the nuchal ligament of the spinous process of the vertebral body. It is a tenacious fascia that resists violation by infection or tumor.

   a. The attachment of the deep layer of deep cervical fascia to the transverse process of the vertebral body divides the PVS into the anterior (prevertebral) and posterior (paraspinal) portions (Fig. 7-2).

   Q#2

   b. The deep layer of deep cervical fascia encircles the PVS. When disease (i.e., infection or tumor) begins within the PVS, it will usually remain confined by this fascia. This is why PVS disease so frequently ends up forced into the deeper recesses of the PVS (i.e., the epidural area).

      1) Only the roots of the brachial plexus pierce this fascia, as they leave the prevertebral portion of the PVS to enter the posterior cervical space on their way to the axillary apex.

   c. Another name used by the surgeons for the deep layer of the deep cervical fascia is the *carpet*. They use the term because approaching this tenacious fascia from a surgical vantage point reveals a smooth, flat, carpetlike surface.

2. Contents. Structures of importance within the PVS include:

   a. Prevertebral portion of the PVS.

      1) Prevertebral muscles.
      2) Scalene muscles.
         a) Anterior, middle, and posterior muscles.
      3) Brachial plexus.
      4) Phrenic nerve.
      5) Vertebral artery and vein.
      6) Vertebral body.

b. Paraspinal portion of the PVS.
   1) Paraspinal muscles.
   2) Posterior elements of the vertebral body.
3. Extent and boundaries.
   a. The PVS extends from the skull base above to approximately the level of T4 in the posterior mediastinum (Fig. 7-1). Some anatomists describe this discrete anatomic area as extending to the level of the coccyx as well.
   b. Bordering spaces.
   1) The prevertebral portion of the PVS sits directly behind the retropharyngeal space (RPS)/danger space throughout the extra-cranial head and neck. Infection or tumor of the RPS can violate the deep layer of deep cervical fascia and enter the PVS, but this occurs only in the most extreme cases. This fascia is sufficiently tough to resist most onslaughts by diseases of the RPS.
   2) Anterolateral to the prevertebral portion of the PVS is the carotid space (Fig. 7-2*A,B*).
   3) The posterior cervical space is directly lateral to the prevertebral and paraspinal portions of the PVS (Fig. 7-2). As a result, normal structures (e.g., transverse process) or masses in the PVS may appear to the clinician as being within the posterior cervical space. Only CT or MRI will place the lesion in the correct space for surgical planning.

C. Imaging issues.

Q#3
1. What radiologic features define a lesion as originating in the PVS?
   a. A mass lesion is primary to the prevertebral portion of the PVS when:
   1) The center of the mass is within the prevertebral muscles or corpus of the vertebral body.
   2) The mass lifts the prevertebral muscles anteriorly (Fig. 7-3). This feature clearly distinguishes a PVS mass from a RPS mass in most cases.

Q#4
   b. A mass is primary to the paraspinal portion of the PVS when:
   1) The center of the mass is within the substance of the paraspinal musculature.
   2) The mass bows the posterior cervical space fat away from the posterior elements of the spine (Fig. 7-4).
   c. Because the vast majority of PVS lesions originate from the vertebral body (infection and metastasis), the vertebral body is usually abnormal at the time of imaging.

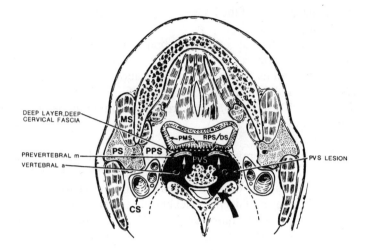

A

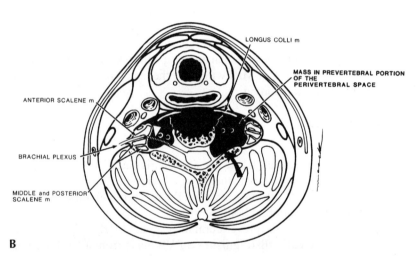

B

Fig. 7-3   Example of prevertebral portion of perivertebral space (*PVS*) masses in the suprahyoid (A) and infrahyoid (B) neck. **A,** In the suprahyoid neck these masses elevate the prevertebral muscles (*white arrows*), pushing the danger space (*DS*)/retropharyngeal space (*RPS*) anteriorly. Tumor is "forced" by the deep layer of deep cervical fascia (*dashed line*) into the epidural area (*curved arrow*). **B,** More inferiorly in the infrahyoid neck, the prevertebral PVS mass again can be seen displacing the prevertebral muscles anteriorly (*straight arrows*). Epidural disease is again depicted as well (*curved*). The brachial plexus roots may be engulfed by such a mass (*white arrowhead*) as in this case. *CS,* Carotid space; *MS,* masticator space; *PMS,* pharyngeal mucosal space; *PPS,* parapharnygeal space; *PS,* parotid space.

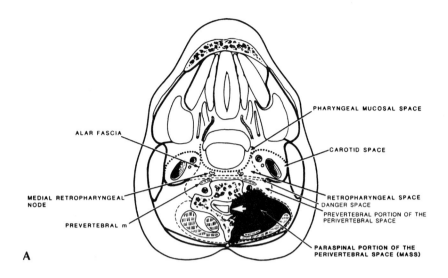

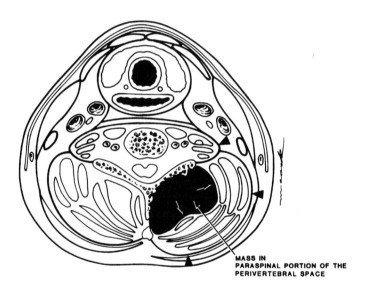

Fig. 7-4   Axial drawing showing a mass in the paraspinal portion of the perivertebral space (*PVS*) in the suprahyoid (A) and infrahyoid (B) neck. **A**, A mass in the suprahyoid, paraspinal PVS (*black area*) displaces the paraspinal musculature away from the spine. An epidural component may be present (*arrow*), which causes cord flattening in this case. The mass remains confined by the deep layer of deep cervical fascia (*dashed line*). **B**, More inferiorly in the infrahyoid neck, a paraspinal PVS mass (*black area*) is seen pushing the paraspinal musculature away from the spine (*arrows*). Note that the deep layer of deep cervical fascia (*arrowheads*) is intact.

    d. At times an infiltrative mass (i.e., malignancy or infection) may traverse the fascial plane separating the prevertebral and paraspinal portions of the PVS (Fig. 7-5). In such a circumstance the lesion will remain confined within the deep layer of deep cervical fascia.

  2. When the lesion has been identified as originating in the PVS, the differential diagnosis unique to the PVS (Table 7-1) should be reviewed. Matching clinical and radiologic features of lesions common to the PVS with the lesion in question often yields a short list of possible diagnoses.

D. Pitfalls in imaging.

1. PVS pseudomasses include:

  a. Anterior vertebral body osteophyte.

    1) Clinical presentation. Incidental; when large, dysphagia.

    2) Imaging features. Bony projection off the anterior vertebral body that may encroach on the digestive tube from the oropharynx to the cervicothoracic junction.

  b. Anterior disc herniation.

    1) Clinical presentation. Patient may have a history of severe head trauma.

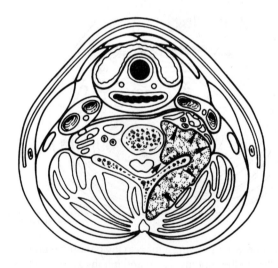

Fig. 7-5 Axial drawing demonstrating the appearance of a pervertebral space (*PVS*) mass that is sufficiently infiltrative to bridge the prevertebral and paraspinal portions of the PVS. The mass displaces the scalene muscles and paraspinal muscles away from the spine (*arrowheads*). Note that the mass remains confined within the deep layer of deep cervical fascia. Epidural disease (*arrow*) is often present and symptomatic in patients with this type of mass long before the lesion has traversed more superficially through the deep layer of deep cervical fascia.

Table 7-1   Differential Diagnosis of Perivertebral Space Lesions

Pseudomass
Vertebral body osteophyte*
Anterior disc herniation
Levator scapulae hypertrophy
Large or asymmetric transverse process
Cervical rib
Hypertrophic facet joint

Vascular
Vertebral artery dissection, aneurysm, or pseudoaneurysm

Inflammatory
Vertebral body osteomyelitis*
   Pyogenic osteomyelitis
   Tuberculous spondylitis

Benign tumor
Schwannoma, neurofibroma (brachial plexus)
Vertebral body benign bony tumors

Malignant tumor
Chordoma*
Vertebral body or epidural metastasis *
Non-Hodgkin lymphoma
Direct invasion of squamous cell carcinoma
Vertebral body primary malignant tumor

*These are common lesions.

    2) Imaging features. Disc material protrudes anteriorly into the pre-vertebral portion of the PVS.
  c. Hypertrophic levator scapulae muscle.
    1) Clinical presentation. Spinal accessory nerve injury, usually at the time of neck dissection, causes atrophy of the sternocleido-mastoid (SCM) and trapezius muscles.
    2) Imaging features. Levator scapulae muscle enlargement with associated SCM and trapezius atrophy. The levator scapulae muscle is usually homogenous internally and may enhance in the early phases of hypertrophy.
    3) Comment. Compensatory hypertrophy of the levator scapulae muscle in spinal accessory neuropathy results from this muscle trying to take up the slack from the atrophic SCM and trapezius muscles. The levator scapulae is working overtime to provide the lift of the arm and shoulder that normally comes from the other two muscles.

    d. Prominent transverse process.

        1) Clinical presentation. Asymptomatic "deep" mass palpated by the referring physician. This usually occurs relative to the question of a parotid space mass. The physician/examiner imagines that a lesion is present deep to the parotid gland.

        2) Imaging features. No mass is seen. Transverse process is identified and presumed to represent the palpated structure. In the parotid space area the offending transverse process is usually seen in the C-2 vertebra.

    e. Cervical rib.

        1) Clinical presentation. Asymptomatic, "deep" mass palpated by the referring physician, usually in the low cervical neck.

        2) Imaging features. No mass is seen. Cervical rib is identified and presumed to represent the palpated structure. Cervical rib is most commonly seen on the C-7 vertebra. Cervical ribs are normally seen in 1% of patients.

        3) In 10% of patients with cervical ribs an associated thoracic outlet compression syndrome also may be present.

    f. Hypertrophic facet joint.

        1) Clinical presentation. Unilateral neck pain. "Deep" mass palpated by the referring physician.

        2) Imaging features. Hypertrophic facet joint is identified.

    g. In the case of the latter three pseudomasses (i.e., prominent transverse process, cervical rib, and hypertrophic facet joint), the examiner perceives a "mass" in the deep tissues of the lateral or posterolateral neck, which is shown to be a nonoperable bony structure or lesion.

E. Common lesions.

1. Vascular.

    a. Vertebral artery dissection.

        1) Clinical presentation. Posttraumatic neck pain with a variety of associated neurologic symptoms depending on the degree of associated vertebral artery thrombosis and embolism. If the vertebral artery thromboses distally to include the posterior inferior cerebellar artery (PICA), a lateral medullary syndrome (Wallenberg's syndrome) may ensue.

        2) Imaging features. MRI shows a crescent of high signal on T1-weighted axial images in the wall of the affected vertebral artery. If the vertebral artery is occluded, lumenal high signal may be seen along with absence of flow. If occlusion extends to involve PICA, lateral medullary and inferior cerebellar infarction will be seen on T2-weighted images as high signal.

2. Inflammatory.
    a. Vertebral body osteomyelitis and PVS abscess.
        1) Clinical presentation. Fever, neck pain, and tenderness signal the onset of cervical spine osteomyelitis. If there is epidural pus, quadriparesis may supervene.
        2) Pathologic findings. In the urban environment the most common cause of vertebral body infection, especially in young patients, is tuberculosis. Bacterial osteomyelitis is most frequently caused by *Staphylococcus aureus*, followed by *Enterobacter* sp. The function of the bone marrow as a "filter for pathogens" makes the spine vulnerable to infection when bacteremia is present.
        3) Radiologic features. Destruction of adjacent vertebral bodies and disc space is seen in conjunction with abscess cavity in the adjacent PVS. If osteomyelitis spreads posteriorly, epidural pus may be visible with associated cord compression. PVS involvement is present in 20% of all cases of vertebral osteomyelitis. Rarely the infection will break through the PVS to extend freely into the RPS/Danger Space.
        4) Comment. Both CT and MRI can readily depict these findings. The sensitivity of MRI to epidural disease and status of the adjacent spinal cord, however, make contrast-enhanced MRI the ideal modality for evaluating suspected cervical spine osteomyelitis with associated PVS or epidural abscess.

3. Benign tumor.
    a. Schwannoma (brachial plexus, cervical roots).
        1) Clinical presentation. Painless, slow-growing mass in the lateral neck, retroclavicular area, or axillary apex. When present in a patient with neurofibromatosis type II, schwannoma may be multiple.
        2) Pathologic findings. Schwannoma is an encapsulated tumor with two components: a cellular component (i.e., Antoni type A tissue); and a loose, myxoid component (i.e., Antoni type B tissue). The presence of these two components allows the pathologist to differentiate schwannoma from neurofibroma.
        3) Imaging features. CT scans show a fusiform, well-encapsulated, tissue-density mass in the course of the brachial plexus anywhere from the epidural space through the cervical neural foramen through the gap between the anterior and middle scalene on into the posterior cervical space to the axillary apex. When the lesion dumb-bells through the cervical neural foramen, any bony change is smoothly scalloped with associated foramenal enlargement. MRI demonstrates the fusiform shape along the course of the brachial plexus better than CT in the coronal

plane. MRI with contrast reveals a uniformly enhancing, well-circumscribed, fusiform mass on T1-weighted images.

  b. Neurofibroma.
  1) Clinical presentation. Symptoms depend on the nerve involved. Only 10% of patients with neurofibromas have von Recklinghausen syndrome (Neurofibromatosis type I). Younger patients (i.e., 20 to 30 years of age) have solitary neurofibromas.
  2) Pathologic findings. Benign, nonencapsulated, well-circumscribed tumor of the peripheral nerves. Histologic studies demonstrate swirls of neuronal elements. Some neurofibromas undergo considerable fatty degeneration.
  3) Imaging features. Similar to those of schwannoma described earlier. At times CT will show a low density lesion when fatty degeneration has occurred.
  c. Vertebral body benign bony tumors.
  1) Aneurysmal bone cyst.
    a) Clinical presentation. Usually a 5- to 20-year-old patient (70% of cases) with posterolateral neck swelling.
    b) Pathologic findings. Expansile, highly vascular lesion of bone with blood-filled cavities. This may be associated with preexisting osseous lesion in 30% to 50% of cases. Trauma is also a commonly associated feature.
    c) Imaging features. CT or MRI will show a multicystic, primary bone lesion of the posterior elements of the spine. The lesion displaces the paraspinal muscles away from the spine. Fluid–fluid levels may be seen within the lesion.
  2) Giant cell tumor.
    a) Clinical presentation. Usually a 20- to 40-year-old patient (70% of cases) with a prevertebral mass on plain-film radiographs emanating from the vertebral body. Root or cord compression may occur.
    b) Pathologic findings. Tumor has multinucleated giant cells in a fibroid stroma. Found in the spine in the sacrum and vertebral body; rarely found in the posterior elements.
    c) Imaging features. Lytic lesion in the vertebral body can be seen on plain-film radiographs with a narrow zone of transition but lacking a sclerotic margin. A soft-tissue component is present in 24% of cases.
  3) Osteoblastoma.
    a) Clinical presentation. Usually a 20- to 40-year-old patient with posterolateral neck swelling. Plain-film radiographs show a lucent or sclerotic expansile mass projecting from the spinal posterior elements.

   b) Pathologic findings. Lesion greater than 2 cm in diameter with same histology as osteoid osteoma.
   c) Imaging features. Nonaggressive, expansile mass emanating from the posterior elements that may be lucent or sclerotic in appearance on plain-film radiographs or CT scans.
4. Malignant tumor.
   a. Chordoma.
   1) Clinical presentation. Headache, facial pain, nasal stuffiness, and progressive cranial nerve malfunction are the most common symptoms of typical clivus chordoma.
   2) Pathologic findings. Low-grade malignant neoplasm that arises from notochordal cell rest and occurs primarily in the spheno-occipital synchondrosis of the clivus and the sacro-coccygeal regions of the spine. Cervical vertebral body chordoma is rare.
   3) Radiologic features. Chordoma appears as a destructive clival mass with early involvement of the nasopharyngeal PVS. On CT scans, 100% of these tumors are calcified.
   4) Comment. CT better delineates tumor calcification. The ability of MRI to show the clivus as the site of origin of this tumor and to depict the full extent of tumor relative to adjacent neurovascular structures, however, makes it the modality of choice in evaluating suspected chordoma.
   b. Vertebral body metastasis.
   1) Clinical presentation. Patient with known malignant tumor and who has neck pain and myelopathy (if epidural tumor is also present).
   2) Pathologic findings. Lung, breast, and prostate gland carcinoma and non-Hodgkin lymphoma are the common malignancies that metastasize to cervical vertebral bodies.
   3) Radiologic features. Vertebral body destruction in association with a PVS mass centered on a single vertebral body. Epidural tumor also may be present if the tumor breaks out posteriorly as well.
   4) Comment. As with osteomyelitis, the superior ability of MRI to depict the true extent of epidural and perivertebral tumors makes it the modality of choice in this setting.
   c. Non-Hodgkin lymphoma.
   1) Clinical presentation. If the PVS is involved with a tissue mass secondary to non-Hodgkin lymphoma, the patient usually has known systemic disease already or is relapsing. Epidural or foramenal soft-tissue mass causes myelopathy, radiculopathy, or brachial plexopathy.

2) Radiologic features. Soft-tissue mass infiltrates the tissue planes of the prevertebral or paraspinal aspect of the PVS. The appearance is indistinguishable from metastatic disease to this area. Epidural disease may be seen if the disease is extensive, because the deep layer of deep cervical fascia confines the tumor to the PVS, forcing it deeper into the epidural area.
  d. Direct invasion of squamous cell carcinoma.
    1) Clinical presentation. Patient is known to have an invasive squamous cell carcinoma in the pharyngeal mucosal space, usually on the posterior wall of the nasopharynx, oropharynx, or hypopharynx.
    2) Radiologic features. The mass is seen extending from the mucosa of the adjacent pharynx through the RPS and danger space to the prevertebral aspect of the PVS. The deep layer of deep cervical fascia is traversed by the tumor. The vertebral body is usually not affected until very late in this process.
  e. Vertebral body primary malignant tumor.
    1) Ewing's sarcoma.
      a) Clinical presentation. Usually a 4- to 25-year-old patient (95% of cases) having a soft-tissue mass emanating from the vertebral body with a highly malignant appearance. One third of patients present with symptoms suggesting infection.
      b) Pathologic findings. Small, round cell lesion.
      c) Radiologic features. Nonmatrix-producing, aggressive, vertebral body lesion, often with an extensive soft-tissue mass.
    2) Osteosarcoma. Osteoid matrix-producing tumor that rarely involves the vertebrae.

SUGGESTED READING

Armington WG, Harnsberger HR, Osborn AG, et al: Radiographic evaluation of brachial plexopathy. *AJNR* 8:361–367, 1987.
Battista RA, Baredes S, Krieger A, et al: Prevertebral space infections associated with cervical osteomyelitis. *Otolaryngol Head Neck Surg* 108:160–166, 1993.
Bilbey JH, Müller NL, Connell DG, et al: Thoracic outlet syndrome: evaluation with CT. *Radiology* 171:381–384, 1989.
Blair DN, Rapoport S, Sostman HD, et al: Normal brachial plexus: MR imaging. *Radiology* 165:763–767, 1987.
Castagno AA, Shuman WP: MR imaging in clinically suspected brachial plexus tumor. *Am J Roentgenol* 149:1219–1222, 1987.
Davis WL, Harnsberger HR, Smoker WRK, et al: Retropharyngeal space: evaluation of normal anatomy and diseases with CT and MR imaging. *Radiology* 174:59–64, 1990.

Davis WL, Smoker WRK, Harnsberger HR: The normal and diseased infrahyoid retropharyngeal, danger and prevertebral spaces. *Semin Ultrasound CT MR* 12:241–256, 1991.

Davis WL, Smoker WRK, Harnsberger HR: The normal and diseased retropharyngeal and prevertebral spaces. *Semin Ultrasound CT MR* 11:520–533, 1990.

George B, Laurian C: Impairment of vertebral artery flow caused by extrinsic lesions. *Neurosurgery* 24:206–214, 1989.

Harnsberger HR: CT and MRI of masses of the deep face. *Curr Probl Diagn Radiol* 16:142–173, 1987.

Harnsberger HR, Bragg DG, Osborn AG, et al: Non-Hodgkin's lymphoma of the head and neck: CT evaluation of nodal and extranodal sites. *Am J Roentgenol* 149:785–791, 1987.

Lusk MD, Kline DG, Garcia CA: Tumors of the brachial plexus. *Neurosurgery* 21:439–453, 1987.

Meyer JE, Oot RF, Lindfors KK: CT appearance of clival chordomas. *J Comput Assist Tomogr* 10:34–38, 1986.

Nyberg DA, Jeffrey B, Brant-Zawadzki M, et al: CT of cervical neck infections. *J Comput Assist Tomogr* 9:788–796, 1985.

Paonessa DF, Goldstein JC: Anatomy and physiology of head and neck infections (with emphasis on the fascia of the face and neck). *Otolaryngol Clin North Am* 9:561–580, 1976.

Posniak HV, Olson MC, Dudiak CM, et al: MR imaging of the brachial plexus. *Am J Roentgenol* 161:373–379, 1993.

Rapoport S, Blair DN, McCarthy SM, et al: Brachial plexus: correlation of MR imaging with CT and pathologic findings. *Radiology* 167:161–165, 1988.

Sze G, Uichanco LS, Brant-Zawadzki MN, et al: Chordomas: MR imaging. *Radiology* 166:187–191, 1988.

Welsh LW, Welsh JJ, Gregor FA: Radiographic analysis of deep cervical abscesses. *Ann Otol Laryngol* 101:854–859, 1992.

8

The Oral Cavity: Emphasizing the Sublingual and Submandibular Spaces

CRITICAL IMAGING QUESTIONS: ORAL CAVITY

1. What are the two major spaces of the oral cavity, and what muscle allows their separation into two distinct spaces? Is there another area that must be considered beyond these two spaces when thinking of pathology arising in the oral cavity?
2. Is the sublingual space a true fascia-lined space? Is there an area where the sublingual and submandibular spaces are contiguous without fascial separation?
3. What structures constitute the neurovascular pedicle of the tongue?
4. Name the principal lesions that traverse the sublingual and submandibular spaces.

Answers to these questions are found beside the question number (Q#) in the margin.

ORAL CAVITY

A. Introduction.

1. The oral cavity (OC) at first glance seems to be an area of the human body that is easily accessible to both visual and manual inspection. Why then does a radiologist need to be familiar with its precise anatomic relationships and forms of pathologic expression?
2. One answer is found in the contribution CT or MRI can make in OC tumor examination. Meticulous imaging of OC squamous cell carcinoma (SCCa) will reveal staging information about the deep tissue extent of tumor, mandibular involvement, perineural spread, and nodal tumor exceeding that derived from a physical examination alone.
3. A second answer is discovered when infection is present in the OC region. These patients often have limited mobility of the jaw and view the friendly, palpating hand of the physician as an enemy. CT can differentiate cellulitis from frank abscess, delineate the extent of pus, determine if the infection is caused by calculus disease or tooth rot, and guide the surgeon on the safest and most cosmetic approach to treatment.
4. Overall, MRI (for tumor) or CT (for infection), focused on the clinical questions, can add considerable information regarding an OC lesion that can be applied to the treatment phase. The radiologist's knowledge of the specific anatomic relationships of the OC and natural history of disease processes of this area has a profound impact on the interpretation quality of the radiologic examination.

B. Anatomic relationships.

1. It is imperative that the OC be differentiated from the oropharynx, because the disease processes of these two areas are very different.
2. The OC is anterior to the oropharynx and separated from it by a ring of structures, including the soft palate, anterior tonsillar pillars, and the circumvallate papillae, which run across the posterior tongue.
   a. The circumvallate papillae divide the tongue into the anterior two thirds, called the *oral tongue*, and the posterior third, called the *tongue base*.
   b. The oral tongue is in the OC. The tongue base is in the oropharynx.
3. The major structures within or forming the boundaries of the OC are:
   a. The hard palate, superior alveolar ridge, and teeth above.
   b. The cheek laterally.
   c. The anterior tonsillar pillars and circumvallate papillae posteriorly.
   d. The mylohyoid muscle (floor of the mouth), inferior alveolar ridge, and teeth inferiorly.
   e. The oral tongue sits as the centerpiece within the OC.

   f. All surfaces of the OC structures are covered with mucosa (i.e., nonkeratinized, stratified, squamous epithelium). Subepithelial collections of minor salivary glands are found throughout the OC.

     1) Any of these mucosal surfaces can serve as a site of origin for SCCa.

     2) Benign mixed tumors or malignant minor salivary gland tumors may arise anywhere from the subepithelial collections of minor salivary glands.

Q#1

4. Within the OC are two major spaces and a third major area: the sublingual space (SLS), the submandibular space (SMS), and the mucosal area. The mylohyoid muscle cleaves the lower OC into the two spaces (Figs. 8-1 through 8-3). The mucosal area is designated separately, because it gives rise to its own set of diseases, which often are different from lesions of the SLS and the SMS.

   a. Lesions of the OC often can be assigned to one of the two spaces based on the location of the center of the lesion relative to the mylo-

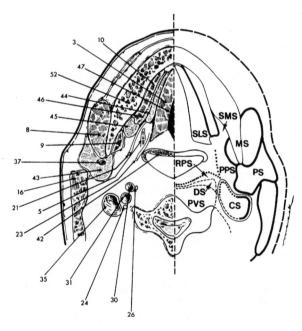

Fig. 8-1 Normal axial anatomy of the oral cavity at the level of the body of the mandible. *Right,* Layers of deep cervical fascia and the spaces they define. *Left,* Normal contents at this level. See key at end of chapter for numbered and lettered structures. (From Hardin CW, Harnsberger HR, Osborn AG, et al: CT in the evaluation of the normal and diseased oral cavity and oropharynx. *Semin Ultrasound CT MR* 7:131–153, 1987. Used by permission.)

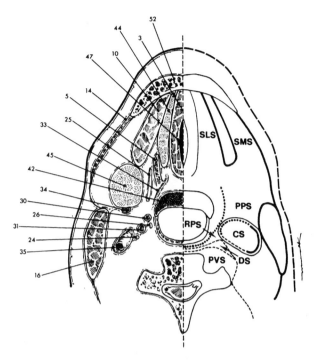

Fig. 8-2   Anatomic drawing depicting normal axial anatomy at the level of the low oral cavity. *Right,* Normal deep cervical fascia and the spaces they define. *Left,* Normal structures at this level. Observe the lack of any fascial barrier separating the posterior sublingual space (*SLS*) and submandibular space (*SMS*) from the inferior parapharyngeal space (*PPS*). See key at end of chapter for numbered and lettered structures. (From Hardin CW, Harnsberger HR, Osborn AG, et al: CT in the evaluation of the normal and diseased oral cavity and oropharynx. *Semin Ultrasound CT MR* 7:131–153, 1987. Used by permission.)

hyoid muscle. Because the differential diagnosis of these spaces is different, this technique can be used to limit the suggested differential diagnosis.

    b. Lesions of the mucosal area usually are obvious to the examining eye and probing finger. Imaging is ordered to evaluate the deep tissue extent of a known lesion, often assessing the lesion's penetration into the SLS or SMS.

C. Terminology. Many terms are used in the literature discussing the anatomy of the OC.

1. *Floor of mouth.* Although it seems to describe multiple structures in the low OC, this term is synonymous with *mylohyoid muscle.* The mylohyoid muscle is the "levator ani" of the OC, serving as a muscular hammock strung between the medial aspects of the mandibular bodies. It separates the SLS from the SMS, except along its posterior margin (Fig. 8-4).

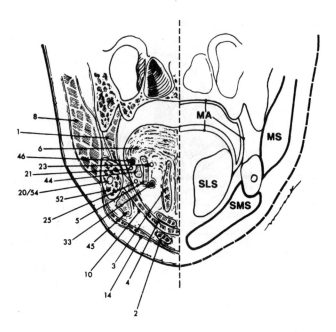

Fig. 8-3   Normal coronal drawing of the oral cavity. *Right*, Fascia and spaces they define. *Left*, Normal structures at this level. There are three areas in the oral cavity to identify: the mucosal area (*MA*), sublingual space (*SLS*), and submandibular space (*SMS*). Note that the SLS is superomedial to the mylohyoid muscle and the SMS inferior to the mylohyoid muscle. See key at end of chapter for numbered and lettered structures. (From Hardin CW, Harnsberger HR, Osborn AG, et al: CT in the evaluation of the normal and diseased oral cavity and oropharynx. *Semin Ultrasound CT MR* 7:131–153, 1987. Used by permission.)

2. *Root of tongue.* This term is used to describe the deep muscles of the OC, including the genioglossus and geniohyoid muscles, and the posterior SLS.
3. *Base of tongue/lingual tonsil.* The posterior third of the tongue (i.e., portion behind the circumvallate papillae) is the *tongue base*, which is primarily made up of the *lingual tonsil*. This term appears in discussions of the OC, but the base of the tongue is in fact part of the oropharynx.
4. *Submaxillary space.* This term has been used to describe the combined areas represented by the SLS and SMS. The term is not used in this chapter, which rather uses the more useful concept of distinct SLS and SMS.

MUCOSAL AREA OF THE ORAL CAVITY

A. Normal anatomic considerations

1. Location. The mucosal area of the OC lines the entire cavity, including the buccal (i.e., cheek), gingival (i.e., gums), palatal, sublingual, and lingual surfaces (Fig. 8-3).

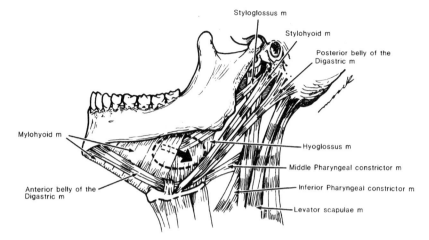

Fig. 8-4   Off-midline sagittal drawing of the oral cavity and floor of the mouth emphasizing the continuous nature of the posterior sublingual and submandibular spaces (*large arrow*). The region circumscribed by the *dotted line* is common ground between the two spaces. Note that no fascial barriers exist between them, permitting masses within the sublingual space to access the submandibular space via this route.

2. Fascial margins. This continuous mucosal sheet is not defined by fascial margins.
3. Contents. The epithelial lining of the OC consists of nonkeratinized, stratified, squamous epithelium. Subepithelial collections of minor salivary glands are found throughout the OC. The most common locations of minor salivary glands in the OC are on the inner surface of the lip, buccal mucosa, and the palate.
4. Extent and boundaries. The depth of the mucosal area of the OC is only a few millimeters. There is no visible separation between the mucosal area of the OC and the adjacent oropharynx.

B. Imaging issues of the mucosal area.

1. When CT or MRI is ordered to evaluate a lesion of the mucosal area of the OC, the most important questions for the clinician to answer are: what is the deep tissue extent of the lesion, and what vital neurovascular structures are involved in the lesion?
2. Because the most common lesion requiring imaging in this area is SCCa, staging of this tumor is the most common task in this area required of the radiologist.
3. Staging SCCa of the OC involves identification of the following:
   a. Does the tumor cross the midline lingual septum?

    b. Is the mandible invaded?

    c. Is the root of the tongue involved (usually via the mylohyoid muscle)?

    d. Are first-order drainage nodes affected? These include the submental and submandibular nodes. The highest deep cervical chain (i.e., jugulodigastric node) may be a first-order node if the lesion is in the posterior OC.

        1) Remember that SCCa of the OC frequently has bilateral nodal spread.

C. Pitfalls in imaging the mucosal area.

1. I prefer MRI in the staging of SCCa, because it is less affected by dental amalgam artifact in the average case and is more sensitive to the true extent of the tumor compared with CT.

2. It is essential that you review your images with the ear, nose, and throat surgeon to incorporate the "mucosal extent" of the tumor as seen by the surgeon into your "deep tissue" extent seen on the radiologic study. Failure to obtain this clinical input will lead to serious errors of interpretation.

D. Lesions of the mucosal area (Table 8-1).

1. Congenital/developmental.

    a. Hemangioma.

        1) With the distinctive vascular hue to the skin overlying a hemangioma and the intense enhancement on CT scans, the diagnosis

Table 8-1   Differential Diagnosis of Mucosal Area Lesions

Congenital/developmental
    Hemangioma
    Lymphangioma/cystic hygroma
    Lingual thyroid tissue

Inflammatory
    Ludwig's angina/cellulitis*
    Odontogenic infection

Benign tumor
    Benign mixed tumor of minor salivary gland origin

Malignant tumor
    Squamous cell carcinoma *
    Minor salivary gland malignancy

*These are more common lesions.

of hemangioma is rarely a significant clinical or radiologic challenge.
  b. Cystic hygroma/lymphangioma.
    1) This lesion involves the SMS more commonly than the SLS. It may project right to the mucosal surface.
    2) See the discussion on cystic hygroma in the congenital lesion section of the SMS later in this chapter.
  c. Lingual thyroid tissue.
    1) Clinical presentation. Lobular mass in the midline involving the tongue base. Can be seen projecting up "like a golf ball" in the midline at the back of the tongue when the tongue is projected anteriorly.
    2) Pathologic findings. Normal, undescended thyroid tissue. Normally the thyroid descends from the foramen cecum area of the tongue base to the lower cervical neck.
    3) Imaging features. CT or MRI scans will show a mass extending from the midline mucosal surface of the tongue base into the medial SLS. CT scans show the lesion as hyperdense with or without administration of intravenous contrast medium.
    4) Comment. Nuclear medicine scans confirm the functioning nature of this ectopic thyroid tissue and help to define whether other thyroid gland tissue is present in the neck. In 80% of cases the removal of all lingual thyroid tissue results in permanent hypothyroidism.
2. Inflammatory/infectious.
  a. Clinical presentation. Sublingual gland or submandibular gland ductal stenosis or calculus precipitates infection of the SLS or SMS. The mucosal area is only involved by proximity. Lower alveolar ridge dental manipulation also may cause infection in these regions.
  b. Imaging features. CT, but not MRI, is recommended in the evaluation of infection. CT is used to identify inciting factors such as calculi or mandibular osteomyelitis and to identify the site of any drainable pus.
3. Benign tumor.
  a. Benign mixed tumor.
    1) Clinical presentation. Pedunculated mass "hanging" into the OC, usually from the palate.
    2) Imaging features. Well-circumscribed, homogenously enhancing mass lesion on both CT and MRI scans.
4. Malignant tumor.
  a. Squamous cell carcinoma.
    1) Clinical presentation. In most cases the diagnosis of SCCa is evident when a mucosal lesion is noted on the physical examina-

tion. Imaging is performed to assess the deep tissue and nodal extent of tumor.

2) Pathologic findings. SCCa is the most common malignancy of the mucosal area of the OC.

3) Imaging features. See B3 of this section.

4) Comment. Further discussion regarding the specifics of staging issues of oral cavity SCCa are found in Chapter 10.

   b. Minor salivary gland malignancy.

1) Clinical presentation. Indistinguishable from that of the far more common SCCa.

2) Pathologic findings. Adenoid cystic carcinoma, acinic cell carcinoma, and mucoepidermoid carcinoma all can occur in the minor salivary glands of the OC mucosal area.

3) Imaging features. Same as those of SCCa.

SUBLINGUAL SPACE

A. Normal anatomy.

1. Location. The SLS is found superomedial to the mylohyoid muscle (Fig. 8-3) in the OC.

Q#2

2. Fascial margins. There is no true fascial lining of the SLS. It is a potential space, with critical contents found within the oral tongue. No fascia separates the posterior SLS from the SMS (Figs. 8-1 through 8-4). As a result, lesions of the SLS readily spread to involve the adjacent SMS.

3. Contents (Figs. 8-1 through 8-3).

Anterior extension of hyoglossus muscle

Nerves

   Lingual nerve (i.e., the sensory branch of cranial nerve V_3 combined with the chorda tympani branch of the facial nerve, which carries the taste fibers of the anterior two thirds of the tongue)

   Cranial nerves IX and XII

Vessels

   Lingual artery and vein

Sublingual glands and ducts

Deep portion of submandibular gland

Submandibular gland duct (i.e., Wharton's duct)

Q#3

   a. The nerves and vessels constitute the neurovascular pedicle of the tongue.

4. Extent and boundaries.

a. The SLS sits in the oral tongue inferior to the intrinsic tongue muscles and between the mylohyoid muscle inferolaterally and the genioglossus–geniohyoid complex medially (Fig. 8-3).

b. The SLS runs into the mandible anteriorly.

c. The SLS empties posteriorly into the posterosuperior aspect of the SMS. No fascia separates these two spaces at this point (Fig. 8-4), allowing free communication of SLS disease into the SMS.

B. Imaging issues.

1. A mass lesion is said to be *primary* to the SLS when its center is within the SLS superomedial to the mylohyoid muscle.

2. At times a lesion will decompress out the backside of the SLS into the SMS, appearing as a mass of the SMS (Figs. 8-4 and 8-5). In this case

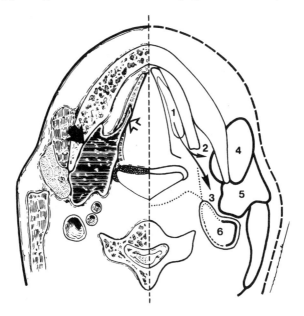

Fig. 8-5   *Left,* Axial diagram of a diving ranula (*large arrow*) as it herniates from the posterior sublingual space into the adjacent cephalad submandibular space and low parapharyngeal space. *Right,* The spaces of the oropharynx and oral cavity. Because no fascial boundary exists at the posterior margin of the mylohyoid muscle, a ranula beginning in the sublingual space (*1*) may dive (*right arrows*) into the adjacent submandibular space (*2*) and parapharyngeal space (*3*). The bulk of the diving ranula is found in the submandibular space, but the "tail sign" (*open arrow*) of residual cyst in the sublingual space suggests the diagnosis. *4,* masticator space; *5,* parotid space; *6,* carotid space. (From Coit WE, Harnsberger HR, Osborn AG, et al: Ranulas and their mimics: CT evaluation. *Radiology* 163:211–216, 1987. Used by permission.)

the majority of the mass is seen in the SMS, with only a tail of the lesion remaining in the SLS. The classic example of this phenomenon occurs with the diving ranula, which begins in the SLS but has the majority of its mass effect in the SMS.

3. When a lesion is identified as originating in the SLS, the differential diagnosis (Table 8-2) should be reviewed. Matching the radiologic features of the lesion with those of diseases that occur in the SLS often will yield a short list of possible diagnoses.

C. Pitfalls in imaging.

1. Perhaps the biggest mistake made in imaging the area of the OC and SLS with CT is that no effort is made to avoid the spray artifact associated with dental amalgam. Using a scan plane parallel to the fillings in the lower teeth ensures that the maximum amount of unobstructed SLS will be imaged.

   a. MRI is less frequently affected by artifacts related to dental amalgam, but the signal occasionally can be seriously distorted by dental amalgam with a high ferrous content.

Table 8-2   Differential Diagnosis of Sublingual Space Lesions

Pseudomass
 Hypoglossal nerve motor atrophy

Congenital/developmental
 Hemangioma
 Lymphangioma/cystic hygroma
 Epidermoid/dermoid*
 Lingual thyroid tissue

Inflammatory
 Ludwig's angina/cellulitis*
 Abscess
 Dilated submandibular gland duct secondary to stenosis or calculus*
 Ranula, simple or diving

Benign tumor
 Benign mixed tumor of sublingual gland origin

Malignant tumor
 Squamous cell carcinoma invading anteriorly from the tongue base or inferiorly
  from the mucosal surface of the oral tongue*
 Sublingual gland malignant tumor
  Adenoid cystic carcinoma
  Mucoepidermoid carcinoma
  Acinic cell carcinoma

*These are more common lesions.

2. Pseudomass. Interpretation errors have been made when the hypoglossal nerve is injured, causing loss of muscle volume and fatty infiltration of the ipsilateral tongue muscles. The CT appearance of hypoglossal atrophy can be mistaken for SLS tumor in the opposite, nonatrophied side of the tongue. Early in the development of motor atrophy of the tongue, MRI scans will show the appearance of infiltrating tumor on the side of the developing atrophy.

D. Lesions (Table 8-2).

1. Congenital/development.
   a. Hemangioma.
      1) With the distinctive vascular hue to the skin overlying a hemangioma and the intense enhancement on CT scans, the diagnosis of hemangioma is rarely a significant challenge.
      2) Imaging features. Both the mucosal area and the deeper SLS are involved by the mass, with a usually displaced, patchy enhancement.
   b. Cystic hygroma/lymphangioma.
      1) This lesion involves the SMS more commonly than the SLS.
      2) See cystic hygroma in the section on congenital lesions of the SMS, later in this chapter.
   c. Epidermoid/dermoid.
      1) Clinical presentation. Slow growing mass under the oral tongue.
      2) Pathologic findings. When lined by simple squamous epithelium, the mass is termed *epidermoid*. If the lesion has an epithelial lining but possesses variable numbers of skin appendages, it is termed *dermoid*.
      3) Imaging features. CT or MRI scans demonstrate a unilocular mass in the SLS or SMS. Epidermoids have fluid density or signal; dermoids are either of mixed density signal or have an area of fat density signal.
      4) Comment. Epidermoids have a propensity for involvement of the SLS. Dermoids seem to involve the SMS more commonly.
   d. Lingual thyroid tissue.
      1) Clinical presentation. Lobular mass in the midline mucosal surface of the tongue base.
      2) Pathologic findings. Normal, undescended thyroid tissue. Normally the thyroid descends from the foramen cecum area of the tongue base to the lower cervical neck.
      3) Imaging features. CT or MRI scans will show a mass that extends from the midline mucosal surface of the tongue base into the medial SLS. CT scans show the lesion as hyperdense with or without administration of intravenous contrast medium.

2. Inflammatory/infectious disease.
    a. Clinical presentation. Sublingual gland or submandibular gland ductal stenosis or calculus precipitates infection of the SLS or SMS. Lower alveolar ridge dental infection or manipulation also may cause infection in these regions.
    b. Cellulitis implies inflammation but no surgically drainable pus collection. The term *abscess* is used only when well-defined areas of fluid (i.e., pus) are identified within the broader cellulitic region. Ludwig's angina is a severe form of cellulitis, occurring 2 to 4 days after dental extraction from the lower alveolar ridge, with abscess in the SLS and SMS.
        1) Imaging features. CT, but not MRI, is recommended in the evaluation of infection of the SLS or SMS. CT is used to identify inciting factors such as calculi or mandibular osteomyelitis and also the site of any drainable pus.
            a) SLS abscess may extend under the frenulum of the tongue anteriorly to become an "upside down," horseshoe-shaped, cystic mass involving both of the SLS under the oral tongue (Fig. 8-6).
        2) Comment. In this era of powerful antibiotics, do not overcall the amorphous, small, fluid areas within cellulitis as "abscess." Instead, err on the side of undercalling surgical disease, allowing the antibiotics to have their maximum effect. Closely spaced follow-up imaging can be done if continued concern over undrained pus arises.
    c. Ranula.
        1) Clinical presentation. Painless swelling of the SLS (i.e., simple ranula) or of both the SLS and SMS (i.e., diving ranula).
        2) Pathologic findings. Simple ranula is a postinflammatory retention cyst of the sublingual glands or the minor salivary glands of the SLS and has an epithelial lining. If the simple ranula becomes large and ruptures out the back of the SLS into the SMS, it is a diving ranula. The diving ranula has no epithelial lining and is actually a pseudocyst.
        3) Imaging features. A unilocular cystic mass of the SLS on CT or MRI scans suggests the diagnosis of simple ranula. Unilocular cystic hygroma and epidermoid cyst, however, cannot be differentiated radiologically from simple ranula. Diving ranula has a characteristic "tail sign" within the SLS, with the bulk of the pseudocyst seen in the SMS (Fig. 8-5).
        4) Comment. The typical appearance of a diving ranula is highly suggestive of the diagnosis.
3. Malignant tumor.

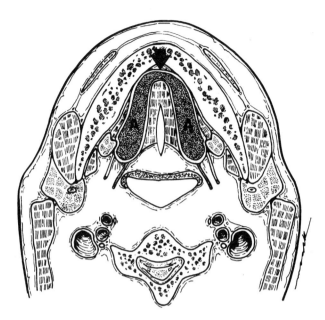

Fig. 8-6   Axial drawing of sublingual space abscess. Larger lesions of the sublingual space may cross the anterior midline under the frenulum of the tongue and become bilobular. In this drawing the abscess is seen in both sublingual spaces, with a thin anterior connection (*arrow*). This type of abscess can be accessed surgically through a sublingual, peroral approach.

    a. Squamous cell carcinoma.
       1) Clinical presentation. In most cases the diagnosis of SCCa is evident when a mucosal lesion is noted on the physical examination. Imaging is performed to assess the deep tissue and nodal extent of tumor.
       2) Pathologic findings. SCCa is the most common malignancy of the SLS.
       3) Imaging features. Both CT and MRI scans show infiltrating tumor mass within the SLS. The part of the SLS involved depends on the site of origin of the primary SCCa. Tongue base SCCa invades the SLS from posterior to anterior; oral tongue SCCa invades it from superior to inferior.
       4) Comment. The specifics of the staging issues of SCCa of the OC are found in Chapter 10.
    b. Sublingual gland or minor salivary gland malignancy. Adenoid cystic carcinoma, acinic cell carcinoma, and mucoepidermoid carcinoma are extremely rare in the glands of the SLS.

SUBMANDIBULAR SPACE

A. Normal anatomy.

1. Location. The SMS is located inferolateral to the mylohyoid muscle (Fig. 8-3) and superior to the hyoid bone.
2. Fascial margins. The superficial layer of deep cervical fascia splits to encircle the SMS, with the deeper slip of fascia running along the external surface of the mylohyoid muscle and the more shallow slip paralleling the deep margin of the platysma (Fig. 8-3).
   a. No fascial margin separates the posterior SMS and SLS from the inferior parapharyngeal space (Figs. 8-1 and 8-4).
3. Contents (Figs. 8-1 through 8-3).
   Anterior belly of digastric muscle.
   Superficial portion of submandibular gland.
   Submandibular and submental lymph nodes.
   Facial vein and artery.
   Inferior loop of hypoglossal nerve (cranial nerve XII).
   Fat.
   a. Comment. The key SMS contents are the bulk of the submandibular gland and the two nodal groups. Primary disease of this space arises from the gland or the nodes in the majority of cases.
4. Extent and boundaries.
   a. The SMS is a horseshoe-shaped space found between the hyoid bone below and the mylohyoid muscle sling above (Figs. 8-4 and 8-7).
   b. The SMS posteriorly runs into the inferior parapharyngeal space and the posterior portion of the SLS. No fascial delineation is found here.

B. Imaging issues.

1. A mass lesion is said to originate in the SMS when its center is within the SMS inferolateral to the mylohyoid muscle.
2. With rare exceptions, lesions of the SMS do not work their way into the SLS, in contrast to the tendency of larger SLS masses to decompress into the SMS.
3. When a lesion is identified as primary to the SMS, the differential diagnosis (Table 8-3) should be reviewed. Matching the radiologic features of the lesion with the list of diseases that occur in the SMS often will lead to a short list of possible diagnoses.

C. Pitfalls in imaging.

1. Pseudomass. Cranial nerve V_3 supplies motor innervation to the muscles of mastication through the masticator branch and to the mylohyoid muscle and anterior belly of the digastric muscles through the mylohyoid branch. When this nerve is injured, the masticator muscles, mylohyoid

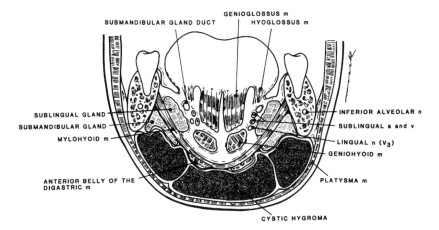

Fig. 8-7   Coronal drawing of submandibular space cystic hygroma. The submandibular space has no midline fascial barrier to the spread of a lesion from side to side. As a result, larger lesions of the submandibular space often take on a "horseshoe shape," filling the space from side to side. In this drawing the lesion is a multilocular cystic hygroma.

muscle, and the anterior belly of the digastric muscle on the side of the injury atrophy.

   a. On first glance the floor of the mouth on the side of the injury looks "normal," whereas the side with the nonatrophied mylohyoid muscle and anterior belly of the digastric muscle appear too large (i.e., like a tumor).

   b. Recognition of the distal aspects of the cranial nerve V_3 atrophy pattern allows the imager to look proximal toward the skull base for the offending lesion and avoid diagnosing tumor on the opposite, normal side of the floor of the mouth.

2. A critical mistake made by imager and clinician alike is to forget that a pedunculated lesion of the parotid tail will present as an angle of mandible mass (i.e., a mass in the posterior SMS). In most cases the lesion will be either benign mixed or Warthin's tumor.

   a. If the lesion is not recognized as parotid in origin by either the clinician or the imager, a submandibular approach will be made to this parotid space lesion. Lack of surgical control of the facial nerve may create partial facial nerve paralysis.

D. Lesions (Table 8-3).

1. Congenital lesions.

   a. Second branchial cleft cysts.

Table 8-3   Differential Diagnosis of Submandibular Space Lesions

Pseudomass

Cranial nerve V_3 motor atrophy (i.e., anterior belly of digastric muscle and mylohyoid muscle are small and infiltrated by fat)

Congenital/developmental

Second branchial cleft cyst*
Suprahyoid thyroglossal duct cyst
Cystic hygroma/lymphangioma*
Hemangioma*

Inflammatory

Ludwig's angina secondary to cellulitis and/or abscess*
Reactive adenopathy*
Submandibular gland inflammation (e.g., ductal stenosis, calculus, tumor)*
Diving ranula

Benign tumor

Lipoma*
Epidermoid/dermoid
Benign mixed tumor of submandibular gland
Tail of parotid pedunculated benign tumor (e.g., benign mixed tumor or Warthin's)

Malignant tumor

Nodal metastasis of squamous cell carcinoma of the face and oral cavity*
Nodal lymphoma*
Submandibular gland malignancy (e.g., adenoid cystic carcinoma, mucoepidermoid carcinoma)
Direct invasion by squamous cell carcinoma of the oral cavity

*These are more common lesions

1) Clinical presentation. Branchial cleft anomalies occur in a bimodal distribution. In a child the mass is most commonly found at the angle of the mandible. If a sinus tract or fistula is associated, the opening is present from birth anteriorly in the neck just above the clavicle (Figs. 8-8 and 8-9). The second peak of incidence is seen in young adults. Trauma or viral infection usually provokes the initial appearance of an angle of mandible mass. In many instances there is a history of "unsuccessful abscess drainage."

2) Pathologic findings. Of all branchial cleft anomalies, 95% arise from the remnant of the second branchial apparatus. The second branchial cleft apparatus normally completely involutes by the

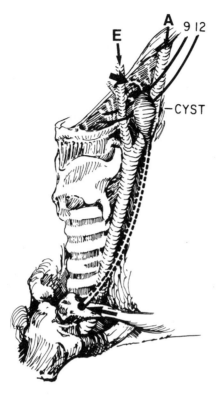

Fig. 8-8   The tract of a second branchial cleft anomaly may stretch from a supra-clavicular cutaneous opening below (*long arrow*) to an oropharyngeal tonsil area internal opening above (*short arrow*). The cystic component is most commonly located at the mandibular angle, just lateral to the glossopharyngeal (*9*) and hypoglossal (*12*) nerves. Because of the potential tract of the cephalad portion of the anomaly passing between the external (*E*) and internal (*A*) carotid arteries, the second branchial cleft cyst sometimes has a characteristic beak pointing toward the oropharynx mucosal space. (From Harnsberger HR, Mancuso AA, Muraki AS, et al: Branchial cleft anomalies and their mimics: CT evaluation. *Radiology* 152:739–784, 1984. Used with permission.)

ninth week of gestation. When the involution phase is incomplete, existence of the remnant tissue creates the potential for growth of a branchial cleft anomaly.

3) Imaging features. CT or MRI scans will reveal a unilocular, "cystic" mass in the posterior SMS at the angle of the mandible (Fig. 8-9). The location is embryologically defined. As the cyst grows it displaces the submandibular gland anteromedially, the sternomastoid muscle posterolaterally, and the carotid space

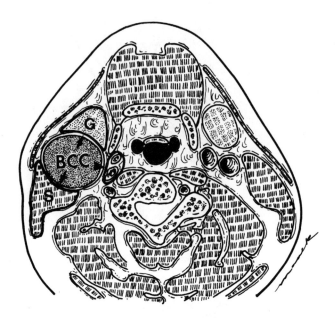

Fig. 8-9   Axial drawing of second branchial cleft cyst (*BCC*). The most common location is in the posterior aspect of the submandibular space. The center of this unilocular cystic mass is embryologically defined. As a result, as the lesion enlarges, a characteristic displacement pattern emerges where the submandibular gland (*G*) is pushed anteromedially, the sternocleidomastoid muscle (*S*) postero-laterally, and the carotid space (*arrowhead*) contents medially.

contents posteromedially in most cases. Only when the cyst is quite large does it begin to break this characteristic pattern of displacement. When present, a beak on the cyst that points medi-ally between the internal and external carotid arteries is pathog-nomonic of second branchial cleft cyst.

   4)   Comment. The most common form of this lesion is a cystic mass without sinus or fistula at the angle of the mandible; however, any combination of cyst, sinus, or fistula is possible. Each lesion should be described individually. When a mass is present, CT or MRI is used to completely define the deep tissue extent of the lesion to facilitate complete surgical resection of the cyst lining. When a cutaneous tract is present without associated mass, sinography is done to delineate its full extent.

 b. Suprahyoid thyroglossal duct cyst (see Chapter 10 for further details).

   1)   Clinical presentation. Midline mass in the suprahyoid region with fullness in the floor of the mouth.

2) Imaging features. Cystic mass in the midline or paramedian location extending from the hyoid bone region upward into the SMS (Fig. 8-10). If the lesion reaches the foramen cecum, it also will have traversed the posterior SLS to reach this mucosal area.

3) Comment. If this unusual form of thyroglossal duct cyst is suspected before imaging, MRI is the better tool for delineation of the deep tissue extent because of its unique ability to display the entire course of this lesion in the sagittal plane.

  c. Cystic hygroma/lymphangioma.

1) Clinical presentation. Fluid-filled cystic mass. It is difficult for the clinician to assess the deep tissue extent of this lesion by palpation.

2) Pathologic findings. Congenital malformation of lymphatic channels. Classified as *capillary* (i.e., small cystic components), *cavernous* (i.e., medium-sized cystic components), and *cystic* (i.e., enormously dilated lymphatic spaces). Sixty-five percent of cystic hygromas are present at birth, and 90% are clinically apparent by 3 years of age.

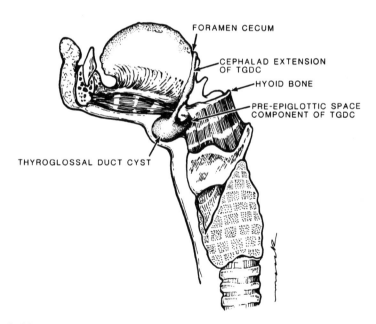

Fig. 8-10 Suprahyoid extension of thyroglossal duct cyst. This is a lateral drawing of such a cyst primarily located just anterior to the hyoid bone but with a cephalic extension through the posterior submandibular space, then penetrating through the mylohyoid muscular sling and posterior sublingual space to access the foramen cecum on the mucosal surface of the tongue.

3) Imaging features. Primarily located in the posterior cervical space (i.e., posterior triangle) and superior mediastinum when found in the infant. In the adult this lesion is more commonly seen in the SLS, SMS, and parotid space (Fig. 8-7).
   a) CT. Fluid density and multilocular mass of the SMS that may cross anteriorly into the opposite SMS.
   b) MRI. Multilocular, fluid-intensity mass.
4) Comment. Cystic hygroma is a tenacious, difficult to remove lesion that at surgery often wraps around and adheres to adjacent structures. In reporting the extent of this lesion a comment should be made concerning the critical neurovascular structures in the surrounding deep tissues. In the case of a SMS lesion its relationship to the neurovascular pedicle of the tongue also should be reported.
5) The SMS is involved by cystic hygroma not uncommonly. When a cystic hygroma involves both the SMS and SLS, it may be impossible to differentiate it from a diving ranula.

Q#4

6) A cystic mass involving the SLS and SMS simultaneously suggests a limited differential diagnosis:
   Diving ranula.
   Cystic hygroma/lymphangioma.
   Abscess.
   a) If unilocular with a "tail sign," diving ranula is most likely. If multilocular, cystic hygroma is most likely. Abscess is best diagnosed with the support of an appropriate clinical history.

2. Inflammatory disease.
   a. Reactive adenopathy.
   1) Clinical presentation. Multiple "masses" are felt in the SMS, often bilaterally. Other associated "masses" are felt in other node-bearing regions of the neck. The lingual, faucial, and adenoidal tonsils are often enlarged and inflamed.
   2) Imaging features. Multiple, oval to round nodes are seen in the SMS in association with nodes in the deep cervical chain and spinal accessory chain.
   3) Comments. Reactive nodes are homogenous internally. If the internal architecture becomes inhomogeneous, suppuration or tumor infiltration is occurring depending on the clinical circumstance. Remember that *no* nodes exist within the submandibular gland itself; therefore if a mass is seen within the gland, it is not nodal in nature.
   b. Cellulitis or abscess.

1) Cellulitis/abscess of the SMS originates from one of three possible sources:
   a) Suppurative adenopathy.
   b) Submandibular gland infection (secondary to ductal stone or stenosis).
   c) Infected teeth/mandible.
2) Imaging features. Cellulitis is readily differentiated from abscess by enhanced CT. In the case of cellulitis there is no walled-off fluid (i.e., abscess). At times the imager may catch the infectious process as it is transforming from cellulitis to abscess, with CT scans showing areas of poorly circumscribed fluid density. It is probably still possible to treat such patients with intravenous antibiotics and follow them clinically (and radiologically) rather than surgically treat this transitional group.

c. Submandibular gland inflammation (e.g., ductal stenosis, calculus, tumor)
   1) Clinical presentation. Unilateral, painful SMS swelling, often associated with eating or psychological gustatory stimulation. This clinical mix is referred to as *salivary colic*. The stone may be palpable in the floor of the mouth, but patient discomfort may prevent adequate examination of this area.
   2) Pathologic findings. Eighty-five percent of stones occur in the submandibular ductal system, while only 15% are found in the parotid ductal system.
   3) Imaging features. Thin-section CT (contiguous, 3 mm slices) directed along the plane of the submandibular ductal system addresses most questions relative to submandibular ductal pathology. Submandibular sialography is a dying art. Stone location can be determined as distal (i.e., toward the ductal opening) or proximal (i.e., toward the hilum of the gland). If ductal stenosis alone is present, a transition in the ductal caliber without stone is seen.
   4) Stones are reported to be radio-opaque in approximately 90% of plain films (occlusal view). With CT the percentage seen must approach the 100% range. Therefore if no stone is seen in the setting of a dilated submandibular duct, floor of mouth tumors must be sought. If no tumor is present either clinically or radiographically, assume that the duct is stenotic.
   5) Comment. Intraoral surgery to remove the stone is completed when a distal stone is removed, whereas it may be necessary to remove the gland and proximal duct if the stone is proximal in the hilum of the submandibular gland.

3. Benign tumor.
   a. Lipoma. When lipoma is present in the SMS during staging of SCCa, it may be clinically labeled a malignant node. CT or MRI can easily correct this clinical misimpression.
   b. Dermoid/epidermoid. See the discussion of benign tumor of the SLS earlier.
   c. Submandibular gland benign mixed tumor.
      1) Clinical presentation. Slow growing mass in the SMS.
      2) Pathologic findings. See the discussion of benign mixed tumor in Chapter 4.
      3) Imaging features. Well-circumscribed mass within an enlarged submandibular gland.
      4) Comment. Results of needle biopsy may be available at the time of imaging, giving the radiologist the diagnosis of benign mixed tumor. Be sure that the mass is intrinsic to the submandibular gland and not pedunculating down from the parotid tail. A submandibular surgical approach to a parotid tail mass can lead to facial nerve injury.
4. Malignant tumor.
   a. Malignant tumor of the SMS is nodal tumor in the vast majority of cases. Because the submandibular gland undergoes early encapsulation in its development, all nodal disease occurs outside the gland.
   b. Malignant adenopathy from squamous cell carcinoma of the face and oral cavity.
      1) Clinical presentation. A known skin or mucosal primary tumor is present on the face or in the OC. A palpable mass is present in the SMS.
      2) Pathologic findings. The submental and submandibular nodal groups receive drainage from the skin of the face, OC structures, and the nose and anterior sinus regions.
      3) Imaging features. Lymph nodes larger than 1.5 cm in diameter or with central inhomogeneity in the situation of known SCCa are considered malignant.
      4) Comment. See Chapter 10 for further discussion.
   c. Nodal non-Hodgkin lymphoma.
      1) Imaging features. Multiple, large, homogeneous lymph nodes in the submental and submandibular groups should suggest the diagnosis of non-Hodgkin lymphoma.
   d. Submandibular gland malignancy.
      1) Malignancy of the submandibular gland is rare. Adenoid cystic carcinoma is the most common malignant tumor seen in this gland.

MANDIBLE

A. Normal anatomy.

1. Gross bony anatomy.
   a. The major parts of the mandible from anterior to posterior include the symphysis, body, angle, ramus, and condyle.
   b. Multiple bony projections off the mandible consist of the coronoid process and the genial tubercles.
   c. Two major foramen allow entrance and exit of the inferior alveolar nerve and vessels: the mandibular foramen, and the mental foramen, respectively.
   d. The mylohyoid sling attaches along the inner table of the mandible to the mylohyoid ridge.
2. Muscular insertions. These are described in Table 8-4.
3. Sensory nerves.
   a. The mandibular division of the trigeminal nerve (cranial nerve V_3) supplies sensory innervation in and around the mandible.
      1) Inferior alveolar nerve. Low gums and teeth.
      2) Mental nerve. Lower lip sensation.
      3) Buccal nerve. Cheek and gums.
      4) Lingual nerve. Floor of mouth and gums.

Table 8-4   Perimandibular Muscular Insertions and Innervations

Muscle	Mandibular Insertion	Innervation
Masseter	Lateral mandibular angle	cranial nerve V_3, masticator nerve
Medial pterygoid	Medial mandibular angle	cranial nerve V_3, masticator nerve
Lateral pterygoid	Medial condyle/skull base	cranial nerve V_3, masticator nerve
Temporalis	Coronoid process	cranial nerve V_3, masticator nerve
Mylohyoid	Mylohyoid ridge	cranial nerve V_3, mylohyoid nerve
Anterior belly, digastric	Digastric fossa	cranial nerve V_3, mylohyoid nerve
Genioglossus	Superior genial tubercle	cranial nerve XII
Geniohyoid	Inferior genial tubercle	cranial nerve XII

        a) The lingual nerve also carries the chorda tympani nerve containing taste fibers from the anterior two thirds of the tongue.

B. Imaging of the mandible.

1. Plain films.
    a. Applications.
        1) Still primarily used in the setting of trauma to look for mandibular fractures.
        2) No role in the assessment of mandibular invasion by SCCa of the oral cavity.

2. CT.
    a. Standard axial CT.
        1) Indications.
            a) Infection in the OC when looking for mandibular osteomyelitis.
            b) Malignant tumor (usually SCCa) in the OC when looking for mandibular invasion.
        2) CT technique.
            a) Soft-tissue and bone reconstructions (i.e., algorithms) are completed in the axial plane in thin, contiguous sections (3 mm).
            b) Bolus/rapid injection technique employed for intravenous contrast to maximize intravascular contrast during scan procedure.
    b. Dentascan.
        1) Indications.
            a) Primary indication is for the assessment of maxillary and mandibular ridges for possible dental implant placement.
        2) CT technique.
            a) Follow the prescribed directions to create the multiple, cross-referenced, axial, cross-sectional, and panoramic images of the mandible and maxilla.
        3) These images allow the oral surgeon to place dental implants safely, because of the presurgical knowledge of the height, width, and contour of the alveolar process as well as the exact location of the neurovascular bundle within the mandible and the floor of the maxillary sinus above the maxilla.

3. MRI.
    a. Indications.
        1) MRI of the mandible is rarely ordered alone. Instead the mandible is included when MRI is focused on staging an OC malignancy.
    b. MRI technique.

1) Fat-saturated, axial, T1-weighted postcontrast images are best for seeing perineural tumor on the inferior alveolar nerve in the mandible.

2) Axial, T1-weighted, noncontrasted images best show mandibular marrow-space change that accompanies mandibular invasion.

C. Lesions.

1. Fracture.
   a. Type of fracture.
      1) Simple. Linear fracture that does not communicate with the oral cavity.
      2) Compound. Any fracture through the alveolar ridge that involves the roots of erupted teeth.
      3) Comminuted. Multiply fragmented.
      4) Complicated. Fracture involves the inferior alveolar artery or nerve.
      5) Pathologic. Fracture occurs at a site of diseased bone, especially bone invaded by tumor.
   b. Fractures of the mandible tend to follow the long axis of the teeth.
   c. Because the mandible simulates a bony ring, bilateral fractures are common and must be searched for.

2. Infection.
   a. Mandibular osteomyelitis most frequently results from tooth infection and less commonly from adjacent deep space infection or dental manipulation.
   b. Because of the variability in appearance of the adult mandible, it is difficult to make a diagnosis of subtle mandibular osteomyelitis with a single CT examination. Sequential CT examinations may be necessary to detect the bone changes of osteomyelitis.
      1) Look for destructive changes and/or periosteal elevation on the axial CT images. Changes on sequential scans should be interpreted as significant evidence for osteomyelitis.
   c. In a patient with recurrent infection in the SLS or SMS, the mandible is one possible site that may harbor inadequately treated microorganisms.
   d. Treatment of deep tissue infection adjacent to the mandible thought to have associated mandibular osteomyelitis consists of a surgical drain in the infected space and a subperiosteal drain.

3. Benign tumor.
   a. Ameloblastoma.
      1) Pathology.
         a) Most common benign mandibular tumor; 1% of all jaw tumors.

   b) Odontogenic tumor comprising epithelial elements. Nonencapsulated, locally invasive.
  2) Radiologic features.
   a) Plain-film radiographic appearance of multilocular, "bubblelike" lucency with no calcification in matrix.
   b) CT/MRI appearance. Multicystic, enhancing mass with aggressive local invasion but no evidence for perineural spread.
  b. There are multiple other benign odontogenic tumors, but a description of all their pathologic and radiologic features is beyond the scope of this publication. They include calcifying epithelial odontogenic tumor, ameloblastic fibroma, adenomatoid odontogenic tumor, dentinoma, calcifying odontogenic cyst, odontogenic ameloblastoma, odontomas, and cementomas.
  c. Other benign nonodontogenic tumors include osteoma, exostosis, osteoid osteoma, chondroma, and hemangioma.
 4. Malignant tumor.
  a. General imaging features.
   1) Usually impossible to tell one malignant tumor from another, unless the tumor matrix is telling. An example is seen when osteogenic sarcoma displays tumorous new bone on plain-film or CT examination.
   2) Soft-tissue extension of these malignant tumors involves the masticator space when the angle, ramus, or condyle is the primary site of involvement. When the body or symphysis is the principal site of tumor, soft-tissue extension involves the SMS or SLS depending on from which side of the mylohyoid muscles the mass originates.
  b. Carcinoma. SCCa may involve the mandible via two mechanism, direct invasion or perineural spread along the inferior alveolar nerve.
  c. Sarcoma.
   1) Sarcoma usually involves younger patients and may arise from bone, cartilage, fibrous tissue, fat, or endothelial tissue.
   2) Osteogenic sarcoma. May see tumorous new bone within tumor matrix that is pathognomonic.
   3) Chondrosarcoma. May see chondroid calcification within tumor matrix that is pathognomonic.
   4) Fibrosarcoma. No tumor matrix is seen.
  d. Multiple myeloma. Poorly defined unilocular or multilocular tumor mass is seen. Serology is key to making the diagnosis.
  e. Metastasis. Usually occurs in the setting of known primary tumor, making diagnosis simple.
 5. Bony cyst.

 a. Odontogenic cysts.
  1) Radicular cyst (referring to the root). Most common cystic lesion of the mandible. Globular cyst at the root or apex of a devitalized tooth.
  2) Dentigerous cyst (follicular cyst). Well-circumscribed radiolucent lesion that develops around the crown of an impacted or unerupted tooth.
  3) Odontogenic keratocyst. Cyst containing keratin. Unilocular or multilocular cyst with sharply demarcated borders. Usually adjacent to the third molar. Rapidly growing.
  4) Calcifying odontogenic cyst. Unilocular or multilocular radiolucent cyst containing variable amounts of calcified material. Occurs in the maxilla in 70% of cases.
  5) Residual cyst. Continues to grow after a tooth is extracted.
  6) Primordial cyst. Develops from the tooth primordia in the third molar location. Indistinguishable from a residual cyst.
 b. Nonodontogenic cysts.
  1) Traumatic bone cyst. Can extend to the alveolar ridge without bone disruption.
  2) Aneurysmal bone cyst. Extremely rare in the mandible.

KEY TO CHAPTER 8 FIGURES

Muscles

1 = buccinator
2 = digastric (anterior belly)
3 = genioglossus
4 = geniohyoid
5 = hyoglossus
6 = intrinsic, of tongue
7 = lateral pterygoid
8 = masseter
9 = medial pterygoid
10 = mylohyoid
11 = palatoglossus (anterior tonsillar pillar)
12 = palatopharyngeus (posterior tonsillar pillar)
13 = paraspinal
14 = platysma
15 = prevertebral
16 = sternocleidomastoid
17 = styloglossus
18 = superior pharyngeal constrictor
19 = trapezius

Nerves

20 = inferior alveolar (branch of cranial nerve V_3)
21 = lingual (branch of cranial nerve V_3)
22 = facial (cranial nerve VII)
23 = glossopharyngeal (cranial nerve IX)
24 = vagus (cranial nerve X)
25 = hypoglossal (cranial nerve XII)
26 = sympathetic plexus

Vessels

30 = external carotid artery
31 = internal carotid artery
32 = internal maxillary artery
33 = lingual artery
34 = facial vein
35 = jugular vein
36 = pharyngeal venous plexus
37 = retromandibular vein

Miscellaneous

40 = adenoids
41 = faucial tonsil
42 = lingual tonsil
43 = parotid gland
44 = sublingual gland
45 = submandibular gland
46 = submandibular gland duct
47 = lingual septum
48 = cartilaginous eustachian tube
49 = soft palate
50 = uvula
51 = hyoid bone
52 = body of mandible
53 = ramus of mandible
54 = mandibular canal

Spaces

CS = carotid space
DS = danger space
MS = masticator space
PCS = posterior cervical space
PPS = parapharyngeal space
PS = parotid space
PVS = perivertebral space
RPS = retropharyngeal space
SLS = sublingual space
SMS= submandibular space

Deep cervical fascia

_____ = superficial layer
.... = middle layer
------- = deep layer

SUGGESTED READING

Abrahams JJ: Anatomy of the jaw revisited with a dental CT software program. *AJNR* 14:979–990, 1993.

Abrahams JJ, Oliverio PJ: Odontogenic cysts: improved imaging with a dental CT software program. *AJNR* 14:367–374, 1993.

Ator GA, Abemayor E, Lufkin RB, et al: Evaluation of mandibular tumor invasion with magnetic resonance imaging. *Arch Otolaryngol Head Neck Surg* 116: 454–459, 1990.

Blaschke DP, Osborn AG: *The mandible and teeth*. In Bergeron RT, Osborn AG, Som PM editors: *Head and neck imaging: excluding the brain*, St. Louis, 1984, Mosby–Year Book.

Coit WE, Harnsberger HR, Osborn AG, et al: Ranulas and their mimics: CT evaluation. *Radiology* 163:211–216, 1987.

Dillon WP, Mancuso AA: *The oropharynx and nasopharynx*. In Newton TH, Hasso AN, Dillon WP, editors: *Computed tomography of the head and neck*, edn 1. New York, 1988, Raven Press.

Hardin CW, Harnsberger HR, Osborn AG, et al: CT in the evaluation of the normal and diseased oral cavity and oropharynx. *Semin Ultrasound CT MR* 7:131–153, 1986.

Harnsberger HR, Mancuso AA, Muraki AS, et al: Branchial cleft anomalies and their mimics: CT evaluation. *Radiology* 152:739–748, 1984.

Minami M, Kaneda T, Yamamoto H, et al: Ameloblastoma in the maxillomandibular region: MR imaging. *Radiology* 184:389–393, 1992.

Muraki AS, Mancuso AA, Harnsberger HR, et al: CT of the oropharynx, tongue base, and floor of mouth: normal anatomy and range of variations, and applications in staging carcinoma. *Radiology* 148:725–731, 1983.

Nguyen VD, Potter JL, Hersh-Schick, MR: Ludwig angina: an uncommon and potentially lethal neck infection. *AJNR* 13:215–219, 1992.

Rothman SLG, Chaftez N, Rhodes ML, et al: CT in the preoperative assessment of the mandible and maxilla for endosseous implant surgery. *Radiology* 168: 171–175, 1988.

Underhill TE, Katz JO, Pope TL Jr., et al: Radiologic findings of diseases involving the maxilla and mandible. *Am J Roentgenol* 159:345–350, 1992.

Vogl TJ, Steger W, Ihrler S, et al: Cystic masses in the floor of the mouth: value of MR imaging in planning surgery. *Am J Roentgenol* 161:183–186, 1993.

Yanagisawa K, Friedman CD, Vining EM, et al: Dentascan imaging of the mandible and maxilla. *Head Neck* 15:1–7, 1993.

9

The Infrahyoid Neck: Normal Anatomy and Pathology of the Head and Neck from the Hyoid Bone to the Clavicles

CRITICAL IMAGING QUESTIONS: INFRAHYOID NECK

1. Describe the principal triangles of the infrahyoid neck as well as their boundaries and contents.
2. Name the spaces of the infrahyoid neck and their fascial boundaries, contents, and interrelationships.
3. Which of the spaces of the infrahyoid neck continue above the hyoid bone cephalad to the skull base? Which of these spaces are confined to the infrahyoid neck?
4. When a lymph node that appears to be malignant is discovered in the lower deep cervical chain of the infrahyoid carotid space, where should the search for a primary tumor be directed? Where should the search be directed if the node is in the upper deep cervical chain or spinal accessory chain?
5. What other normal structure besides the brachial plexus passes between the anterior and middle scalene muscles? Why does it matter that this anatomic detail should be known to the radiologist during an imaging search for a brachial plexus lesion?

The answers to these questions are found in the text beside the question number (Q#) in the margin.

INFRAHYOID NECK

A. Introduction.

1. Traditionally, the infrahyoid neck has been taught from the perspective of surgical and gross anatomic *triangles*. As most imaging of this area is done in a transaxial plane, this triangular orientation does not easily translate into the CT or MRI axial images viewed by the radiologist. Another method of learning about the infrahyoid neck, based on *spaces*, permits a more direct imaging approach to the anatomy of this region. This method is simply adapted to the axial CT and MRI scans.

2. To this end, the normal anatomy of the infrahyoid neck is presented here primarily from the point of view of spaces. Triangles are discussed as well, because the triangular terminology is used in the older radiologic literature and present-day clinical discussions. Where possible, however, triangles are converted to spaces to bridge this gap in terminology.

3. Even though the radiologic perspective is spatial to accommodate axial images, the fact that clinicians localize lesions relative to the longitudinal perspective of triangles of the neck makes it imperative that the radiologist be conversant with both terminologies.

4. The second part of this chapter discusses diseases of the infrahyoid neck. The major focus in this section is the identification of the space the lesion occupies, normal contents of the space, and the space-specific differential diagnosis.

B. Normal anatomy.

1. Triangles.

Q #1

   a. The cervical neck from the mandible to the clavicles is divided by the sternocleidomastoid muscle into two large triangles: the anterior and posterior triangles. These triangles are subdivided into six smaller triangles (Fig. 9-1): the carotid, muscular, submental, and submandibular triangles in the anterior triangle, and the occipital and subclavian triangles in the posterior triangle.

   b. Anterior triangle. The anterior triangle constitutes everything in the cervical neck anteromedial to the sternocleidomastoid muscle (Fig. 9-1). It is subdivided at the hyoid bone into the suprahyoid and infrahyoid components. The suprahyoid portion is subdivided by the anterior belly of the digastric muscle into the submental and submandibular triangles. Because these triangles are above the hyoid bone and functionally related to the oral cavity, they are discussed in Chapter 8.

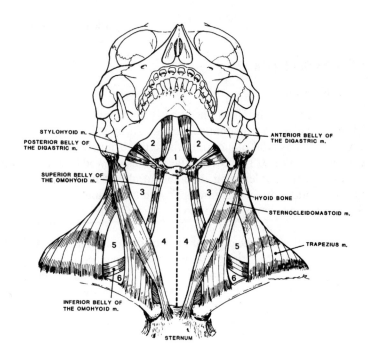

A

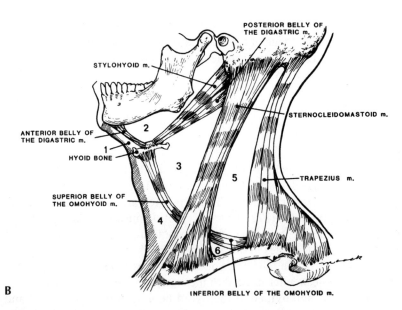

B

Fig. 9-1 Anterior (A) and lateral (B) drawings of the triangles of the cervical neck. The anterior triangle is subdivided into the submental (*1*) and submandibular (*2*) triangles in its suprahyoid component and the carotid (*3*) and muscular (*4*) triangles in its infrahyoid component. The posterior triangle is subdivided into the occipital (*5*) and subclavian (*6*) triangles by the inferior belly of the omohyoid muscle.

c. Infrahyoid component of anterior triangle. The infrahyoid anterior triangle is subdivided by the superior belly of the omohyoid muscle into muscular and carotid triangles (Fig. 9-1).
  1) Muscular triangle.
    a) Boundaries.
      i)   Superior. Superior belly of omohyoid muscle.
      ii) Inferolateral. Sternocleidomastoid muscle.
      iii) Midline. No medial boundary; these paramedian triangles meet in the midline.
    b) Contents.
       Infrahyoid strap muscles.
       Hypopharynx and larynx.
       Cervical trachea and esophagus.
       Thyroid and parathyroid glands.
       Recurrent laryngeal nerve (vagus nerve branch).
    c) Spatial correlation. The muscular triangle occupies the area called the *visceral space* (discussed later).
  2) Carotid triangle.
    a) Boundaries.
      i)   Inferior. Superior belly of omohyoid muscle.
      ii) Lateral. Sternocleidomastoid muscle.
      iii) Superior. Posterior belly of digastric muscle.
    b) Contents.
       Common carotid artery.
       Internal jugular vein.
       Vagus nerve (cranial nerve X).
       Cervical sympathetic trunk.
       Lymph nodes (deep cervical or internal jugular chain).
    c) Spatial correlation. The carotid triangle occupies the area called the *carotid space* (discussed later).
d. Posterior triangle. The posterior triangle comprises the region of the cervical neck posterolateral to the sternocleidomastoid muscle and anteromedial to the trapezius muscle (Fig. 9-1).
  1) This area of the posterolateral cervical neck is subdivided by the inferior belly of the omohyoid muscle into the occipital and subclavian triangles (Fig. 9-1).
  2) Occipital triangle.
    a) Boundaries (Fig. 9-1).
      i)   Anteromedial. Sternocleidomastoid muscle.
      ii) Posterolateral. Trapezius muscle.
      iii) Inferior. Inferior belly of omohyoid muscle.
    b) Contents.
       Fat.

Spinal accessory nerve (cranial nerve XI).
Dorsal scapular nerves.
Transverse cervical veins and arteries.
Lymph nodes (spinal accessory chain).

c) Spatial correlation. The occipital triangle represents the majority of what is called the *posterior cervical space* (discussed later).

3) Subclavian triangle.
   a) Boundaries (Fig. 9-1).
     i) Superior. Inferior belly of omohyoid muscle.
     ii) Anteromedial. Sternocleidomastoid muscle.
     iii) Posterolateral. Trapezius muscle.
   b) Contents.
     Third portion of subclavian artery.
     Transverse cervical artery and vein.
     Cervical portion of brachial plexus.
   c) Spatial correlation. The subclavian triangle describes the area of the cervical neck called the *lower portion of the posterior cervical space.*

2. Fascia-defined spaces.
  a. The spaces of the infrahyoid neck are defined by the deep cervical fascia of the region. To understand the spaces, at least a rudimentary understanding of the fascial anatomy of the infrahyoid neck is necessary.

   1) The three layers of deep cervical fascia divide the infrahyoid neck into spaces. They cannot be seen on normal CT or MRI scans but nonetheless define the spaces of this area and provide barriers to the spread of disease in this region.

   2) If axial images of the infrahyoid neck are inspected with foreknowledge of the fascial boundaries in this area, the ability of the radiologist to correctly define anatomic landmarks and the extent of disease is vastly enhanced.

  b. Deep cervical fascia.
   1) Three layers of deep cervical fascia cleave the infrahyoid neck into fascia-defined spaces (Figs. 9-2 and 9-3):
    a) Superficial (investing) layer.
    b) Middle (visceral) layer.
    c) Deep (prevertebral) layer.

   2) These fascial names are the same as in the suprahyoid neck, with the exception of the middle layer of deep cervical fascia, called the *buccopharyngeal fascia in the suprahyoid neck* (see Chapter 1).

   3) These three layers of deep cervical fascia allow identification of each area on an axial image by space. A lesion within one

of these spaces allows consideration of what are the critical contents of the space and construction of a space-specific, differential diagnosis for the lesion based on its space of origin.

    a) Because the infrahyoid neck is so tightly packed compared with the suprahyoid neck, this spatial analysis process is considerably more effective above the level of the hyoid bone.

    b) Even though the assignment of space and space-specific diagnosis is more difficult in the infrahyoid neck, it still provides an important starting point for analysis of the CT or MRI scans.

c. Superficial (investing) layer of deep cervical fascia.

    1) This fascia "invests" the entire extracranial head and neck region from the skull base above to the clavicle below. Chapter 1 described its suprahyoid course, where it splits to enclose the parotid, masticator, and submandibular spaces.

    2) In the infrahyoid neck the superficial layer of deep cervical fascia encircles the neck completely (Fig. 9-2A). Significant attachments include:

       a) Superior. Hyoid bone.

       b) Inferior. Sternum, clavicle, acromion, and spine of the scapula.

       c) Posterior. Nuchal ligament

    3) This fascia splits as it runs posteriorly to encircle the sternocleidomastoid and trapezius muscles. A slip of this fascia also contributes to the carotid sheath (Figs. 9-2B and 9-3).

d. Middle layer of deep cervical fascia.

    1) Alternative terms used to describe the middle layer include the *visceral fascia* (infrahyoid neck) and *buccopharyngeal fascia* (suprahyoid neck).

    2) The middle layer of deep cervical fascia encircles the "viscera" of the neck, including the larynx, trachea, esophagus, thyroid and parathyroid glands, recurrent laryngeal nerves, and the paraesophageal (paratracheal) lymph nodes. This fascia circumscribes and defines the visceral space (Fig. 9-2C).

    3) The middle layer runs on the deep surface of the strap muscles, but it merges anteriorly with the superficial layer of deep cervical fascia. It splits to encapsulate the thyroid gland.

    4) The posterior margin of the middle layer of the deep cervical fascia constitutes the anterior border of the retropharyngeal space. Its lateral and posterior borders are formed by the deep layer of deep cervical fascia (discussed later).

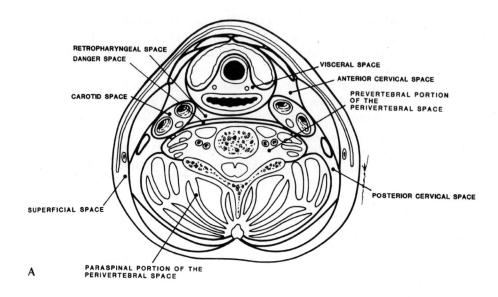

RETROPHARYNGEAL SPACE
DANGER SPACE

VISCERAL SPACE

ANTERIOR CERVICAL SPACE

CAROTID SPACE

PREVERTEBRAL PORTION
OF THE
PERIVERTEBRAL SPACE

POSTERIOR CERVICAL SPACE

SUPERFICIAL SPACE

A

PARASPINAL PORTION OF THE
PERIVERTEBRAL SPACE

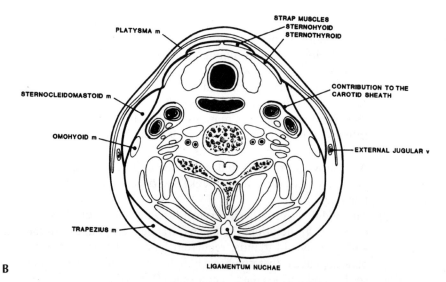

STRAP MUSCLES
STERNOHYOID
STERNOTHYROID

PLATYSMA m

CONTRIBUTION TO THE
CAROTID SHEATH

STERNOCLEIDOMASTOID m

OMOHYOID m

EXTERNAL JUGULAR v

TRAPEZIUS m

B

LIGAMENTUM NUCHAE

Fig. 9-2 Axial drawings through the thyroid bed depicting the fascia and the spaces they define. **A**, Spaces defined by the three layers of deep cervical fascia in the infrahyoid neck. **B**, Superficial layer of deep cervical fascia (i.e., investing layer). This transaxial drawing at the level of the thyroid bed shows the superficial layer splitting to enclose the sternomastoid and trapezius muscles. Only the external jugular vein and platysma lie external to this "investing fascia." **C**, Middle layer of deep cervical fascia (i.e., visceral layer). This axial drawing at the level of the thyroid bed shows the middle layer contributing to the formation of the

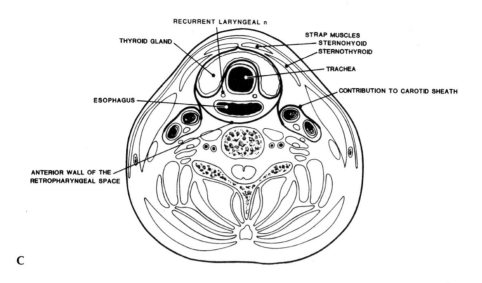

RECURRENT LARYNGEAL n

THYROID GLAND

STRAP MUSCLES
STERNOHYOID
STERNOTHYROID

TRACHEA

CONTRIBUTION TO CAROTID SHEATH

ESOPHAGUS

ANTERIOR WALL OF THE
RETROPHARYNGEAL SPACE

C

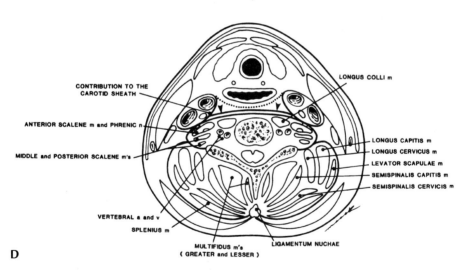

CONTRIBUTION TO THE
CAROTID SHEATH

ANTERIOR SCALENE m and PHRENIC n

MIDDLE and POSTERIOR SCALENE m's

LONGUS COLLI m

LONGUS CAPITIS m
LONGUS CERVICUS m
LEVATOR SCAPULAE m
SEMISPINALIS CAPITIS m
SEMISPINALIS CERVICIS m

VERTEBRAL a and v
SPLENIUS m

MULTIFIDUS m's
(GREATER and LESSER)

LIGAMENTUM NUCHAE

D

carotid sheath. This layer completely circles the visceral space of the infrahyoid neck. Its posterior margin also serves as the anterior wall of the retropharyngeal space. **D**, Deep layer of deep cervical fascia. This axial drawing through the thyroid bed shows the deep layer encircling the prevertebral and scalene muscle to attach to the transverse processes. The deep layer continues posteriorly to meet at the nuchal ligament. The perivertebral space is subdivided into prevertebral and paraspinal areas. A second slip of fascia (i.e., alar fascia) forms the lateral walls of the retropharyngeal space and contributes to formation of the carotid sheath.

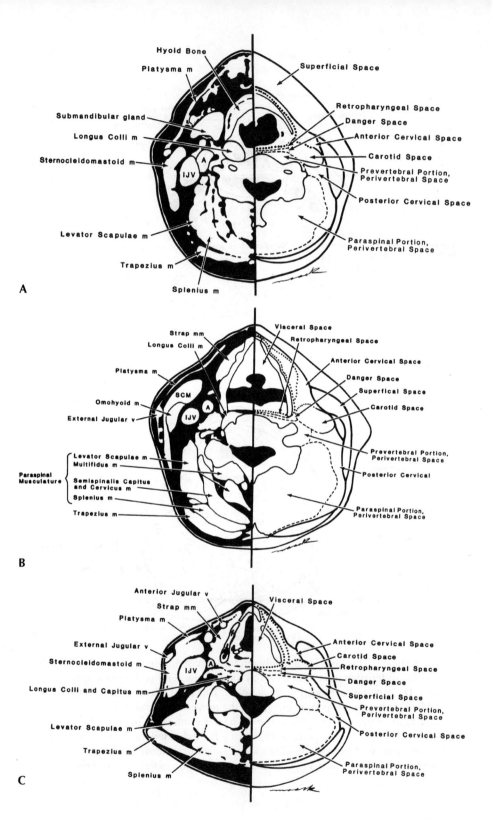

A

Hyoid Bone

Platysma m

Submandibular gland

Longus Colli m

Sternocleidomastoid m

Levator Scapulae m

Trapezius m

Splenius m

Superficial Space

Retropharyngeal Space

Danger Space

Anterior Cervical Space

Carotid Space

Prevertebral Portion, Perivertebral Space

Posterior Cervical Space

Paraspinal Portion, Perivertebral Space

IJV

A

B

Strap mm

Longus Colli m

Platysma m

Omohyoid m

External Jugular v

Paraspinal Musculature {
Levator Scapulae m
Multifidus m
Semispinalis Capitus and Cervicus m
Splenius m
Trapezius m
}

Visceral Space

Retropharyngeal Space

Anterior Cervical Space

Danger Space

Superfical Space

Carotid Space

Prevertebral Portion, Perivertebral Space

Posterior Cervical

Paraspinal Portion, Perivertebral Space

SCM

IJV

A

C

Anterior Jugular v

Strap mm

Platysma m

External Jugular v

Sternocleidomastoid m

Longus Colli and Capitus mm

Levator Scapulae m

Trapezius m

Splenius m

Visceral Space

Anterior Cervical Space

Carotid Space

Retropharyngeal Space

Danger Space

Superficial Space

Prevertebral Portion, Perivertebral Space

Posterior Cervical Space

Paraspinal Portion, Perivertebral Space

IJV

A

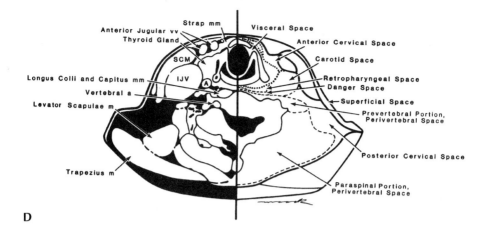

D

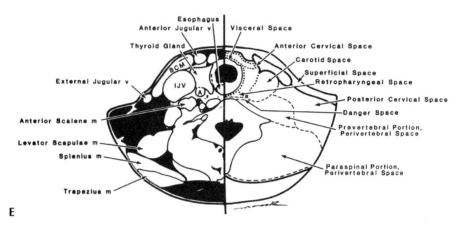

E

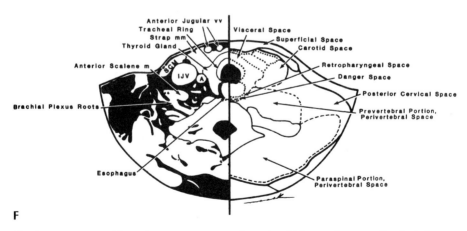

F

◄ **Fig. 9-3** Axial line-diagram sequence from hyoid bone above to the first rib below illustrating the important anatomy of the infrahyoid neck typically seen on CT or MRI scans. Each drawing has the critical contents of the spaces on the left and the fascial lines/spaces on the right. **A,** Hyoid bone level. **B,** Supraglottic level. **C,** Glottic level. **D,** Cricoid (i.e., subglottic) level. **E,** First tracheal ring level. **F,** First rib level.

5) A slip of the visceral layer contributes to the carotid sheath (Fig. 9-2*C*).

6) Other significant attachments of the visceral fascia include superiorly to the skull base and inferiorly with the deep layer of deep cervical fascia to the pericardium.

e. Deep layer of deep cervical fascia.

1) The deep layer of deep cervical fascia encircles the prevertebral and paraspinal muscles, scalene muscles, vertebrae, vertebral artery and vein, phrenic nerve, and trunks of the brachial plexus (Fig. 9-2*D*). The deep layer circumscribes and defines the perivertebral space.

a) In the first edition of this book and much of the supporting radiologic literature, the perivertebral space has been referred to as the *prevertebral space*. The name is changed here, because one quick look at the space beneath the deep layer of the deep cervical fascia reveals that only the anterior portion is indeed *prevertebral* (Latin for "in front of the vertebral body").

b) The paraspinal portion of this space is to the side and behind the vertebrae in the cervical neck (Fig. 9-2*A*). Calling this area the paraspinal portion of the *pre*vertebral space simply is not appropriate; hence the change to *peri*vertebral space.

c) Renaming this space the *perivertebral* (Greek for "around") *space* is an attempt to regain the moral "high ground" in this discussion. Henceforth this book refers to prevertebral and paraspinal portions of the perivertebral space (Fig. 9-2*A*).

d) This discussion is further confused by the fact that the anatomic literature freely refers to the deep layer of the deep cervical fascia as the *prevertebral fascia*. Again, only the anterior portion of this fascia is *pre*vertebral; the remainder encloses the paraspinal area posterolaterally. To keep the confusion to a minimum this book refers to the *deep layer of deep cervical fascia* only and dispenses with the term *prevertebral fascia*.

2) Laterally, the deep layer of the deep cervical fascia attaches to the transverse process (Figs. 9-2 and 9-3), subdividing the perivertebral space into anterior and posterior areas. In this discussion the entire area is referred to as the *perivertebral space*.

a) The anterior area is called the *prevertebral aspect of the perivertebral space*, whereas the posterior area is called the *paraspinal aspect of the perivertebral space*. Some authors prefer to call the posterior area the *paraspinal space*.

3) A slip of the deep layer contributes to the carotid sheath (i.e., alar fascia). All three layers of the deep cervical fascia contribute to the carotid sheath.

   a) The alar fascia also flares anteriorly to form the lateral wall of the retropharyngeal space (Fig. 9-2*D*).

4) Other significant attachments of the deep layer of deep cervical fascia include superiorly to the skull base and inferiorly with the middle layer of the deep cervical fascia to the pericardium of the mediastinum.

3. Spaces and their contents (Figs. 9-2 and 9-3, Table 9-1).

   a. When the radiologist looks at a CT or MRI scan of the infrahyoid neck, the major problem is creating a method by which to analyze the images and draw conclusions from this analysis. An understanding of the spaces and their contents allows the construction of a differential diagnosis unique to each space. As in the suprahyoid neck, this spatial analysis of a lesion found in the infrahyoid neck gives the radiologist a rational method of approach rather than a frustrating sense of inadequacy when confronted with a lesion in this area.

Q#2

   b. Five major spaces are easily identified in the infrahyoid neck: the visceral, carotid, posterior cervical, retropharyngeal, and perivertebral spaces (Fig. 9-2*A*). This section reviews each of these spaces and their fascia, contents, extent, and corresponding triangle relationship. The subsequent section on diseases of the infrahyoid neck is organized along the same spatial lines.

Q#3

   c. Of the five spaces only the visceral space is unique to the infrahyoid neck (Fig. 9-4). The carotid, posterior cervical, retropharyngeal, and perivertebral spaces all traverse both the suprahyoid and infrahyoid neck.

1) Visualizing these spaces as tubes or columns of circumscribed tissue gives the radiologist a conceptual advantage when interpreting CT or MRI scans. As axial images merely represent a 90° slice through these columns of tissue, the axial and cranial–caudal relationships can be assessed simultaneously.

2) For the most part there are no horizontal fascia in either the suprahyoid or infrahyoid neck. Consequently, disease processes tend to spread in a "north–south" dimension.

   d. Visceral space.

1) Fascia. Completely enclosed by the middle layer of deep cervical fascia (Figs. 9-5 and 9-6).

Table 9-1 Space and Contents of the Infrahyoid Neck

Space	Fascia	Extent	Contents
Carotid space	Carotid sheath: composed of all three layers of deep cervical fascia	Skull base (jugular foramen) to aortic arch	Common carotid artery Internal jugular vein Vagus nerve (cranial nerve X) Sympathetic chain Deep cervical lymph nodes
Posterior cervical space	Complex fascial margins: lies between layers of deep cervical fascia Anteriorly: contacts carotid sheath Medially: contacts deep layer of deep cervical fascia Posterolaterally: contacts superficial layer of deep cervical fascia	Skull base to clavicle	Fat Spinal accessory nerve (cranial nerve XI) Spinal accessory lymph nodes Pre-axillary brachial plexus
Visceral space	Middle layer of deep cervical fascia	Hyoid bone to mediastinum	Thyroid gland Parathyroid glands Larynx Trachea Hypopharynx Trachea Esophagus Recurrent laryngeal nerves Lymph nodes (paratracheal)

Table 9-1 *(continued)*

Space	Fascia	Extent	Contents
Retropharyngeal space	Anterior wall: middle layer of deep cervical fascia Lateral walls: alar slips from deep layer of deep cervical fascia Posterior wall: deep layer of deep cervical fascia	Skull base to mediastinum (T3)	Fat *Note:* Remember no lymph nodes found in infrahyoid RPS.
Perivertebral space	Deep layer of deep cervical fascia	Skull base to mediastinum	Prevertebral portion: Prevertebral and scalene muscles Brachial plexus roots Phrenic nerve Vertebral artery and vein Vertebral body and pedicle Paraspinal portion: Paraspinal muscles Posterior elements

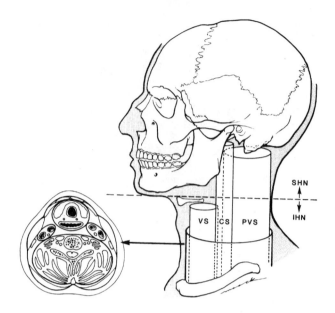

A

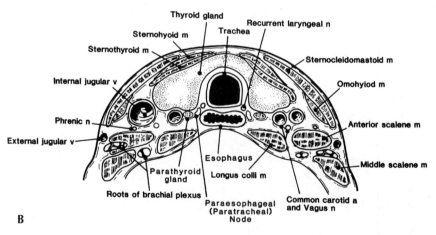

B

Fig. 9-4 **A,** Cranial–caudal nature of the spaces of the neck. Note that only the visceral space (*VS*) is solely infrahyoid. The other spaces of the infrahyoid neck (*IHN*) are also found in the suprahyoid neck (*SHN*). These include the carotid space (*CS*), perivertebral space (*PVS*), posterior cervical space, and retropharyngeal space. **B,** Axial drawing through the thyroid bed emphasizing the normal structures seen at this level.

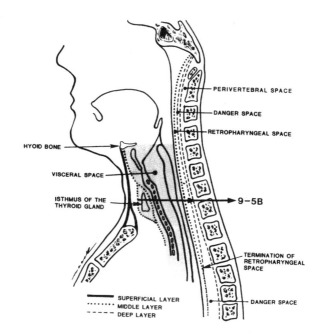

PERIVERTEBRAL SPACE

DANGER SPACE

RETROPHARYNGEAL SPACE

HYOID BONE

VISCERAL SPACE

ISTHMUS OF THE
THYROID GLAND

9-5B

TERMINATION OF
RETROPHARYNGEAL
SPACE

DANGER SPACE

SUPERFICIAL LAYER
MIDDLE LAYER
DEEP LAYER

A

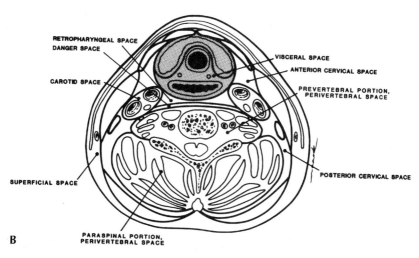

RETROPHARYNGEAL SPACE
DANGER SPACE

VISCERAL SPACE

ANTERIOR CERVICAL SPACE

CAROTID SPACE

PREVERTEBRAL PORTION,
PERIVERTEBRAL SPACE

POSTERIOR CERVICAL SPACE

SUPERFICIAL SPACE

PARASPINAL PORTION,
PERIVERTEBRAL SPACE

B

Fig. 9-5 Sagittal (A) and axial (B) drawings of the cervical neck highlighting the visceral space. **A,** Sagittal drawing of the neck showing the visceral space surrounded by the middle layer of deep cervical fascia (....). It terminates at the hyoid bone above and does not have a distinct fascial margin inferiorly, where it blends with the superior mediastinum. **B,** Axial drawing emphasizing the visceral space and showing its central position in the neck. The middle layer of deep cervical fascia circumscribes this space. The visceral space contains the viscera (thyroid gland, parathyroid glands, larynx, trachea, esophagus), recurrent laryngeal nerve, and paraesophageal lymph nodes.

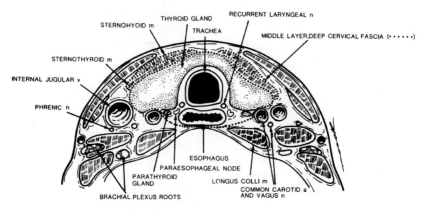

Fig. 9-6 The middle layer of deep cervical fascia (....) is drawn into this axial illustration to emphasize the margins of the visceral space. Note that this fascia splits around the infrahyoid strap muscles anteriorly. Structures that normally may be found in the tracheoesophageal groove include the recurrent laryngeal nerve, paraesophageal nodes, and parathyroid glands.

2) Contents (Fig. 9-6).
   Thyroid gland.
   Parathyroid glands.
   Hypopharynx, larynx and trachea.
   Esophagus.
   Recurrent laryngeal nerve.
   Paraesophageal (paratracheal) lymph nodes.
3) Extent. Hyoid bone to mediastinum.
4) Corresponding infrahyoid neck triangle. Muscular triangle.
   e. Carotid space.
   1) Fascia. Completely encircled by the carotid sheath, which is composed of all three layers of deep cervical fascia.
   2) Contents (Fig. 9-7).
      Common carotid artery.
      Internal jugular vein.
      Vagus nerve proper.
      Sympathetic chain.
      Deep cervical lymph nodes.
   3) Extent. Skull base (jugular foramen) to the aortic arch.
   4) Corresponding infrahyoid neck triangle: Carotid triangle.
   f. Posterior cervical space.
   1) Fascia. Complex fascial boundaries (Fig. 9-8).
      a) Superficial. Superficial layer of deep cervical fascia.
      b) Deep. Deep layer of the deep cervical fascia.

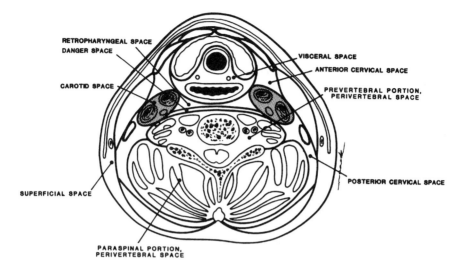

Fig. 9-7   The carotid spaces are circumscribed by a mixture of all three layers of deep cervical fascia (i.e., carotid sheath). This paired set of tissue tubes runs from the arch below to the skull base (i.e., jugular foramen) above. In the infrahyoid neck it is the common carotid artery, jugular vein, and vagus trunk that are found within the carotid space. Although not within the carotid space, the deep cervical nodal chain is intimately associated with it.

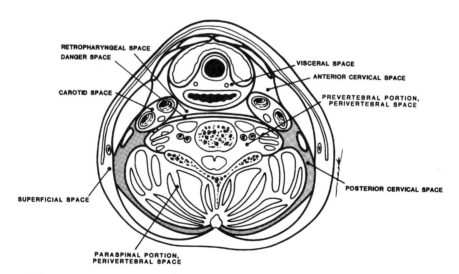

Fig. 9-8   The posterior cervical space shaded in this drawing contains only fat, spinal accessory lymph nodes, and the spinal accessory nerve. Lesions from the deeper perivertebral space often mimic masses of the posterior cervical space clinically.

      c) Anterior (ventral). Carotid sheath.

  2) Contents. (Fig. 9-9).

     Fat.

     Spinal accessory nerve (cranial nerve XI).

     Spinal accessory lymph node chain.

     Preaxillary brachial plexus.

     Dorsal scapular nerve.

  3) Extent. The posterior cervical space extends from a small superior tip at the skull base to the clavicle.

  4) Corresponding infrahyoid neck triangles: Occipital and subclavian triangles.

  g. Retropharyngeal space.

    1) Fascia (Figs. 9-2*D* and 9-10). Complex fascial boundaries:

      a) Anterior (ventral). Middle layer of deep cervical fascia.

      b) Posterior (dorsal). Anterior slip of the deep layer of deep cervical fascia.

      c) Lateral. Alar fascia, which is a slip of the deep layer of deep cervical fascia.

    2) Contents.

     Fat.

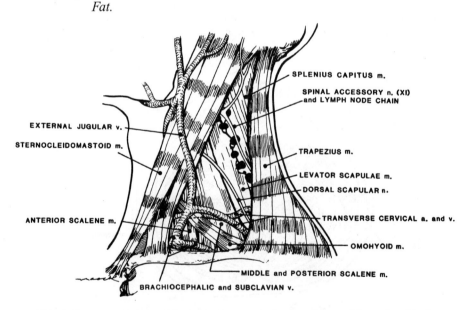

Fig. 9-9 Lateral view of the posterior cervical space. Viewed from the side the posterior cervical space is a posteriorly leaning triangle containing the spinal accessory nerve, posterior cervical lymph node chain, and fat. The floor of this space is comprised of a series of muscles covered by the deep layer of deep cervical fascia.

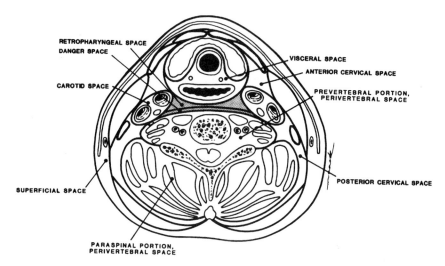

Fig. 9-10   Axial drawing highlighting the more anterior retropharyngeal space and the immediately posterior danger space. The retropharyngeal space in the infrahyoid neck contains only fat. As a result only lesions spreading down from the suprahyoid neck are found in this space, the most common being abscess and squamous cell carcinoma.

Retropharyngeal lymph nodes (suprahyoid retropharyngeal space only).

3) Extent. Skull base to level of the T-3 vertebral body.
4) Corresponding infrahyoid neck triangle: None.
5) Danger space.
    a) The danger space can be found directly behind the retropharyngeal space. It is fat filled and cannot be distinguished from the retropharyngeal space by CT or MRI.
    b) The danger space has complex fascial boundaries:
        i) Anterior (ventral). Anterior slip of the deep layer of deep cervical fascia.
        ii) Posterior (dorsal). Posterior slip of the deep layer of deep cervical fascia.
        iii) Lateral. Alar fascia, which is a lateral slip of the deep layer of deep cervical fascia.
    c) The purpose of mentioning this lackluster space is that the danger space represents the inferior conduit for retropharyngeal space infection or tumor to reach the mediastinum (Figs. 9-2*A,D*).
    d) Because it is not possible to distinguish a lesion in the retropharyngeal space from one in the danger space, this

book uniformly describes lesions in this area as being in the retropharyngeal space. Inclusion of the danger space here is mainly for completeness. It has little clinical relevance.

i. Perivertebral space.

   1) Fascia. Completely enclosed by the deep layer of deep cervical fascia (Figs. 9-11). This fascia attaches to the transverse process as it passes posteriorly. In so doing it cleaves the perivertebral space into anterior and posterior areas.

     a) The anterior area is referred to as the *prevertebral portion of the perivertebral space,* and the posterior area is called the *paraspinal portion of the perivertebral space.*

   2) Contents of the prevertebral portion of perivertebral space (Figs. 9-2*A,D*):

     a) *Prevertebral muscles, longus colli muscle.*

     b) *Scalene muscles* (anterior, middle, posterior).

     c) *Proximal brachial plexus.*

     d) *Phrenic nerve* (C3, C4, C5).

     e) *Vertebral artery and vein.*

     f) *Vertebrae and pedicles.*

   3) Contents of the paraspinal portion of perivertebral space (Figs. 9-2*A,D*):

     a) *Paraspinal muscles.*

     b) *Posterior vertebral body elements* (including lamina and spinous process).

   4) Extent. Skull base to mediastinum at approximately the T3 level.

   5) Corresponding infrahyoid neck triangle: None.

   6) Brachial plexus (Fig. 9-12). The brachial plexus is a structure that traverses multiple contiguous spaces (transpatial). It begins in the prevertebral portion of the perivertebral space and passes between the anterior and middle scalene muscles to enter the posterior cervical space. From there it passes inferolaterally into the axillary apex.

     a) Because most diseases that affect the brachial plexus occur in the prevertebral portion of the perivertebral space, the discussion of the normal and diseased brachial plexus is included in the perivertebral space sections.

C. Diseases.

1. Introduction.

  a. With radiologic evaluation now being done earlier in the clinical work-up, lesions of the infrahyoid neck are being imaged earlier in their natural history, when they are smaller and less extensive.

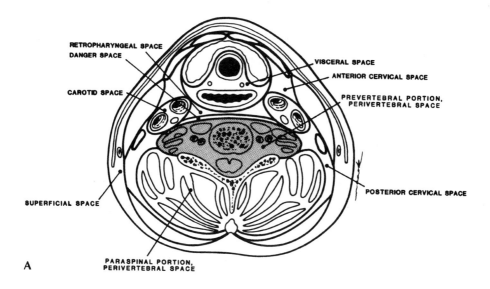

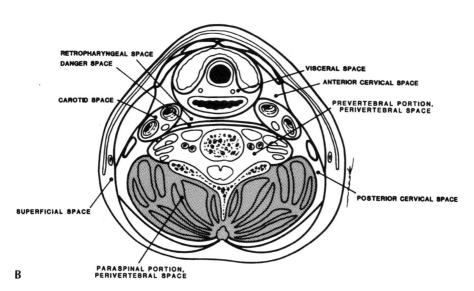

Fig. 9-11 At the level of the thyroid bed these drawings depict the two parts of the perivertebral space. **A,** Anteriorly the prevertebral aspect of the perivertebral space contains the more important structures, including the phrenic nerves, brachial plexus roots, scalene and prevertebral muscles, vertebral arteries and veins, and the vertebral body. **B,** The more posterior paraspinal aspect of the perivertebral space is of much less interest, as it contains only the posterior spinal elements and the paraspinal muscles.

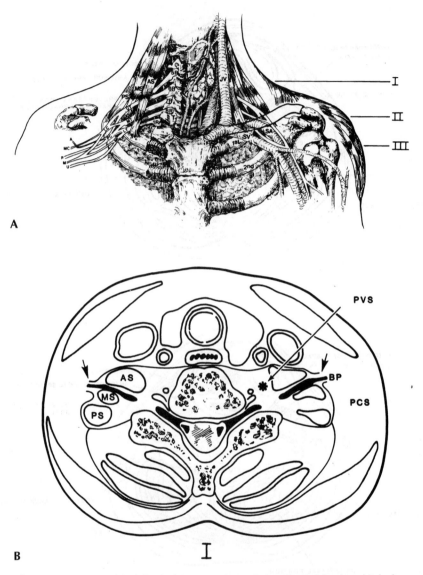

Fig. 9-12 Normal brachial plexus. **A,** Frontal drawing of the brachial plexus shows the C5–T1 roots (*R*) traveling through the prevertebral aspect of the periver-tebral space, then leaving this space between the anterior (*AS*) and middle (*MS*) scalene muscles. The brachial plexus trunks (*T*) then traverse the posterior cervi-cal space on their way to the axillary apex. The subclavian artery (*SA*) also follows this course. *JV*, jugular vein; *MT*, middle trunk; *LT*, lower trunk; *PS*, posterior sca-lene muscle; *SV*, subclavian vein; *UT*, upper trunk. **B,** Axial drawing through the thyroid bed shows the roots of the brachial plexus (*BP, dark lines*) passing through

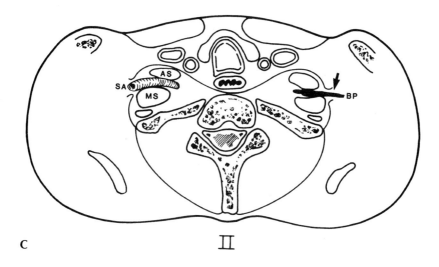

C   II

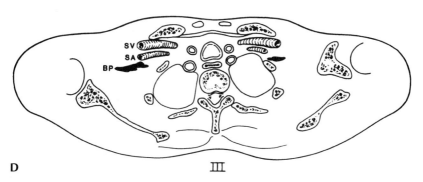

D   III

the prevertebral aspect of the perivertebral space (*asterisk, PVS*). The roots exit the PVS between the anterior (*AS*) and middle (*MS*) scalene muscles, where they perforate the deep layer of deep cervical fascia (*short arrows*) to enter the posterior cervical space (*PCS*). PS = posterior scalene muscle. **C,** Axial drawing at the level of the first rib demonstrates the brachial plexus (*BP, dark lines*) on the right passing through the deep layer of deep cervical fascia (*arrow*) into the posterior cervical space. Note on the left that the subclavian artery (*SA*) also follows this course between the anterior (*AS*) and middle (*MS*) scalene muscles. **D,** Transaxial drawing at the level of the axillary apex reveals the brachial plexus (*BP, dark lines*) posterior to the subclavian vein (*SV*) and subclavian artery (*SA*). The high axillary aspect of the brachial plexus may be involved by nonpalpable disease, especially apical lung carcinoma (Pancoast's tumor). (With permission from Armington WG, Harnsberger HR, Osborn AG, et al: Radiographic evaluation of brachial plexopathy. *AJNR* 8:361–367, 1987.)

    b. As a result even aggressive infections and invasive malignancies are usually confined to a single space when initially imaged.

    c. Now that we can recognize and identify these spaces, we can use them as a foundation on which to build space-specific differential diagnoses.

    d. The exercise is simple once the spatial anatomy is mastered. The method of image analysis for lesions of the infrahyoid neck is:

        1) First the lesion is identified and determined to be real and not a pseudomass. Many things in the extracranial head and neck that can be seen or felt clinically are found to be pseudomasses on radiologic evaluation.

        2) Next the mass lesion is assigned to a space of origin according to the characteristic displacement pattern of the normal surrounding structures and the center of the lesion.

        3) Finally the radiologic features of the specific lesion are matched with the known possible diseases of the space to create a space-specific differential diagnosis.

    e. Abbreviated, this method is:

        1) Decide mass vs. pseudomass.

        2) If mass, assign it a space of origin.

        3) Match radiologic features with differential diagnosis for space.

        4) Generate a differential diagnosis unique to the lesion and space.

2. Lesions of the visceral space

    a. Imaging clues help to determine that a mass lesion is primary to the visceral space (VS) (Fig. 9-13).

        1) Each major area of the VS has different imaging clues suggesting that the mass originated within it. Major areas within the VS are the laryngeal, thyroid, parathyroid, and esophageal areas.

        2) Thyroid lesions. The center of the mass is within the thyroid gland, with the thyroid tissue seen surrounding the mass lesion (Fig. 9-13). The carotid space is displaced laterally, and the trachea and esophagus are displaced to the side opposite the lesion.

        3) Parathyroid lesions. When large parathyroid lesions usually displace the thyroid gland anteriorly and carotid space laterally. The center of a parathyroid mass is between the thyroid gland anteriorly and the longus colli muscle posteriorly.

            a) Alternatively, parathyroid lesions may be within the thyroid gland or in "ectopic" locations from the hyoid bone to the carina.

        4) Laryngeal lesions. Easily identified within the cartilaginous edifice of the larynx.

        5) Esophageal lesions. The mass is centered in the middle of the posterior visceral space, abutting or surrounding the esophagus.

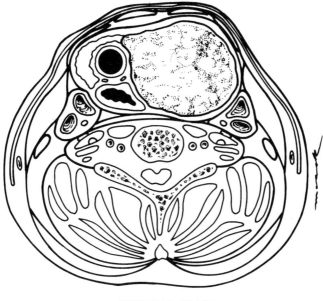

VISCERAL SPACE

Fig. 9-13   Visceral space mass. Such masses may arise from the thyroid, parathyroid, esophagus, or larynx. This intrathyroid visceral space mass, with thyroid tissue surrounding it, displaces the carotid space laterally and the trachea contralaterally.

In most cases the mass is directly behind the trachea and displaces it anteriorly.

6) In general when a VS lesion is malignant (i.e., invasive appearing), the only clue to its visceral space origin is the loss of soft-tissue planes within the structures of the visceral space (larynx, trachea, esophagus, thyroid).

a) Esophageal malignancy often tracks along the esophagus longitudinally much more often than it breaks out into the surrounding tissues.

b) Thyroid malignancy usually spreads throughout the thyroid bed before invading the surrounding spaces.

7) Once the lesion is identified as in the VS, the differential diagnosis (Table 9-2) should be reviewed.

b. Congenital/developmental.

1) Thyroglossal duct cyst when infrahyoid is found in the anterior aspect of the VS.

2) For all details regarding this congenital mass, see Chapter 10.

Table 9-2 Differential Diagnosis of Visceral Space Lesions

Pseudomass
Pyramidal lobe of thyroid gland
Prominent thyroid isthmus
Posttraumatic larynx
Patulous esophagus in tracheoesophageal groove (parathyroid adenoma mimic)

Congenital/developmental
Infrahyoid thyroglossal duct cyst

Laryngeal lesions
Squamous cell carcinoma
Chondrosarcoma
Laryngocele

Thyroid lesions
Colloid cyst
Goiter
Adenoma
Carcinoma (papillary, follicular, mixed)
Anaplastic carcinoma
Non-Hodgkin lymphoma
Metastasis

Parathyroid lesions
Adenoma
Cyst

Esophageal lesions
Zenker's diverticulum
Carcinoma

Paraesophageal (paratracheal) nodal lesions
Thyroid carcinoma metastases
Squamous cell carcinoma metastases (treated neck)
Lymphoma
Other metastases

Visceral space inflammation
Abscess
Hashimoto's thyroiditis

---

    c. Laryngeal lesions.
        1) Squamous cell carcinoma (SCCa) and laryngocele are commonly imaged laryngeal lesions. See Chapter 11 for details.
    d. Thyroid lesions.

1) Imaging issues. Ultrasound and radionuclide scanning are the first studies ordered to evaluate a suspected thyroid mass. CT or MRI follow when these studies leave unanswered questions.
   a) Clinical indications that may lead to ordering ultrasound or radionuclide scanning of the thyroid are:
      i) History of radiation exposure.
      ii) Family history of multiple endocrinopathy syndrome.
      iii) Solitary nodule when demonstration of multiple nodules may alter treatment.
      (iv) Palpable low neck mass when it is questionable whether it is thyroidal or extrathyroidal.
   b) CT or MRI is used secondarily to evaluate the deep tissue extent of a mass that is to be surgically removed.
2) An important generalization in thyroid imaging with CT or MRI is that neither tool can differentiate benign thyroid adenoma from thyroid malignancy based on primary imaging findings. Calcification or cystic areas within the mass have no predictive value in making this differentiation. Ancillary findings such as nodal tumor, cartilaginous or bony destruction, and vagus nerve malfunction allow the identification of malignancy.
3) Colloid cyst.
   a) Radiologic appearance. Single cystic mass within the thyroid gland. Cannot be differentiated from goiter or carcinoma that has undergone cystic degeneration.
4) Goiter.
   a) Etiology. Familial; iodine deficiency.
   b) Clinical presentation. Long history of lower neck mass. When very large, they can cause tracheal and esophageal compression. Breathing and/or swallowing problems may result. Pressure on the recurrent laryngeal nerve may cause vocal cord malfunction.
   c) Pathology. Goiter may be diffuse or nodular. Thyroid enlargement results from an increase in thyrocytes, from adenomas, or from degenerative changes with cyst formation.
   d) Radiologic appearance. Mixed-density, well-circumscribed mass involving both lobes of the thyroid gland that may extend well into the mediastinum. These lesions may raise concern for malignancy, but the crisp margins and complete involvement of both lobes of the enlarged thyroid gland signal their benign nature.
5) Thyroid adenoma.
   a) Radiologic appearance. Inhomogeneous mass, 1 to 4 cm in diameter, with the thyroid gland. Margins are well circum-

scribed. May have multiple amorphous calcifications within it. Cannot be differentiated radiologically from thyroid carcinoma.

6) Thyroid carcinoma.
   a) Five types. Papillary (50% of cases), follicular (20%), medullary (10%), giant cell or anaplastic (3%), and Hürthle cell (2%) carcinomas.
   b) Prognosis depends on cell type (papillary has the best prognosis, giant cell the worst), gender (better in female patients), age (better in younger patients), and extent of tumor at presentation.
   c) MRI is the preferred cross-sectional imaging tool when evaluation of thyroid malignancy is required as a presurgical guide. Surgery is usually anticipated to remove maximum tumor volume before therapy with iodine-131. In this setting MRI is used to define the tumor or nodal extent.
   d) CT is *not recommended* in this setting, because the iodine administered during the CT examination can takes months to clear from the patient's system. Contrast-enhanced CT scanning can postpone iodine-131 therapy for up to 6 months. This problem can be avoided by using MRI exclusively in this clinical setting.
   e) Comment. Careful evaluation of the thyroid gland is necessary in any patient with a cystic mass in the lower neck. Nodal metastases of thyroid carcinoma often appear cystic at presentation. It is not uncommon for a lesion thought clinically to be a branchial cleft cyst to be found to be a cystic thyroid metastasis on pathologic examination.
   f) Radiologic appearance. Unilateral intrathyroidal mass with infiltrating margins obscuring adjacent soft-tissue planes. Calcifications are present in up to 35% of patients. They may have associated adenopathy. A mass with well-defined margins does not necessarily exclude thyroid malignancy.

7) Thyroid non-Hodgkin lymphoma.
   a) The thyroid gland is an unusual site for extranodal, extralymphatic lymphoma of the extracranial head and neck.
   b) From an imaging point of view thyroid lymphoma cannot be differentiated from anaplastic thyroid carcinoma. In both cases an infiltrating mass within the thyroid and with indistinct margins is seen.
   c) The clinical presentation of both non-Hodgkin lymphoma and anaplastic carcinoma are also very similar. In both cases a rapidly growing thyroid mass is present.

e. Parathyroid adenoma.
1) Imaging issues. As with thyroid masses, ultrasound and radionuclide imaging are the first studies ordered by the clinician in search of a parathyroid adenoma.
   a) Ultrasound is the most inexpensive and direct method to search for the presence of adenoma in the thyroid bed. Ectopic parathyroid adenoma will not be seen with ultrasound.
   b) Radionuclide scanning is recommended when ectopic parathyroid adenoma is suspected (i.e., after surgery when no adenoma was found in the thyroid bed). Some authors recommend radionuclide scanning as the initial imaging study in all patients with suspected adenoma. They argue that both the thyroid bed and ectopic adenoma will be identified without the need for ultrasound. In my experience, however, the radionuclide success rate is operator dependent.
   c) CT and MRI usually are reserved to search for ectopic parathyroid adenoma, either to locate precisely a lesion found by radionuclide study or as the primary examination. CT is less operator dependent, but MRI is probably the best tool if meticulous protocol and image inspection are employed.
2) Important facts about parathyroid adenoma.
   a) The number of normal parathyroid glands varies from two to six.
   b) The usual anatomic arrangement is two pairs of glands nestled behind the lateral upper and lower poles of the thyroid gland.
   c) Atypically located or ectopic lower parathyroid glands are not uncommon, and they are related to the variable degree of caudal migration of these glands during embryogenesis.
   d) The inferior parathyroid glands may be located some distance below the lower poles of the thyroid gland in the cervicothoracic junction or in the upper mediastinum.
3) Imaging features.
   a) Ultrasound. Parathyroid adenoma in the thyroid bed is diagnosed when ultrasound demonstrates an oval sonolucent mass, larger than 5 mm in diameter, typically between the longus colli posteriorly and the upper or lower pole of the thyroid gland anteriorly.
      i) Ultrasound may miss the more medial adenomas, because they are obscured by tracheal air shadowing. It also is unable to detect ectopic adenomas.

       b) Radionuclide scanning with thallium-201 and technetium-99m. Thallium focal uptake outside the thyroid gland is diagnostic of parathyroid adenoma. Sensitivity of this scan is 80% to 90%.

       c) CT. CT shows a moderately enhancing mass with well-circumscribed borders either in the thyroid bed or an ectopic location. When small and ectopic, the adenoma may be difficult to distinguish from enhancing vessel or paratracheal lymph node. Asymmetric esophageal protrusion also may be difficult to distinguish from parathyroid adenoma. CT esophageal contrast can help in such a circumstance.

       d) MRI. T1-weighted images usually show parathyroid adenoma as isointense to muscle. Fat in the neck provides ample contrast on T1-weighted images. T2-weighted images show parathyroid adenoma to have hyperintense signal.

  f. Esophageal carcinoma.

    1) The diagnosis of esophageal carcinoma is made by barium swallow followed by endoscopy and biopsy.

    2) CT and MRI are reserved for evaluation of the deep tissue extent of the tumor and examination of the mediastinum and abdomen for nodal disease.

  g. Paraesophageal nodal lesions.

    1) The paraesophageal or paratracheal nodal chain runs along the lateral esophagus in the VS into the mediastinum below.

    2) The most common neck tumor to follow this chain is thyroid carcinoma. Upper aerodigestive tract SCCa does not follow this path. Hence it is critical to image to the arch when staging thyroid carcinoma, while the exam can be terminated at the cervical–thoracic junction when staging squamous cell carcinoma.

    3) Thyroid carcinoma enters the mediastinum along this nodal chain. This route of spread is responsible for the higher propensity of thyroid malignancy to spread into the mediastinum compared with the extremely rare occurrence of SCCa spreading into the mediastinum.

    4) Comment. Beware of esophageal pseudomass in this area. The esophagus can pouch out from its normal, retrotracheal location into the tracheoesophageal groove and mimic a paraesophageal nodal mass. A small amount of esophageal contrast medium during CT will clear any confusion as to the nature of a mass in this area.

  h. Visceral space inflammation.

    1) Abscess.

      a) Abscess originating in the VS of the neck is rare, because the usual inciting factors (salivary gland calculus, poor dentition, and Waldeyer's ring inflammation) are not present in this area.

    b) Abscess in the VS is usually secondary to penetrating trauma or superinfection of a hematoma.

  2) Acute thyroiditis.

    a) Clinical presentation. Sudden onset of pain and swelling in the thyroid gland. Redness in the overlying skin also is present with exhaustion.

    b) Pathogenesis. Viral infection is the most common etiology.

  3) Subacute thyroiditis.

    a) Hashimoto's thyroiditis. Familial autoimmune thyroiditis. Nontender, thyroid enlargement. Diagnosis based on thyroglobulin and microsomal antibodies in the serum.

3. Lesions of the carotid space.

  a. Two imaging clues identify a lesion as originating in the infrahyoid carotid space (CS) (Fig. 9-14):

    1) The mass abuts the carotid artery or the jugular vein (i.e., its center is in close association with the carotid artery and the jugular vein).

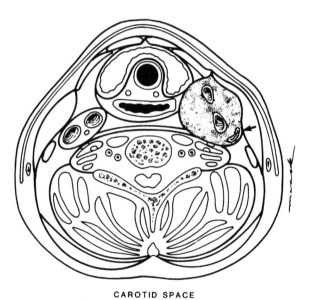

CAROTID SPACE

Fig. 9-14 Carotid space mass in the infrahyoid neck. Such a mass is typically centered in the region of the carotid artery. This axial drawing shows a carotid space mass splaying the external and internal carotid arteries and compressing the internal jugular vein (*arrow*). These masses are usually fusiform or tubular when viewed on multiple axial sections or on sagittal or coronal MRI scans.

     2) The mass is tubular or fusiform.
- b. Once the lesion is identified as being within the infrahyoid CS, the differential diagnosis (Table 9-3) should be considered.
  - 1) Note that many of the lesions presented in Table 9-3 are the same as those found in the suprahyoid CS (Table 5-1).
- c. Pseudomass.
  - 1) Carotid bulb asymmetry.
    - a) In older patients the atherosclerotic carotid bulb can become prominent. If there is clinical suspicion of a carotid body tumor (paraganglioma), CT or MRI is done.
    - b) CT or MRI reveals an atherosclerotic, enlarged carotid bulb. Do not mistake an associated area of subintimal hematoma as necrotic malignant adenopathy.

Table 9-3   Differential Diagnosis of Infrahyoid Carotid Space Lesions

Pseudomass
    Carotid bulb asymmetry
    Carotid artery ectasia
    Jugular vein asymmetry

Congenital/development
    Infrahyoid second branchial cleft cyst

Inflammatory
    Abscess
    Deep cervical chain
      Reactive adenopathy
      Suppurative adenopathy
      Tuberculous adenitis

Vascular
    Jugular vein thrombosis/thrombophlebitis
    Carotid artery posttraumatic pseudoaneurysm

Benign tumor
    Carotid body tumor (paraganglioma)
    Neural sheath tumor (schwannoma, neurofibroma)

Malignant tumor
    Deep cervical chain
      Squamous cell carcinoma
      Thyroid carcinoma
      Non-Hodgkin lymphoma
      Hodgkin lymphoma
      Metastasis (lung, abdomen)

2) Jugular vein asymmetry.
    a) The internal jugular veins are normally asymmetric. In fact, either jugular vein may be normally absent.

d. Congenital/developmental.
    1) Infrahyoid second branchial cleft cyst.
        a) The typical second branchial cleft cyst is seen at the angle of the mandible wedged between the submandibular space and the CS.
        b) When seen below the hyoid bone, this lesion is found just anterior to the infrahyoid CS to the level of the clavicle.
        c) A cystic, tubular mass is seen along the anterior border of the common carotid artery. It may be difficult to differentiate this lesion from cystic metastasis or from thyroid carcinoma · in the deep cervical chain.
        d) Large lesions protrude posteriorly into the posterior cervical space as well.

e. Inflammatory lesions.
    1) Deep cervical chain nodal inflammation.
        a) The deep cervical lymph node chain is in close approximation with the structures of the CS. As a result this book discusses the deep cervical nodal chain as if it is within the CS. Elaboration on the staging of squamous cell adenopathy can be found in Chapter 13.
        b) When these nodes react to inflammation of the head and neck, they enlarge and are referred to as *reactive adenopathy.*
            i) This term is used only for nodes less than 1.5 cm in maximum dimension, oval, and with homogeneous internal architecture.
            ii) When nodes exceed 1.5 cm in diameter, malignancy (either SCCa, lymphoma, or metastatic adenopathy) is suspected.
        c) When microorganisms invade the lymph node and cause an intranodal abscess, the term *suppurative adenopathy* is used.
            i) Suppurative nodes have fluid density in the center on CT scans.
            ii) Caution must be exercised when interpreting a CT scan in a patient having known SCCa with concurrent head and neck infection. Suppurative adenopathy and malignant adenopathy can be indistinguishable radiologically.
            iii) Abscess of the CS most commonly arises from an extracapsular spread of infection from the suppurative lymph nodes.

    d) Tuberculous adenitis occurs when mycobacteria invade the nodes of the deep cervical chain.

      i) Radiologic features. Tuberculous nodes have a somewhat unique appearance. Multiple, mixed, high- and low-density nodes with globular calcifications on enhanced CT scans should suggest the diagnosis.

  f. Vascular lesions.

    1) Jugular vein thrombosis/thrombophlebitis.

      a) Patients often have a history of central venous catheter placement, drug abuse, or malignancy.

      b) In the acute thrombophlebitic phase the neck mass is tender and mimics abscess. In the chronic thrombotic phase the mass is hard and nontender, imitating a tumor.

      c) CT appearance. In the acute thrombophlebitic phase CT scans show loss of soft-tissue planes surrounding the enlarged, thrombus-filled jugular vein. In the chronic thrombotic phase the jugular vein appears as a well-marginated, tubular mass without loss of the surrounding soft-tissue planes.

      d) MRI appearance. In the subacute phase (i.e., >36 hours) jugular vein thrombosis is seen as a high signal, tubular mass on T1 weighted sequences. This is thought to result from the paramagnetic nature of methemoglobin.

  g. Benign tumor.

    1) Paraganglioma.

      a) The only paraganglioma occurring in the infrahyoid CS is paraganglioma of the carotid bifurcation, or carotid body tumor.

      b) Clinical presentation. This tumor presents as a slowly growing mass at the level of the carotid bifurcation. It may be difficult to differentiate clinically from atherosclerotic, carotid bulb ectasia in its early phase.

      c) Pathologic features. Benign tumor arising from neural crest paraganglion cells.

      d) Imaging characteristics.

        i) CT scans show a characteristic, intensely enhancing mass that splays the carotid bifurcation. Smaller tumors may be mistaken for vascular loops (see Fig. 5-2).

        ii) Angiography is not necessary for diagnosis and should be undertaken only when preoperative embolization for operative hemostasis is anticipated.

        iii) MRI scans also show a characteristic mass in the carotid bifurcation, with multiple serpiginous flow

voids within its parenchyma signaling the degree of tumor vascularity.
2) Neural sheath tumors.
   a) Schwannoma, neurofibroma. These lesions are thoroughly discussed in Chapter 5.
   h. Malignant tumor.
   1) Malignancy of the infrahyoid CS occurs in the lymph nodes of the deep cervical chain.
   2) SCCa adenopathy. Squamous cell malignant adenopathy is suspected in a patient without infection but with a known, primary SCCa when CT or MRI scans demonstrate nodes larger than 1.5 cm in diameter with or without central nodal inhomogeneity.

Q#4

   a) When such a lymph node mass is located in the upper deep cervical chain in a patient without a visible primary site, the primary tumor should be sought in the common SCCa sites (i.e., nasopharynx, tongue base, faucial tonsil, and pyriform sinus).
   b) See Chapter 13 for further discussion.
   3) Nonsquamous malignant adenopathy.
      a) When a lymph node mass is found in the low deep cervical chain of the CS, the primary tumor should be sought in the thyroid, thorax, or abdomen.
      b) As a rule, spread of SCCa into the nodes of the neck does not occur in a skipping fashion. If nodes are seen only in the low deep cervical or spinal accessory chains, the primary site is not in the neck.
      c) The left supraclavicular area is most commonly affected in this manner, because the metastatic tumor comes up the thoracic duct from the abdomen. Local lymphatic involvement in the low left neck then results.
   4) Lymphomatous adenopathy.
      a) Both Hodgkin and non-Hodgkin lymphoma may present as adenopathy in the deep cervical chain of the neck.
      b) With non-Hodgkin lymphoma the nodes are usually large, nonnecrotic, and often bilateral on CT and MRI scans. More aggressive non-Hodgkin lymphoma (especially the AIDS-related variety) may present with necrotic adenopathy.
4. Lesions of the posterior cervical space.
   a. When viewed from the side (Fig. 9-9), the posterior cervical space (PCS) is a posteriorly tilted triangle containing the spinal accessory

nerve (cranial nerve XI), spinal accessory lymph nodes (posterior cervical chain), and fat.

b. Given the paucity of significant contents in this space, it is not surprising that the differential diagnosis of lesions in the PCS is short (Table 9-4).

c. The majority of the PCS is below the hyoid bone, although the very top of this space extends well into the suprahyoid neck.

d. Criteria for defining a mass as primary to the PCS (Fig. 9-15) are:
  1) The center must be within the fat of the PCS.
  2) A strip of fat usually separates the mass from the carotid artery–jugular vein complex (i.e., CS) anteriorly.
    a) At the very apex of the PCS the structures of the CS and the PCS come close together. In this area it may become difficult to determine the space of origin of the mass. Unless a fat plane exists between the mass and the CS, it is prudent to consider the mass as originating from the CS and not the PCS.

e. Congenital/development.
  1) Cystic hygroma–lymphangioma spectrum.
    a) Clinical presentation. It is difficult for the clinician to assess the deep tissue extent of these fluid-filled cystic masses with

Table 9-4   Differential Diagnosis of Posterior Cervical Space Lesions

Congenital/development
  Cystic hygroma, lymphangioma
  Hemangioma

Inflammatory
  Abscess
  Posterior cervical chain
    Reactive adenopathy
    Suppurative adenopathy
    Tuberculous adenitis

Benign tumor
  Lipoma
  Neural sheath tumor (schwannoma, neurofibroma)

Malignant tumor
  Posterior cervical chain
    Squamous cell carcinoma (nasopharynx)
    Non-Hodgkin lymphoma
    Hodgkin lymphoma
  Liposarcoma

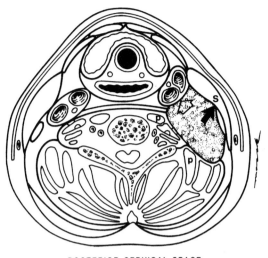

POSTERIOR CERVICAL SPACE

Fig. 9-15 Posterior cervical space mass in the infrahyoid neck. This axial drawing at the level of the thyroid bed demonstrates a generic posterior cervical space mass. The lesion is centered in the fat of the posterior cervical space. Note that the mass displaces the sternocleidomastoid muscle (*s*) outward (*arrow*), flattens the deeper perivertebral space muscles, and displaces the carotid space (*open arrow*) anteromedially.

palpation. Cross-sectional imaging is critical to complete presurgical assessment of these lesions.

b) Pathologic findings. There is a pathologic spectrum of these lesions that is defined by the size of their internal cystic matrix. These lesions are congenital malformations of lymphatic channels. They are classified as *capillary* (i.e., small cystic components), *cavernous* (i.e., medium-sized cystic components), and *cystic* (i.e., enormously dilated lymphatic spaces). Sixty-five percent of cystic hygromas are present at birth; 90% are clinically apparent by 3 years of age. The remaining 10% present as neck masses in young adults.

c) Imaging features. Cystic hygromas are primarily located in the PCS and superior mediastinum in the infant. In the adult, they are more commonly seen in the submandibular and parotid spaces. CT scans show a fluid density, multilocular mass of the PCS. MRI scans demonstrate a multilocular, fluid intensity mass. The margin of these lesions usually shows a characteristic lobular contour.

       d) Comment. Cystic hygroma is a tenacious, difficult to remove lesion that at surgery often wraps around and adheres to adjacent structures. In reporting the extent of this lesion some comment should be made concerning the critical neurovascular structures in the surrounding deep tissues. In the case of a PCS lesion its relationship to the adjacent carotid artery and vagus nerve should be addressed.

   f. Inflammatory lesions.

     1) Inflammatory lesions originate in the posterior cervical nodal chain. This nodal chain runs down the PCS along the course of the spinal accessory nerve (Fig. 9-9). Another name for this nodal chain is the *spinal accessory nodal chain.*

     2) Reactive adenopathy, suppurative adenopathy, and tuberculous adenitis occur in this nodal chain just as in the deep cervical nodal chain associated with the CS.

     3) PCS abscess begins as a suppurative process in the nodes of the spinal accessory chain, extending into the PCS itself by breaking through the node capsule.

   g. Benign tumor.

     1) Lipoma.

       a) Larger lipomas in the head and neck region are almost always found within the PCS.

       b) Clinical presentation. The slowly growing mass is often thought by the examining physician to be a cystic hygroma or other cystic lesion.

       c) Radiologic features. CT and MRI scans both show a fatty mass in the PCS with a thin capsule having convex margins. Internal architecture is minimal. If there is significant internal stranding or inhomogeneity of signal, liposarcoma should be considered; however, liposarcoma is exceedingly rare in this area.

   h. Malignant tumor.

     1) Malignant tumor of the PCS is nodal malignancy of the spinal accessory nodal chain.

     2) When SCCa malignant adenopathy is seen, the primary tumor is usually in the nasopharynx or high oropharynx. The primary tumor may be "unknown" to the clinician because of its location in the crypt of the nasopharyngeal adenoids or oropharyngeal tonsil.

     3) Both Hodgkin and non-Hodgkin lymphoma can present in the nodes of the spinal accessory chain.

5. Lesions of the retropharyngeal space.

   a. The infrahyoid retropharyngeal space (RPS) is identical to the suprahyoid RPS, except there are no retropharyngeal lymph nodes in this portion.

    b. Because of this absence of nodes, the infrahyoid RPS has only fat within it. It serves as a channel for infection and tumor to travel from the neck into the mediastinum. A tumor or infection empty inferiorly into the danger space on their way to the mediastinum below (see Fig. 6-1). Few lesions arise primarily from this part of the RPS.

    c. Criteria for a mass lesion to be primary to the infrahyoid RPS (Fig. 9-16) are:

        1) The mass is in the shape of a horizontal rectangle or "bow tie."

        2) The center of the mass is anterior to the prevertebral muscles.

        3) The mass displaces the prevertebral muscles posteriorly.

    d. See Chapter 6 for a differential diagnosis of lesions of the RPS and description of their clinical, pathologic, and radiologic features.

6. Lesions of the perivertebral space.

    a. The bordering fascia of the infrahyoid perivertebral space (PVS) are identical to those of the suprahyoid PVS. The contents are also the same except for the brachial plexus, which is found only in the infrahyoid PVS.

    b. The vast majority of lesions of the PVS, both infection and tumor alike, arise in the vertebral body then spread into the adjacent PVS.

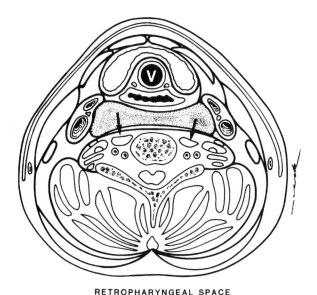

RETROPHARYNGEAL SPACE

Fig. 9-16 Transaxial drawing at the level of the thyroid bed showing retropharyngeal space mass in the infrahyoid neck. Note the central location of this "bow tie"–shaped lesion. Retropharyngeal space masses characteristically are found anterior to the prevertebral strap muscles (*arrows*) and posterior to the visceral space (*V*).

 c. Criteria for a lesion to originate in the prevertebral portion of the perivertebral space (see Fig. 7-3*B*) are:
  1) The center is within the prevertebral muscles or the vertebral body.
  2) The lesion displaces the prevertebral muscles anteriorly.
 d. Criteria for a lesion to originate in the paraspinal portion of the perivertebral space (see Fig. 7-4*B*) are:
  1) The mass is centered in the paraspinal muscles or arises from the posterior elements of the cervical spine.
  2) The mass displaces the paraspinal muscles away from the spine.
 e. When a lesion of the PVS is particularly aggressive, it will violate the fascia that attaches to the transverse process. In such a case the lesion involves both the prevertebral and paraspinal parts of the PVS (Fig. 9-17).
 f. See Chapter 7 for a differential diagnosis of lesions that occur in the PVS and description of their clinical, pathologic, and radiologic features.
 g. Pseudomass

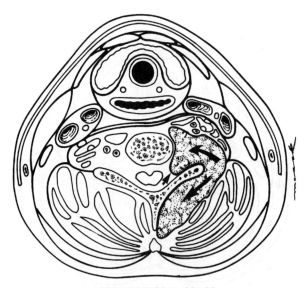

PERIVERTEBRAL SPACE

Fig. 9-17 This axial drawing at the level of the thyroid bed reveals the features of an invasive perivertebral space mass in the infrahyoid neck. The lesion involves both the prevertebral (*curved arrow*) and paraspinal (*large straight arrow*) portions of the perivertebral space. The slip of fascia that normally separate these two areas has been violated, and epidural disease is evident (*short arrow*).

1) On palpation, pseudomass of the PVS is perceived as arising in the posterior cervical space, because it displaces the fat of the PCS toward the palpating hand. On radiologic examination, however, such pseudomass is seen beneath the deep layer of deep cervical fascia within the PVS.
2) Prominent transverse process and cervical rib.
   a) Both of these bony projections may be perceived by the examining physician as a mass in the PCS.
   b) Radiologic features. CT or MRI scans show these two bony pseudomasses in the absence of any other abnormality.
3) Hypertrophy of the levator scapulae muscle.
   a) Clinical presentation. Injury of the spinal accessory nerve, usually at the time of neck dissection, causes atrophy of the sternocleidomastoid and trapezius muscles. In most cases the patient has had a SCCa treated and is undergoing follow-up CT or MRI to search for recurrent tumor.
   b) Radiologic features. CT or MRI scans show sternocleidomastoid and trapezius muscle atrophy, with levator scapulae muscle homogeneous enlargement.
   c) Comment. The levator scapulae muscle enlarges as a result of being used to lift the shoulder after sternocleidomastoid and trapezius muscle denervation.

Q#5
4) Subclavian artery pseudomass.
   a) Clinical presentation. Arm symptoms suggesting brachial plexus malfunction.
   b) Radiologic features. CT is ordered to evaluate the brachial plexus. A prominent "enhancing mass" is seen passing between the anterior and middle scalene muscles.
   c) Comment. The subclavian artery normally passes between the anterior and middle scalene muscle (Fig. 9-18). Do not mistake this for an "enhancing mass." Surgical exploration of a normal subclavian artery is not considered "good form."
h. Brachial plexopathy.
1) The brachial plexus is a neural structure that is transpatial. That is, it crosses from one space (i.e., PVS) to the next (i.e., PCS) (Fig. 9-12).
2) Its course from the spinal cord (C5–T1 roots) to the axillary apex makes it particularly difficult to image properly. Overmagnification of images will exclude the axillary apex as well as disease affecting the brachial plexus in this area.
3) Clinical presentation.

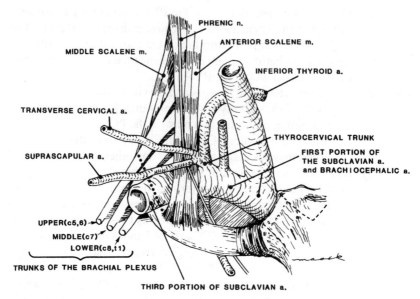

Fig. 9-18 Subclavian artery pseudomass. This frontal drawing of the supraclavicular fossa shows the normal subclavian artery passing to the axillary apex through the gap between the anterior and middle scalene muscles. The brachial plexus also follows this course. The normal subclavian artery often has been mistaken for a "vascular tumor" by novice observers on CT imaging.

> a) Symptoms of brachial plexus dysfunction are quite variable. Unilateral arm and shoulder pain, paresthesia, or numbness suggest a more distal (e.g., PVS, PCS, axillary apex) lesion. Bilateral arm and shoulder symptoms associated with cord compression symptoms signal a more proximal lesion (e.g., cord, epidural space).
> b) In patients with trauma and brachial plexopathy, root avulsion is suspected.
> c) On clinical examination a mass may be palpable in the area of the PCS and/or PVS. Mass lesions behind the clavicle or in the cephalad part of the axillary apex, however, may be beyond the perception of the examiner.
> 4) Root avulsion.
>> a) Myelography or high resolution MRI is best suited to assess nerve root avulsion.
>> b) Radiologic findings.
>>> i) Acute phase. In the acute phase, contrast extravasation is seen through the avulsed nerve root on myelography

with CT. MRI scans show fluid in the adjacent soft tissue with T2- or T2*-weighted images.

   ii) Subacute phase. An "empty socket" is evident with CT–myelography. A *pseudomeningocele* also may be present at the affected levels.

   iii) It is possible for nerve root avulsion to occur even with a "normal" MRI scan. In these cases CT scans using intrathecal contrast will show an "empty socket" only.

5) Malignant tumor.
  a) Tumors that may involve the brachial plexus include vertebral body metastases, infiltrating breast carcinoma, lymphoma, and apical lung carcinoma.
  b) Involvement of the distal brachial plexus with infiltrating tumor can go undiagnosed for months if careful attention to the imaging details does not occur. In such cases the retroclavicular and axillary apex portions of the brachial plexus are not included in the CT scan or are obscured by motion or coil selection on MRI.

6) Imaging issues.
  a) If CT is used to image the brachial plexus, the following imaging guidelines are recommended:
    i) Scan extent. Hyoid bone to aortic arch.
    ii) Slice thickness and increment. 5 mm, contiguous slices.
    iii) Maximize the mAs settings through cervicothoracic junction.
    iv) Sequential demagnification in a stepwise fashion so that axillary apical contents are included on the lower scan.
    v) Contrast strategy. Bolus-drip technique with a 50 mL bolus of 60% contrast followed by rapid infusion of 150 mL of 60% contrast. Maximize the intravascular contrast phase during scanning.
  b) When MRI is used to image the brachial plexus, the following guidelines are recommended:
    ii) Scan planes. Axial and coronal.
    ii) Scan thickness and increment: 3 or 4 mm, contiguous slices, or skip 1 mm.
    iii) Parameters. T1 and T2 in the axial plane; T1 only in the coronal plane.
    iv) Contrast. T1-weighted contrast scan with fat saturation.
    v) Coil technique. Dedicated neck coil is essential.
    vi) Miscellaneous. Flow compensation on. Water bags on neck to create a more uniform magnetic environment. Use a larger field of view (i.e., 28 cm) for coronal images.

7. Transpatial and multispatial disease processes
   a. Transpatial diseases.
      1) When diseases of the extracranial head and neck involve multiple contiguous spaces, the term *transpatial* is used (Fig. 9-19).
      2) Benign congenital lesions that often originate during development of the extracranial head and neck frequently traverse multiple contiguous spaces.
      3) The larger or more aggressive infections and tumors seen in their later stages also may present in a transpatial manner.
      4) Transpatial diseases can be divided into three broad categories: developmental, infections, and tumors (both benign and malignant).
         a) Developmental lesions. Cystic hygroma, hemangioma, thyroglossal duct cyst, branchial cleft cyst.
         b) Infectious lesions. Large, transpatial abscess, diving ranula.
         c) Benign tumors. Lipoma, nerve sheath (schwannoma, neurofibroma), juvenile angiofibroma.
         d) Malignant tumors. SCCa, non-Hodgkin lymphoma, rhabdomyosarcoma, and other head and neck malignancies.

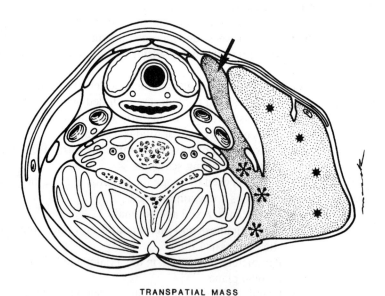

TRANSPATIAL MASS

Fig. 9-19 Axial drawing of a transpatial mass seen in the posterior cervical space (*asterisks*), superficial space (*stars*), and anterior cervical space (*arrow*). When a mass is found in multiple contiguous spaces simultaneously, the term *transpatial* is applied.

b. The term *multispatial* is applied to disease that involves multiple noncontiguous spaces of the head and neck (Fig. 9-20).
   1) Because of the extensive chains of lymph nodes draining the head and neck spaces, any systemic disease involving this region can manifest itself as a multispatial nodal disease.
   2) Inflammatory processes as well as malignancy involving the lymph nodes are the most common multispatial diseases encountered.
   3) The parotid, submandibular, carotid, retropharyngeal, posterior cervical, and visceral spaces are the node-bearing spaces of the neck.
   4) As a result these are the spaces involved with multispatial processes in the neck.
   5) Multispatial disease processes in the extracranial head and neck include:
      a) Nodal disease, inflammatory adenopathy. Reactive adenopathy from upper respiratory infection, mononucleosis, tularemia, tuberculosis, cat scratch fever

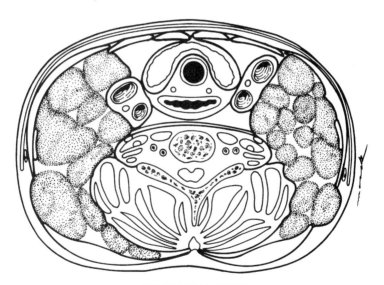

MULTISPATIAL / NODAL

Fig. 9-20 A multispatial disease process. This axial drawing shows bilateral, multiple nodal masses in the deep cervical chain (associated with the carotid space) and the spinal accessory chain (found within the posterior cervical space). When multiple noncontiguous spaces are involved by a disease process, the term *multispatial* can be applied.

b) Nodal disease, other. Sarcoidosis, malignant adenopathy (SCCa, non-Hodgkin lymphoma)
c) Nonnodal diseases. Neurofibromatosis, nonnodal hematogenous metastases

SUGGESTED READING

Armington WG, Harnsberger HR, Osborn AG, et al: Radiographic evaluation of brachial plexopathy. *AJNR* 8:361–367, 1987.

Babbel RW, Smoker WRK, Harnsberger HRH: The visceral space: The unique infrahyoid space. *Semin Ultrasound CT MR* 12:204–223, 1991.

Benson MT, Dalen K, Mancuso AA, et al: Congenital anomalies of the branchial apparatus: embryology and pathologic anatomy. *RadioGraphics* 12:943–960, 1992.

Bryan RN, Miller RH, Ferreyro RI, et al: Computed tomography of the major salivary glands. *Am J Roentgenol* 139:547–554, 1982.

Coit WE, Harnsberger HR, Osborn AG, et al: Ranulas and their mimics: CT evaluation. *Radiology* 163:211–216, 1987.

Curtin HD: Separation of the masticator space from the parapharyngeal space. *Radiology* 163:195–204, 1987.

Davis WL, Harnsberger HR, Smoker WRK, et al: Retropharyngeal space: evaluation of normal anatomy and diseases with CT and MR imaging. *Radiology* 174:59–64, 1990.

Davis WL, Smoker WRK, Harnsberger HR: The normal and diseased infrahyoid retropharyngeal, danger, and prevertebral spaces. *Semin Ultrasound CT MR* 12:241–256, 1991.

Endicott JN, Nelson RJ, Saraceno CA: Diagnosis and management decisions in infections of the deep fascial spaces of the head and neck utilizing computerized tomography. *Laryngoscope* 92:630–633, 1982.

Fruin ME, Smoker WRK, Harnsberger HR: The carotid space of the infrahyoid neck. *Semin Ultrasound CT MR* 12:224–240, 1991.

Glasier CM, Stark JE, Jacobs RF, et al: CT and ultrasound imaging of retropharyngeal abscesses in children. *AJNR* 13:1191–1195, 1992.

Hardin CW, Harnsberger HR, Osborn AG, et al: CT in the evaluation of the normal and diseased oral cavity and oropharynx. *Semin Ultrasound CT MR* 7:131–153, 1986.

Hardin CW, Harnsberger HR, Osborn AG, et al: Infection and tumor of the masticator space: CT evaluation. *Radiology* 157:413–417, 1985.

Harnsberger HR: CT and MR of masses of the deep face. *Curr Probl Diagn Radiol* 16:147–173, 1987.

Hollinshead WH: *Anatomy for surgeons,* ed 2, *vol 1, The head and neck.* New York, 1968, Harper & Row.

Kellman GM, Kneeland JB, Middleton WD, et al: MR imaging of the supraclavicular region: normal anatomy. *Am J Roentgenol* 148:77–82, 1987.

Kulkarni MV, Patton JA, Price RR: Technical considerations for the use of surface coils in MRI. *Am J Roentgenol* 147:373–378, 1986.

Langman J: *Medical embryology*. Baltimore, 1969, Williams & Wilkins.

Larsson SG, Mancuso AA, Hanafee W: Computed tomography of the tongue and floor of the mouth. *Radiology* 143:493–500, 1982.

Last RJ: *Anatomy: regional and applied*. New York, 1978, Churchill Livingstone.

Lloyd GAS, Phelps PD: The demonstration of tumors of the parapharyngeal space by magnetic resonance imaging. *Br J Radiol* 59:675–683, 1986.

Lufkin RB, Hanafee W: MRI of the head and neck. *Magn Reson Imaging* 6:69–88, 1988.

Lufkin RB, Votruba J, Reicher M, et al: Solenoid surface coils in magnetic resonance imaging. *Am J Roentgenol* 146:409–412, 1986.

Mancuso AA, Harnsberger HR, Muraki AS, et al: Computed tomography of cervical and retropharyngeal lymph nodes: normal anatomy, variants of normal, and applications in staging head and neck cancer. *Radiology* 148:709–714, 1983.

Miller MB, Rao VM, Tom BM: Cystic masses of the head and neck: pitfalls in CT and MR interpretation. *Am J Roentgenol* 159:601–607, 1992.

Montgomery RL: *Head and neck anatomy with clinical correlations*. New York, 1981, McGraw-Hill.

Moore KL: *The developing human*. Philadelphia, 1974, WB Saunders.

Nyberg DA, Jeffrey RB, Brandt-Zawadzki M, et al: Computed tomography of cervical infections. *J Comput Assist Tomogr* 9:288–296, 1985.

Ohnishi T, Noguchi S, Murakami N, et al: MR imaging in patients with primary thyroid lymphoma. *AJNR* 13:1196–1198, 1992.

Paff GH: *Anatomy of the head and neck*. Philadelphia, 1981, WB Saunders.

Parker GD, Harnsberger HR: Radiologic evaluation of the normal and diseased posterior cervical space. *Am J Roentgenol* 157:161–165, 1991.

Parker GD, Harnsberger HR: Smoker WRK: The anterior and posterior cervical spaces. *Semin Ultrasound CT MR* 12:257–273, 1991.

Posniak HV, Olson MC, Dudiak CM, et al: MR imaging of the brachial plexus. *Am J Roentgenol* 161:373–379, 1993.

Reede DL, Bergeron RT: The CT evaluation of the normal and diseased neck. *Semin Ultrasound CT MR* 7:181–201, 1986.

Reede DL, Bergeron RT, Som PM: CT of thyroglossal duct cysts. *Radiology* 157:121–125, 1985.

Reede DL, Whelan MA, Bergeron RT: CT of the soft tissue structures of the neck. *Radiol Clin North Am* 22:239–250, 1984.

Romanes GJ: *Cunningham's manual of practical anatomy* (rev), *vol 3: Head, neck, and brain*. London, 1971, Oxford University Press.

Shaha AR, LaRosa CA, Jaffe BM: Parathyroid localization prior to primary exploration. *Am J Surg* 166:289–293, 1993.

Silver AJ, Ganti SR, Hilal SK: The carotid region. Normal and pathologic anatomy on CT. *Radiol Clin North Am* 22:219–238, 1984.

Silver AJ, Mawad ME, Hilal SK, et al: Computed tomography of the carotid space and related cervical spaces. I: anatomy. *Radiology* 150:723–728, 1984.

Smoker WRK: Normal anatomy of the infrahyoid neck: an overview. *Semin Ultrasound CT MR* 12:192–203, 1991.

Smoker WRK, Gentry LR: Computed tomography of the nasopharynx. *Semin Ultrasound CT MR* 7:107–130, 1986.

Smoker WRK, Harnsberger HR: Differential diagnosis of head and neck lesions based on their space of origin. 2. The infrahyoid neck. *Am J Roentgenol* 157:155–159, 1991.

Smoker WRK, Harnsberger HR, Osborn AG: The hypoglossal nerve. *Semin Ultrasound CT MR* 8:301–312, 1987.

Som PM: Lymph nodes of the neck. *Radiology* 165:593–600, 1987.

Som PM, Biller HF, Lawson W: Tumors of the parapharyngeal space. Preoperative evaluation, diagnosis, and surgical approaches. *Ann Otol Rhinol Laryngol* 90:1–15, 1981.

Som PM, Biller HF, Lawson W, et al: Parapharyngeal space masses: an updated protocol based upon 104 cases. *Radiology* 153:149–156, 1984.

Som PM, Braun IR, Shapiro MD, et al: Tumors of the parapharyngeal space and upper neck: MR imaging characteristics. *Radiology* 164:823–829, 1987.

Stevens SK, Chang J-M, Clark OH, et al: Detection of abnormal parathyroid glands in postoperative patients with recurrent hyperparathyroidism: sensitivity of MR imaging. *Am J Roentgenol* 160:607–612, 1993.

Stiernberg CM: Deep-neck space infections. Diagnosis and management. *Arch Otolaryngol* 112:1274–1279, 1986.

Takashima S, Morimoto S, Ikezoe J, et al: Primary thyroid lymphoma: comparison of CT and US assessment. *Radiology* 171:439–443, 1989.

Unger JM: Computed tomography of the parapharyngeal space. *CRC Crit Rev Diagn Imaging* 26:265–290, 1987.

Vogelzang P, Harnsberger HR, Smoker WRK: Multispatial and transpatial diseases of the extracranial head and neck. *Semin Ultrasound CT MR* 12:274–287, 1991.

Vogl T, Brüning R, Schedel H, et al: Paraganglioma of the jugular bulb and carotid body: MR imaging with short sequences and Gd-DTPA enhancement. *AJNR* 10:823–827, 1989.

Zadvinskis DP, Benson MT, Kerr HH, et al: Congenital malformations of the cervicothoracic lymphatic system: embryology and pathogenesis. *RadioGraphics* 12:1175–1189, 1992.

10

Cystic Masses of the Head and Neck: Rare Lesions with Characteristic Radiologic Features

CRITICAL IMAGING QUESTIONS: CYSTIC MASSES OF THE HEAD AND NECK

1. Describe the characteristic location and displacement pattern of the most common form of second branchial cleft cyst. What other normal anatomic structure "lives" in this location?
2. Are cystic hygromas usually unispatial or transpatial? What imaging features help to differentiate cystic hygromas from other lesions of the head and neck?
3. Is CT or MRI the modality of choice in the setting of head and neck abscess? Why?
4. Is a simple ranula a pseudocyst or a retention cyst? Is a diving ranula a retention cyst or a pseudocyst?

Answers to these questions are found in the text beside the question number (Q#) in the margin.

CYSTIC MASSES OF THE HEAD AND NECK

A. Introduction.

1. The gamut of cystic lesions of the extracranial head and neck is not long (Table 10-1). Many of these lesions are rare, but their radiologic features often permit definitive histopathologic diagnoses to be rendered by the radiologist.

Table 10-1   Cystic Masses of the Extracranial Head and Neck

Congenital cystic neck masses
  Branchial cleft cysts
    First (periparotid)
    Second (posterior submandibular space)
    Third (posterior cervical space)
  Thyroglossal duct cyst
  Lymphangioma–cystic hygroma spectrum
  Tornwaldt cyst

Inflammatory cystic masses
  Abscess
  Suppurative adenopathy
  Granulomatous adenopathy
  Ranula
  Retention cyst (vallecular, tonsillar, adenoidal)

Vascular cystic masses
  Jugular venous thrombosis–thrombophlebitis
  Carotid artery, vertebral artery aneurysm

Visceral saccular cysts
  Laryngocele
  Zenker's diverticulum

Parenchymal cysts
  Thyroid cyst
  Parathyroid cyst
  Thymic cyst

Cystic benign tumors
  Neural sheath tumors (schwannoma, neurofibroma)
  Lipoma (clinically "cystic")

Cystic malignant tumors
  Primary squamous cell carcinoma
  Nodal squamous cell carcinoma
  Primary or nodal thyroid carcinoma

2. Because the radiologist often functions as a repository of experience regarding the appearances of these lesions, he or she will find that their understanding of these diseases may far exceed that of their clinical colleagues, who only may have seen one in their lifetime.

3. Foreknowledge of the clinical and radiologic characteristics of these cystic neck masses puts the radiologist in the enviable position of describing both the deep tissue extent and the probable histopathology to the referring physician.

4. This chapter does not follow the space oriented differential diagnosis discussion followed in the chapter on the infrahyoid neck. Rather, it includes a differential diagnosis list (Table 10-2) describing the cystic masses by the space where they are most commonly found.

B. Congenital cystic neck masses

1. The most common congenital cystic neck masses include:
   a. Branchial cleft cyst (BCC)
   1) First BCC.
   2) Second BCC.
   3) Third BCC.
   b. Thyroglossal duct cyst.
   c. Cystic hygroma–lymphangioma.
   d. Dermoid/epidermoid.
   e. All masses in this group arise from a rest of tissue left behind after formation of the structures in the neck.

2. First branchial cleft cyst.
   a. Clinical presentation. The typical patient with a first BCC is a middle-aged female with a history of "multiple parotid abscesses unresponsive to drainage and antibiotics." Otorrhea is present when the cyst connects to the bony–cartilaginous junction of the external auditory canal. When present, a cutaneous opening is seen from birth at or around the angle of the mandible.
   b. Imaging features. CT or MRI scans will show a cystic mass superficial to, within, or deep to the parotid gland. Wall thickness varies with the degree of inflammation. When the lesion occurs in the deep margin of the parotid space, it may extend into the adjacent parapharyngeal space.
   c. Comment. Pathologists have trouble with this diagnosis, as it is a rare entity that appears to them as an "epithelium-lined cyst" they may label as "ectatic duct" or "parotid cyst."

3. Second branchial cleft cyst.
   a. Clinical presentation. Second BCC anomalies occur in a bimodal distribution. In the infant a mass is found at the angle of the mandible. If a sinus tract or fistula is associated, the opening is pres-

Table 10-2   Cystic Masses of the Neck by Space and Area

Parotid space: suprahyoid neck–periparotid area
  First branchial cleft cyst
  Cystic hygroma
  Abscess, suppurative node
  Obstructed parotid duct, sialocele
  Warthin's tumor
  Cystic schwannoma, neurofibroma
  Malignant necrotic adenopathy
  Mucoepidermoid carcinoma

Posterior submandibular space: angle of the mandible
  Second branchial cleft cyst
  Cystic hygroma
  Dermoid
  Mixed (external) laryngocele
  Submandibular gland mucocele
  Abscess, suppurative node (SMC)
  Diving ranula
  Lipoma
  Malignant necrotic adenopathy (SMC)

Sublingual space: oral cavity
  Epidermoid
  Simple ranula
  Obstructed submandibular duct; sialocele

Carotid space
  Jugular vein thrombosis
  Carotid artery aneurysm, pseudoaneurysm
  Abscess, suppurative adenopathy (DCC)
  Malignant necrotic adenopathy (DCC)

Visceral space: midline neck
  Thyroglossal duct cyst
  Internal (simple) laryngocele
  Cystic benign thyroid or parathyroid tumor
  Malignant laryngeal squamous cell carcinoma
  Cystic malignant thyroid tumor

Posterior cervical space: posterior triangle area
  Cystic hygroma
  Abscess, suppurative adenopathy (SAC)
  Cystic schwannoma, neurofibroma
  Malignant necrotic adenopathy (SAC)

DCC, Deep cervical chain; *SAC*, Spinal accessory chain; *SMC*, Submandibular nodal chain.

ent from birth anteriorly in the neck just above the clavicle (Fig. 10-1). The second peak of incidence is seen in the young adult. Usually trauma or viral infection provokes the initial appearance of a mass at the angle of mandible, and in many instances there is a history of "unsuccessful abscess drainage."

   b. Pathology. Of all branchial cleft anomalies, 95% arise from the remnant of the second branchial apparatus. Normally the second branchial

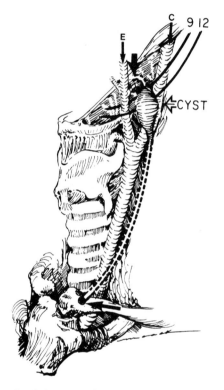

Fig. 10-1 Longitudinal drawing of second branchial cleft anomalies. The tract of a second branchial cleft anomaly may stretch from a supraclavicular cutaneous opening below (*long arrow*) to an oropharyngeal tonsil area internal opening (*short arrow*). The cystic component is most commonly located at the mandibular angle just lateral to the glossopharyngeal (*9*) and hypoglossal (*12*) nerves in the posterior submandibular space. Because the potential tract of the cephalad portion of the anomaly passes between the external (*E*) and internal (*C*) carotid arteries, the second branchial cleft cyst sometimes will have a characteristic "beak" pointing toward the oropharynx. (With permission from Harnsberger HR, Mancuso AA, Muraki AS, et al: Branchial cleft anomalies and their mimics: CT evaluation. *Radiology* 152:739–748, 1984.)

cleft apparatus completely involutes by the ninth fetal week. When the involution phase is incomplete, existence of the remnant tissue creates the potential for growth of a branchial cleft anomaly.

Q#1

   c. Imaging features. CT or MRI scans will reveal a unilocular "cystic" mass in the posterior submandibular space at the angle of the mandible. The location is embryologically defined (Fig. 10-2). In most cases the cyst displaces the submandibular gland anteromedially, the sternomastoid muscle posterolaterally, and the carotid space contents posteromedially as it grows. Only when the cyst becomes quite large does it begin to break this characteristic pattern of displacement.

      1) When present on the cyst, a beak that points medially between the internal and external carotid artery is pathognomonic of second BCC. In my experience this "beak sign" is rarely present.

      2) The jugulodigastric node "lives" in the same location of the most common form of second BCC. Clinicians may mistake an

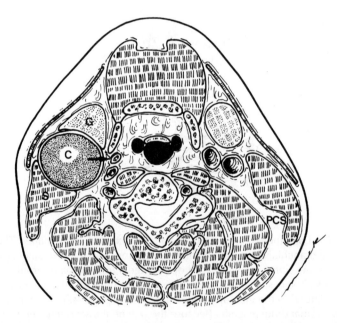

Fig. 10-2 Axial drawing of a classic second branchial cleft cyst. Note the embryologically defined location of the cyst (*C*) posterolateral to the submandibular gland (*G*), lateral to the carotid artery (*arrow*), and anteromedial to the sternocleidomastoid muscle (*S*). When large, these cysts may herniate into the posterior cervical space (*PCS*).

enlarged suppurative, reactive, or tumor-infiltrated jugulodigastric node for this lesion.

d. Comment. The most common form of this lesion is a cystic mass without sinus or fistula at the angle of the mandible; however, any permutation of cyst, sinus, or fistula is possible. Each lesion should be described individually. When a mass is present, CT or MRI is used to define completely the deep tissue extent of the lesion, which will facilitate complete surgical resection of the cyst lining. Sinography is performed when a cutaneous tract is present to delineate its full extent.

4. Third branchial cleft cysts.

a. Clinical presentation. Painless, fluctuant mass in the posterior triangle (posterior cervical space) area.

b. Pathologic considerations. Rare congenital cyst arising from the third branchial apparatus.

c. Radiologic features. Unilocular cystic mass centered in the posterior cervical space. The third BCC must be distinguished from the large second BCC, which often protrudes posteriorly into the posterior cervical space. If the lesion is centered in the posterior cervical space, it is probably a third BCC.

5. Thyroglossal duct cyst.

a. Clinical presentation.

  1) A patient with a thyroglossal duct cyst presents with a midline neck mass, usually at the level of the hyoid bone. There often is a history of previous incision and drainage of an "abscess" in this area.

  2) Of patients with this lesion, 50% present before the age of 10 years. A second group of patients present in young adulthood (i.e., 20 to 30 years of age).

b. Pathogenesis.

  1) During embryogenesis the anlage of the thyroid/parathyroid glands descends from the foramen cecum at the tongue base to its final position in the anterior visceral space of the infrahyoid neck (Fig. 10-3).

  2) During this caudal migration the thyroid/parathyroid anlage passes just anterior to the precursor tissue of the hyoid bone, leaving a tract of epithelial tissue called the *thyroglossal duct.*

    a) The normal thyroglossal tract involutes by the eighth fetal week.

  3) Thyroid elements remain in the thyroglossal duct in 5% of cases. These residua may give rise to thyroglossal duct cysts, fistulae, or solid nodules of thyroid tissue.

    a) Thyroglossal duct cysts most commonly occur in the region of the hyoid bone.

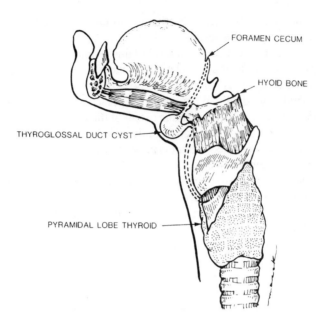

FORAMEN CECUM

HYOID BONE

THYROGLOSSAL DUCT CYST

PYRAMIDAL LOBE THYROID

Fig. 10-3   Migration of a thyroglossal duct cyst. This is a sagittal view of the embryonic tract (thyroglossal duct) taken by the thyroid anlage as it migrates from the foramen cecum of the tongue base through the area of the hyoid bone to the final, adult, lower neck location of the pyramidal lobe of the thyroid gland. When the tract does not completely involute, thyroglossal duct cyst results. The most common location of thyroglossal duct cyst is the midline at or just below the hyoid bone level.

        b) Thyroid nodules most commonly are found in the region of the foramen cecum (lingual thyroid).

    4) The thyroglossal duct cyst wall is comprised of squamous cell mucosa. However, inflammatory changes may obliterate this mucosa, making the pathologic diagnosis difficult. Thyroid tissue is *not* usually present in the wall of the cyst.

  c. Radiologic features.

    1) In most cases the thyroglossal duct cyst is located at (15%) or just below (65%) the hyoid bone. The cyst is suprahyoid in location only 20% of the time.

    2) CT or MRI scans will show a characteristic midline or paramedian cystic mass at the level of the hyoid bone (Fig. 10-4). The cyst is usually 2 to 4 cm in diameter.

        a) The cyst is nestled in the infrahyoid strap muscles with the muscles appearing to "beak" over the edges of the cyst.

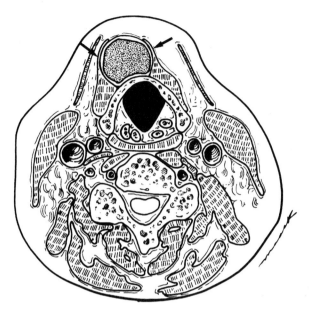

Fig. 10-4   Axial thyroglossal duct cyst at the level of the hyoid bone. The features marking this cystic lesion as a thyroglossal duct cyst include its midline location, proximity to the hyoid bone, and "beaking" of the strap muscles over the surface of the cyst (*arrows*).

3) When the cyst extends inferiorly, the key to the radiologic diagnosis remains its midline location and relationship to the infrahyoid strap muscles.
   a) The more inferior the cyst, the more likely it is to be off the midline (Fig. 10-5). This is not surprising given the paramedian location of the lobes of the thyroid gland.
4) Superior extension is unusual. The cyst splits the muscles in the floor of the mouth as it projects toward the foramen cecum of the tongue base along a midline course.
   a) MRI is an ideal tool to evaluate the cephalad course of a suprahyoid thyroglossal duct cyst, as this is best demonstrated on a direct sagittal image. T2-weighted imaging is best to demonstrate this cystic tract as it passes through muscle and fat.
d. Treatment options.
   1) Surgical removal of the entire squamous epithelial lining of the thyroglossal duct cyst is the only sure cure for this lesion.

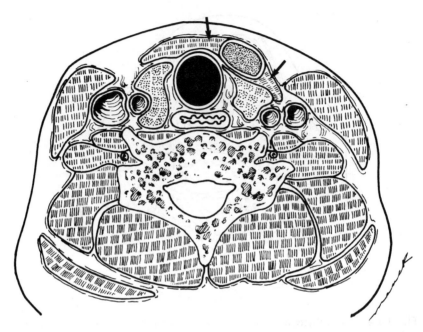

Fig. 10-5   Axial thyroglossal duct cyst of the infrahyoid paramedian type. The infrahyoid thyroglossal duct cyst is uncommon but still may be identified by the radiologist because of its unilocular cystic nature and characteristic location within the infrahyoid strap muscles (*arrows*). As a rule, the further down the neck the cyst is located, the further from the midline it is found.

   2) If even a small area of residual cyst lining is left, the lesion will recur.
6. Cystic hygroma–lymphangioma spectrum
   a. Clinical presentation. Because it is a fluid-filled cystic mass, it is difficult for the clinician to palpate the deep tissue extent of this lesion. Sixty-five percent of cystic hygromas present at birth, with 90% becoming clinically apparent by 2 years of age. The remaining 10% present as neck masses in young adults.
   b. Pathology. Congenital malformation of lymphatic channels. Classified as *capillary* (i.e., small cystic components), *cavernous* (i.e., medium-size cystic components), and *cystic* (i.e., enormously dilated lymphatic spaces).

Q#2
   c. Imaging features. Most cystic hygromas are transpatial (i.e., found in multiple contiguous spaces) but seem to fill one primary space and

spill into the adjacent spaces. The most common primary space site is the posterior cervical space (Fig. 10-6), followed in descending order by the submandibular, parotid, and sublingual spaces. When the lesion is small, it may be unispatial. In the infant, a large combined, cervical neck–thoracic lesion may be seen.

1) CT scans show a fluid density, multilocular, transpatial cystic mass that may insinuate in and around normal structures.

2) MRI scans demonstrate a multilocular, transpatial, fluid intensity mass. Careful attention to the margin of this lesion often will reveal a crinkled appearance.

3) Because lymphatic and vascular rests may occur together, creating a hemangiolymphangioma, a tissue component that may enhance can be seen with the previously described imaging features.

d. Comment. Cystic hygroma is a tenacious, difficult to remove lesion that at surgery often wraps around and adheres to the adjacent structures. In reporting the extent of this lesion, comment should be made regarding the critical neurovascular structures in the surrounding deep tissues. In the case of a lesion in the posterior cervical space, its

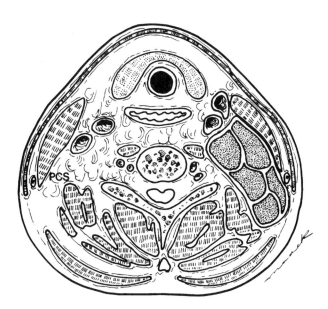

Fig. 10-6   Axial drawing of a classic cystic hygroma in the posterior cervical space of the infrahyoid neck. The features marking this lesion as a cystic hygroma include its *multilocular* nature and typical location in the posterior cervical space (*PCS*).

relationship to the adjacent carotid artery and vagus nerve should be addressed.
7. Dermoid/epidermoid.
    a. Clinical presentation. Slow-growing mass under the oral tongue (i.e., epidermoid) or in the soft tissues under the chin (i.e., dermoid).
    b. Pathologic considerations. When the mass is lined by a simple squamous epithelium, the term *epidermoid* is used. If the lesion has an epithelial lining but possesses variable numbers of skin appendages, it is called *dermoid*.
    c. Imaging features. CT or MRI scans demonstrate a unilocular mass in the sublingual or submandibular space. Epidermoids have fluid density (CT) or signal (MRI), while dermoids are either of mixed density and signal or have an area of fat density or signal.
    d. Comment. Epidermoids tend to involve the sublingual space. Dermoids seem to involve the submandibular space more commonly.

C. Inflammatory cystic lesions of the neck.

1. Abscess.
    a. Clinical presentation: The type of symptoms experienced by the patient depend on the space of origin of the infection.
        1) Pharyngitis usually precedes pharyngeal mucosal space abscess (also referred to as a *peritonsillar abscess*). Pharyngitis is the source of one third of all neck infections.
        2) Dental infection or manipulation can create masticator space infection with subsequent involvement of the parapharyngeal space. This also is the source of one third of all neck infections. Trismus signals involvement of the masticator space.
        3) Parotid duct calculus disease may result in parotid space abscess, which may present as a cheek mass with facial nerve paralysis.
        4) Organism seeding of nodes in the carotid space (deep cervical chain), posterior cervical space (spinal accessory chain), or retropharyngeal space (retropharyngeal nodes) creates suppurative adenopathy. With nodal capsular rupture, this creates abscess in the space occupied by the node.

Q#3
    b. Imaging features. Enhanced CT is still the modality of choice in evaluating head and neck abscess because of its ability to identify associated calculus disease and mandibular or maxillary osteomyelitis.
        1) Abscess is differentiated from cellulitis when a pocket of fluid density material is seen within the enhancing cellulitic soft tissues. The abscess is usually thick walled and may have multiple septations.

2) If only one abscess pocket is identified, it should be described according to its space of involvement.

3) If multiple spaces are involved, they must be described carefully to the surgeon, because in most cases a drain must be placed in each affected space.

4) Calculus disease, osteomyelitis, and tooth infections seen on CT scans should be reported so that these causal processes can be dealt with at the time of abscess drainage. Failure to recognize these causal processes will result in recurrence of the infection.

2. Suppurative adenopathy.
   a. Clinical presentation. When head and neck infection spreads to nodes, a "reactive" process initially occurs. Untreated microorganisms cause an intranodal abscess, which is termed *suppurative adenopathy.*
   b. Radiologic features. Enhanced CT scans will reveal single or multiple nodal distribution masses with fluid density centers.
      1) Caution must be exercised when interpreting a CT scan in a patient with known squamous cell carcinoma and concurrent head and neck infection. Suppurative adenopathy and malignant adenopathy can be indistinguishable radiologically.

3. Granulomatous adenopathy.
   a. Tuberculous adenitis occurs when mycobacteria invade the nodes of the deep cervical chain.
      1) Radiologic features. Tuberculous nodes may have a somewhat unique appearance, suggesting this diagnosis. Multiple, mixed, high and low density nodes with globular calcifications on enhanced CT scans should suggest this diagnosis to the radiologist.

4. Glandular retention cyst/mucocele.
   a. Any of the many glandular tissues of the extracranial head and neck may have a postinflammatory retention cyst form as a result of stenosis or occlusion of mucous-producing gland.
   b. Different names are given to these retention cysts depending on where they are found.
      1) Retention cyst of the sublingual gland is termed a *ranula.*
      2) Retention cyst of the submandibular gland is called a *submandibular gland mucocele.*
      3) Retention cyst of the faucial or adenoidal tonsil is termed a *retention cyst.*
      4) Retention cyst of the low lingual tonsil is called a *vallecular cyst.*
      5) Retention cyst of the paranasal sinus is termed a *retention cyst.*
   c. Radiologic features. CT scans show the retention cyst as a thin-walled, fluid density structure in immediate proximity to the obstructed glandular tissue.

5. Ranula.
   a. Clinical presentation. Painless swelling of the sublingual space (i.e., simple ranula) or of both the sublingual and the submandibular spaces (i.e., diving ranula).

Q#4
   b. Pathologic considerations. The simple ranula is a postinflammatory retention cyst of the sublingual glands or the minor salivary glands of the sublingual space with an epithelial lining. If the simple ranula becomes large and ruptures out the back side of the sublingual space into the submandibular space, it is called a *diving ranula* (Fig. 10-7). The diving ranula has no epithelial lining and is really a pseudocyst.
   c. Imaging features. A unilocular cystic mass of the sublingual space on CT or MRI scans suggests the diagnosis of simple ranula. Unilocular cystic hygroma and epidermoid cyst, however, cannot be differentiated radiologically from simple ranula. Diving ranula has a characteristic "tail sign" within the sublingual space, with the bulk of this pseudocyst seen in the submandibular space (Fig. 10-7).

D. Vascular lesions.

1. Jugular vein thrombosis/thrombophlebitis.
   a. Clinical presentation.
      1) Patients with this entity often have a history of central venous catheter placement, drug abuse, or malignancy.
      2) In the acute thrombophlebitic phase the neck mass is tender and mimics abscess. In the chronic thrombotic phase the mass is hard and nontender, imitating a tumor.
   b. Radiologic features.
      1) CT appearance. In the acute thrombophlebitic phase the CT scan shows a loss of soft-tissue planes surrounding the enlarged thrombus-filled jugular vein (Fig. 10-8). In the chronic thrombotic phase the jugular vein appears as a well-marginated, tubular mass without loss of the surrounding soft-tissue planes.
      2) MRI appearance. In the subacute phase (> 36 hours) jugular vein thrombosis is seen as a high-signal tubular mass on T1-weighted sequences.

E. Visceral saccular cysts.

1. Laryngocele.
   a. Clinical presentation. Symptoms resulting from laryngocele depend on its size and location. Internal laryngocele may present with hoarseness or stridor. Mixed (external) laryngocele presents with an

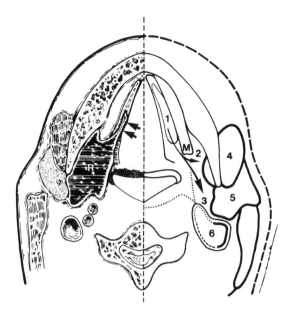

Fig. 10-7   Diving ranula. *Left*, Axial diagrammatic representation of a diving ranula (*R*) as it herniates from the posterior sublingual space into the adjacent cephalad submandibular and low parapharyngeal spaces. The bulk of the diving ranula is found in the submandibular space, but the "tail sign" (*short arrows*) of residual cyst in the sublingual space is very suggestive of the diagnosis. *Right*, Spaces of the oropharynx and oral cavity. As no fascial boundary exists at the posterior margin of the mylohyoid muscle (*M*), a ranula beginning in the sublingual space (*1*) may dive (*arrows*) into the adjacent submandibular space (*2*) and parapharyngeal space (*3*). *4*, Masticator space; *5*, parotid space; *6*, carotid space. (With permission from Coit WE, Harnsberger HR, Osborn AG, et al: Ranulas and their mimics: CT evaluation. *Radiology* 163:211–216, 1987.)

anterior neck mass just below the angle of the mandible that may expand with Valsalva maneuver.

   b. Pathogenesis. Laryngocele occurs when the laryngeal ventricle or its more distal sacculus (i.e., appendix) is functionally obstructed from increased intraglottic pressures arising from excessive coughing, playing an instrument, or blowing glass (Fig. 10-9). Obstruction of the proximal saccule by postinflammatory stenosis, trauma, or tumor is a less common cause of laryngocele. This cystic mass may be filled with air, fluid, or pus. With continued growth the laryngocele penetrates the thyrohyoid membrane to enter the neck in the lower submandibular space.

   c. Radiologic features.

      1) Internal (simple) laryngocele.

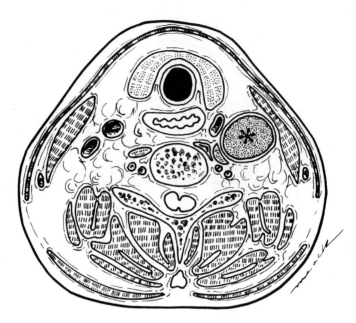

Fig. 10-8 Drawing in the axial plane of jugular vein thrombosis of the internal jugular vein of the infrahyoid neck. The diagnosis of jugular vein thrombosis is made when the internal jugular vein cannot be identified normally. Instead, a "linear cystic lesion" (*asterisk*) is seen on multiple axial images where the jugular vein should reside.

    a) An air- or fluid-filled cystic mass is identified in the paralaryngeal (paraglottic) space of the supraglottis and can be followed down to the level of the ventricle (Fig. 10-10).

  2) Mixed (external) laryngocele.

    a) An air- or fluid-filled, well-circumscribed, cystic mass is seen in the lower submandibular space directly adjacent to the thyrohyoid membrane (Fig. 10-11).

    b) The isthmus (or waist) through the perforation in this membrane usually is readily identifiable, although the internal component of the mixed laryngocele may be completely collapsed.

  3) Pyolaryngocele.

    a) Pyolaryngocele is a superinfected laryngocele.

    b) Laryngocele wall thickening suggests the diagnosis of pyolaryngocele. Clinical manifestations of infection are not subtle.

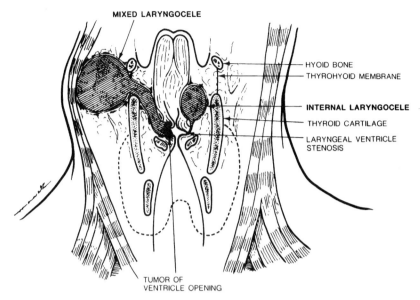

MIXED LARYNGOCELE

HYOID BONE
THYROHYOID MEMBRANE

INTERNAL LARYNGOCELE
THYROID CARTILAGE
LARYNGEAL VENTRICLE
STENOSIS

TUMOR OF
VENTRICLE OPENING

Fig. 10-9   Laryngocele. Coronal drawing of the larynx demonstrates a simple internal laryngocele on the right and a mixed (external) laryngocele on the left. Note that the internal laryngocele projects cephalad in the paralaryngeal space in a submucosal fashion. The mixed laryngocele has penetrated through the thyrohyoid membrane to enter the soft tissues of the neck. In this case the mixed laryngocele on the left is secondary to a small, squamous cell carcinoma of the laryngeal ventricle of the supraglottis.

    4) Secondary laryngocele.
      a) Secondary laryngocele refers to the group of laryngoceles that form secondary to tumor obstruction at the opening to the ventricle in the supraglottis (Fig. 10-9).
      b) Presence of an infiltrating mass in the supraglottis associated with an internal or mixed laryngocele makes this diagnosis.
      c) Comment. Any laryngocele that occurs in an adult who smokes should have the lower supraglottis clinically and radiologically searched for squamous cell carcinoma.
2. Zenker's diverticulum.
  a. Clinical presentation. Dysphagia; halitosis.
  b. Radiologic features.
    1) Outpouching of the posterior wall of the upper esophagus, usually diagnosed by esophagram.
    2) May appear on CT scans as an oval mass in the posterior visceral space with "foamy" material within it.

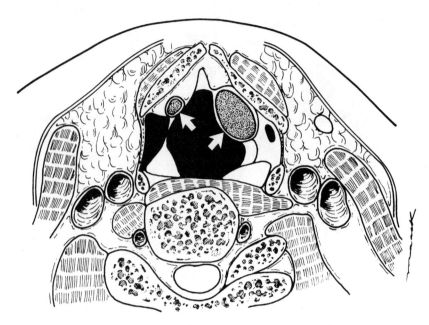

Fig. 10-10   Bilateral internal (simple) laryngoceles. Bilateral laryngoceles (*arrows*) are seen in this axial drawing through the supraglottic larynx. Note that the mucosal surface overlying the laryngoceles is convexed but otherwise normal.

F. Parenchymal cysts.

1. Thyroid cyst (colloid cyst with or without hemorrhage)
   a. Clinical presentation. Colloid cysts present as rapidly enlarging, tense, lower neck masses that may be painful and tender if hemorrhage has occurred.
   b. Pathologic considerations.
      1) Cyst fluid has increased T3 and T4 but low parathyroid hormone levels.
      2) At surgery the cyst plane separating it from the thyroid gland itself is indistinct, making surgical removal a laborious task.
   c. Radiologic features.
      1) When small, the mass is clearly thyroidal in origin, because thyroid tissue can be seen on all sides. The cyst is well defined, with a thin wall and low-density center (i.e., 10–20 HU).
      2) When larger, the cystic mass may not be entirely surrounded by thyroid tissue but still can be identified as thyroidal in origin by the characteristic displacement of the surrounding structures. The trachea is deviated contralaterally, while the carotid space

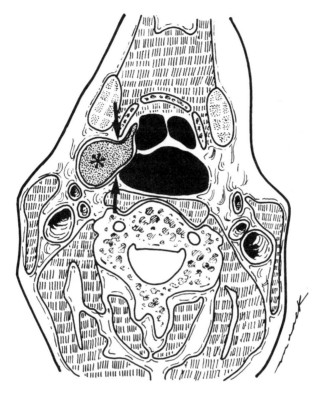

Fig. 10-11   Axial drawing of mixed (external) laryngocele, seen on the right. When a laryngocele herniates through the thyrohyoid membrane (*arrows*), it transforms from an internal (simple) laryngocele to a mixed (external) laryngocele (*asterisk*).

      (i.e., carotid artery and jugular vein) is deviated laterally (Fig. 10-12).

     3) Colloid cyst may be difficult to differentiate from goiter or carcinoma that has undergone cystic degeneration.

2. Parathyroid cysts.
    a. Clinical presentation.
      1) Dependent on size and whether the cyst is "functional."
      2) Large parathyroid cysts compress the adjacent trachea, esophagus, and recurrent laryngeal nerve, producing hoarseness.
      3) Functional cysts, which are a minority of cases, create a state of hyperparathyroidism.
    b. Pathologic considerations.
      1) Most commonly found in the area of the inferior parathyroid gland behind or just below the lower pole of the thyroid lobes.

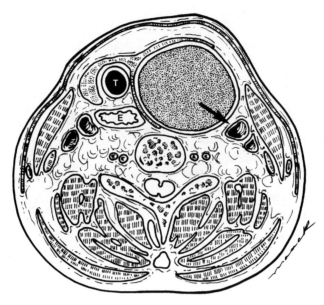

Fig. 10-12   Axial drawing of a thyroid colloid cyst. Cystic masses of the thyroid such as this will displace the carotid space structures laterally (*arrow*) and the trachea (*T*) and esophagus (*E*) in a contralateral direction.

      2) Encapsulation makes surgical removal straightforward.

      3) Fluid within the cyst has high parathyroid hormone but low T3 and T4 levels.

   c. Radiologic features.

      1) A thin-walled, 1- to 10-cm diameter, cystic mass compressing the ipsilateral thyroid lobe anteriorly.

      2) The center of the mass is usually located behind the thyroid lobe, displacing the lobe anteriorly (Fig. 10-13).

3. Thymic cysts.

   a. Clinical presentation.

      1) Slowly enlarging mass in the lower anterior cervical neck.

      2) Two thirds of cases occur in the first decade of life, with the remaining one third occurring in the second and third decades.

   b. Pathologic considerations.

      1) Very rare lesion. When congenital, thought to arise from thymopharyngeal duct. When acquired, thought to develop as either inflammation or cystic degeneration of thymic cells.

      2) Histologic diagnosis is made when the cyst wall contains respiratory epithelium with Hassall's corpuscles.

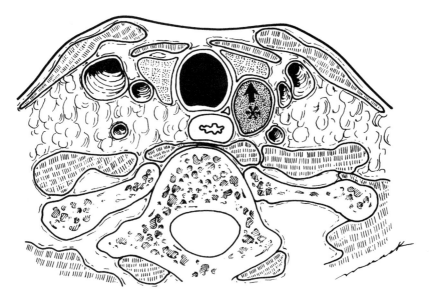

Fig. 10-13   This axial drawing of a parathyroid cyst demonstrates its typical posterior location relative to the ipsilateral thyroid lobe. Note the anterior displacement of this thyroid lobe by the cyst (*asterisk*).

   c. Radiologic features.
      1) Large, unilocular cystic mass is seen on CT scans extending parallel to the sternomastoid muscle.
      2) The thymic cyst may be confined to the cervical neck or course into the anterior mediastinum.

G. Cystic benign tumor.

1. Multinodular goiter.
   a. Etiology. Familial; iodine deficiency
   b. Clinical presentation. Long history of lower neck mass. When very large, they can cause tracheal compression.
   c. Radiologic appearance. Bilobed, mixed-density, well-circumscribed thyroid mass that may extend well into the mediastinum. These lesions may look malignant but the crisp margins and complete involvement of both lobes of the enlarged thyroid gland are key features signaling their benign nature.
2. Thyroid adenoma.
   a. Radiologic appearance. Inhomogeneous mass 1 to 4 cm in diameter within the thyroid gland. Margins are well circumscribed. They may

have multiple, amorphous calcifications within it. Cannot be differentiated radiologically from thyroid carcinoma.

3. Cystic schwannoma/neurofibroma.
   a. Clinical presentation.
      1) Schwannoma. Slow-growing, painless neck mass. Produces pain only when it has grown large enough to compress the surrounding structures.
      2) Neurofibroma. Same as schwannoma.
   b. Pathologic considerations.
      1) Schwannoma. Benign *encapsulated* tumor arising from Schwann cells of the nerve sheath. Larger tumors frequently undergo cystic degeneration. Cervical spinal rootlets, vagus nerve, and cervical sympathetics are most commonly affected.
      2) Neurofibroma. Benign *non-encapsulated* tumor involving peripheral nerves. Of all cases, 10% occur with von Recklinghausen's syndrome. Larger tumors frequently do not undergo cystic degeneration but instead demonstrate fatty degeneration.
   c. Radiologic features.
      1) Schwannoma. CT scans show a well-demarcated, mildly enhancing mass that may demonstrate central cystic degeneration. MRI scans reveal a fusiform mass without significant flow voids. Uniform contrast enhancement on MRI is the rule.
      2) Neurofibroma. Well-circumscribed, solid, low density mass on CT involving a peripheral nerve. The low density is probably a function of diffuse fatty degeneration.

4. Lipoma.
   a. Larger lipomas in the head and neck region are almost always found within the posterior cervical space. They may, however, be found in any space in the head and neck area.
   b. Clinical presentation. The slowly growing mass often is felt by the examining physician to be a cystic hygroma or other cystic lesion.
   c. Radiologic features. Both CT and MRI scans show a fatty mass within the affected space, with a thin capsule having convex margins. Internal architecture is minimal. If there is significant internal stranding or inhomogeneity of signal, liposarcoma should be considered. Remember, however, that liposarcoma is exceedingly rare in this area.

H. Cystic malignant tumor.

1. Squamous cell carcinoma.
   a. In the primary or nodal state, more advanced squamous cell carcinoma may appear cystic (necrotic) on either CT or MRI scans.

b. When the tumor is necrotic (cystic), the primary tumor site along the mucosal surface of the extracranial head and neck presents little imaging problem, as the lesion ordinarily is already known to be squamous cell carcinoma by mucosal biopsy.

c. When the primary is not visible either by clinical examination or by imaging (i.e., setting of the "unknown primary"), necrotic adenopathy may be mistaken for one of the other cystic neck masses by the unwary radiologist.

    1) Generalized, central necrosis in nodes of the neck commonly is seen in only two pathologic settings: squamous cell carcinoma adenopathy, and adenopathy involved with aggressive infection (i.e., suppurative adenopathy).

2. Thyroid carcinoma.

    a. Five types. Papillary (50% of cases), follicular (20%), medullary (10%), giant cell or anaplastic (3%), and Hurthle cell (2%) carcinomas.

    b. Prognosis of a given patient depends on the cell type (papillary has the best prognosis and giant cell the worst), gender (females have a better prognosis), age (younger patients have a better prognosis), and extent of tumor at presentation.

    c. MRI is useful in evaluating a patient with thyroid malignancy when surgery is anticipated to remove maximum tumor volume before therapy with iodine-131. In this setting MRI is used to define the tumor/nodal extent.

    d. Comment. A patient that presents with a cystic lower neck mass needs careful evaluation of the thyroid gland. Nodal metastases of thyroid carcinoma often appear quite cystic on CT or MRI scans at presentation. The patient story of a lesion thought clinically to be a BCC but turning out pathologically to be a cystic thyroid metastases is not uncommon.

    e. Radiologic appearance. Unilateral, intrathyroidal mass with infiltrating margins obscuring adjacent soft-tissue planes. Calcifications present in up to 35% of cases. May have associated adenopathy. A mass with well-defined margins does not necessarily exclude thyroid malignancy.

    1) A cystic neck mass in the area of the deep cervical chain with calcifications or hemorrhage seen on CT or MRI scans should elicit a search for the primary in the thyroid gland.

    2) When a "BCC" is seen in the wrong location or has atypical imaging features, consider the diagnosis of malignant thyroid adenopathy.

    3) MRI may show the cystic mass to be high signal on T1-weighted images, again suggesting the diagnosis of thyroid malignant adenopathy.

3. Metastases.
   a. When a necrotic lymph node mass is found in the low deep cervical chain of the carotid space, the primary tumor should be sought in the thyroid, thorax, or abdomen.
4. Non-Hodgkin lymphoma.
   a. Undifferentiated or AIDS lymphoma in nodes of the neck may present as necrotic cystic masses. In typical non-Hodgkin lymphoma of neck nodes, necrosis is not seen at presentation.
   b. During or following therapy (chemotherapy and/or radiotherapy), nodes with non-Hodgkin lymphoma often will be seen as cystic.

SUGGESTED READING

Albertyn LE, Alcock MK: Diagnosis of internal jugular vein thrombosis. *Radiology*, 162:505–508, 1987.

Allard R: The thyroglossal cyst. *Head Neck Surg* 5:134–146, 1982.

Braun IF, Hoffman JC, Malko JA, et al: Jugular vein thrombosis: MR imaging. *Radiology*, 157:357–360, 1985.

Cinberg JZ, Silver CE, Molnar JJ, Vogl SE: Cervical cysts: cancer until proven otherwise? *Laryngoscope* 92:27–30, 1982.

Coit WE, Harnsberger HR, Osborn AG, et al: Ranulas and their mimics: CT evaluation. *Radiology* 163:211–216, 1987.

Harnsberger HR, Mancuso AA, Muraki AS, et al: Branchial cleft anomalies and their mimics: computed tomographic evaluation. *Radiology* 152:739–748, 1984.

Holt GR, Holt JE, Weaver RG: Dermoids and teratoma of the head and neck. *Ear Nose Throat J* 58:520–531, 1979.

Karmody CS, Forston JK, Calcaterra VE: Lymphangiomas of the head and neck in adults. *Otolaryngol Head Neck Surg* 9:283–288, 1982.

Nyberg DA, Jeffrey RB, Brandt-Zawadzki M, et al: Computed tomography of cervical infections. *J Comput Assist Tomogr* 9:288–296, 1985.

Parker GD, Harnsberger HR, Smoker WRK: The anterior and posterior cervical spaces. *Semin Ultrasound CT MR* 12:257–273, 1991.

Reede DL, Bergeron RT: Cervical tuberculous adenitis: CT manifestations. *Radiology* 154:701–704, 1985.

Reede DL, Bergeron RT, Osborn AG: CT of the soft tissues of the neck. In Bergeron RT, Osborn AG, Som PM, editors. *Head and neck imaging excluding the brain.* St. Louis: 1984, Mosby–Year Book.

Reede DL, Bergeron RT, Som PM: CT of thyroglossal duct cysts. *Radiology* 157:121–125, 1985.

Reede DL, Whelan MA, Bergeron RT: CT of the soft tissue structures of the neck. *Radiol Clin North Am* 22:239–250, 1984.

Silverman PM, Korobkin M, Moore AV: CT diagnosis of cystic hygroma of the neck. *J Comput Assist Tomogr* 7:519–520, 1983.

Silverman PM, Korobkin M, Moore AV: CT of cystic neck masses. *J Comput Assist Tomogr* 7:498–502, 1983.

Som PM: Cystic lesions of the neck. *Postgrad Radiol* 7:211–236, 1987.

Som PM, Sacher M. Lanzieri CF, et al: Parenchymal cyst of the lower neck. *Radiology* 57:399–406, 1985.

Vogl TJ, Steger W, Ihrler S, et al: Cystic masses in the floor of the mouth: value of MR imaging in planning surgery. *Am J Roentgenol* 161:183–186, 1993.

Wallace MP, Betsill WL: Papillary carcinoma of the thyroid gland seen as lateral neck cyst. *Arch Otolaryngol* 110:408–411, 1984.

11

The Larynx and Hypopharynx

CRITICAL IMAGING QUESTIONS:
LARYNX AND HYPOPHARYNX

Larynx

1. What are the three principal cartilages of the larynx? Which cartilage is the only complete ring?
2. What is the name of the anterior projection of the arytenoid cartilage where the posterior margin of the true vocal cord attaches?
3. What are the two spaces of the endolarynx where submucosal squamous cell carcinoma most frequently hides? Are these two spaces separated by a fascial border?
4. Name the clinical blind spots in clinical staging of supraglottic carcinoma.

Hypopharynx

5. What anatomic structure divides the pyriform sinus from the larynx? Is it considered to be a part of the larynx or the hypopharynx?
6. The pyriform sinus is one of three major sites where unknown primary carcinoma hides from the eye of the clinician. What are the other two sites?
7. Describe the most common pattern for spread of pyriform sinus carcinoma.

Answers to these questions are found in the text beside the question number (Q#) in the margin.

LARYNX

A. Introduction.

1. The larynx is examined radiologically when it is involved by squamous cell carcinoma (SCCa), laryngocele, thyroglossal duct cyst, and trauma (postintubation or blunt). Other indications for laryngeal imaging are extremely rare.

2. Clinical endoscopic examination of the laryngopharynx provides a clear understanding of the mucosal extent of laryngeal involvement by tumor. When combined with the deep tissue extent derived from a radiologic study, this information gained by visual inspection creates a complete, pretreatment picture of tumor of the larynx.

   a. Imaging of the larynx performed without prior knowledge of the endoscopic mucosal impression is perilous. Only when the clinical and radiologic information are combined is a complete picture of the lesion gained.

3. The radiologic examination of the larynx involved with SCCa can be done with either CT or MRI. In choosing between these modalities, the following factors should be weighed:

   a. MRI is slightly better for determining laryngeal cartilage invasion.

   b. MRI better delineates transglottic tumor in the coronal plane compared with the obligate axial plane of CT.

   c. At times MRI can differentiate between subglottic tumor spread and inferior displacement of the vocal cord by tumor because of the unique perspective gained in the coronal view.

   d. Twenty percent of patients are inadequately imaged by MRI in the area of the larynx because of patient motion from breathing, coughing, and swallowing.

   e. In most facilities MRI is significantly more expensive than CT.

   f. Spiral/helical CT allows high detail, single breath hold data set acquisition.

   g. Comment. Although MRI has some unique advantages over CT, I recently have begun using CT almost exclusively since the arrival of our spiral unit.

4. In the clinical setting of nonmalignant disease of the larynx (e.g., laryngocele, thyroglossal duct cyst, trauma), CT is the preferred method for laryngeal radiologic examination.

B. Normal anatomy of the larynx.

Q#1

1. The soft tissues of the larynx are draped over the supporting cartilaginous framework of the cricoid, thyroid, and arytenoid cartilages (Figs. 11-1 through 11-3). The epiglottic cartilage serves as a lid to the laryngeal "box."

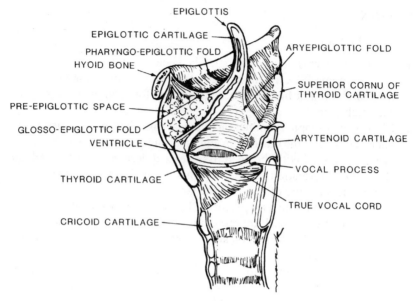

Fig. 11-1 Lateral (sagittal) drawing of the normal larynx. The upper borders of the larynx are formed by the glossoepiglottic fold and the pharyngoepiglottic fold. The inferior margin is at the lower edge of the cricoid cartilage.

2. The upper larynx (i.e., supraglottis) ends at the level of the glossoepiglottic and pharyngoepiglottic folds (Figs. 11-1 and 11-4*A*). Above these folds is the oropharynx (i.e., tongue base and valleculae).

3. The hypopharyngeal pyriform sinus is separated from the supraglottis by the aryepiglottic folds (Fig. 11-4*C, D, E, F*).

4. Ossification of the laryngeal cartilages increases with age. Eventually the laryngeal cartilages ossify, with cortex and marrow visible on radiologic examination.

   a. The adolescent larynx mimics a soft-tissue mass because of its complete lack of ossification.

   b. The well-ossified laryngeal cartilages make determination of tumor invasion significantly easier than in the case of incomplete ossification.

5. Thyroid cartilage.

   a. The thyroid cartilage is the largest laryngeal cartilage. Two anterior laminae meet at an acute angle in the anterior midline.

   b. The superior aspect of the thyroid cartilage is indented by a V-shaped thyroid notch, called the *superior thyroid notch* (Fig. 11-4*D, E*).

      1) This notch can appear on axial imaging to represent destroyed cartilage if laryngeal tumor is present.

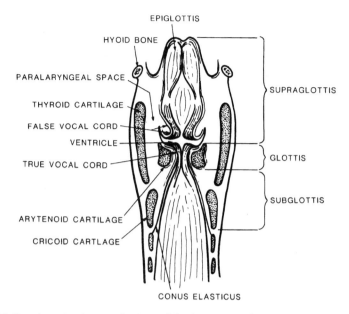

Fig. 11-2   Anterior (coronal) view of the larynx emphasizing the three major laryngeal subdivisions (i.e., supraglottis, glottis, subglottis) on the right. Note that the paraglottic (paralaryngeal) space spans the entire larynx from the subglottis below to the pre-epiglottic space above. A tumor may access the paraglottic space by either direct invasion from the mucosal surface of the false vocal cord or budding from the laryngeal ventricle.

    c. Posteriorly the laminae are elongated superiorly and inferiorly to form the superior and inferior cornua.

        1) The superior cornua are elongated and narrow, providing attachment to the thyrohyoid ligament.

        2) The inferior cornua are short and thick, articulating medially with the sides of the cricoid cartilage at the cricothyroid joint.

    d. Ossification of the thyroid cartilage progresses with age. Although usually symmetric, the variability of ossification can cause trouble for the radiologist trying to determine whether thyroid cartilage invasion by SCCa is present.

6. Cricoid cartilage.

Q#1

    a. The cricoid cartilage is the only complete ring in the endolarynx and trachea. It provides stability to the cartilaginous edifice of the larynx with its structural integrity.

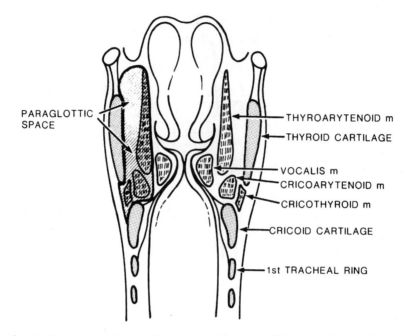

Fig. 11-3   Anterior (coronal) drawing of the larynx illustrating the cranial–caudal extent of the paraglottic space. Tumors beneath intact mucosal can run up and down in the paraglottic space without clinical detection. A second laryngeal feature depicted is the endolaryngeal muscles (i.e., thyroarytenoid, vocalis, cricoarytenoid, and cricothyroid muscles). High-resolution MRI scans can differentiate these individual muscles, making their recognition more important.

     1) The cricoid cartilage must be uninvolved by SCCa for conservative surgical therapy to be successful.
  b. The cricoid cartilage has two portions: the posterior lamina, and the anterior arch. It has been described as a "signet ring," with its band pointing anteriorly and its "signet" posteriorly (Fig. 11-1).
  c. The lower border of the cricoid cartilage is the junction between the larynx above and the trachea below.
7. Arytenoid cartilage.
  a. Arytenoid cartilages are paired, pyramidal cartilages that sit atop the posterior cricoid cartilage lamina.

Q#2
  b. The vocal processes are anterior projections of the arytenoid cartilage (Fig. 11-1). The posterior margins of the vocal cords attach to the vocal processes.

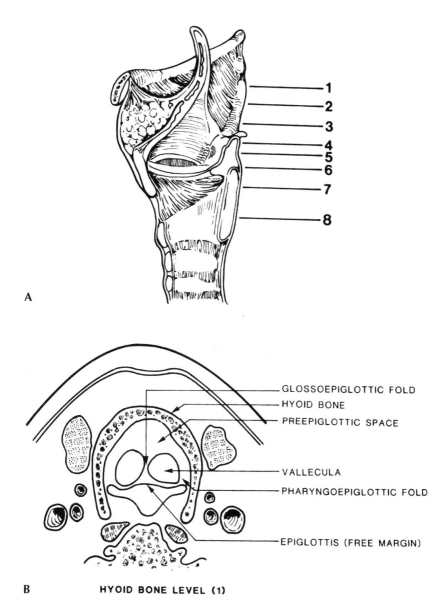

Fig. 11-4   **A**, Lateral view of the larynx. Subsequent axial drawings progress caudally, from the cephalad edge of the larynx (level 1) through the larynx to the subglottic area (level 8). **B**, Axial drawing through the roof of the larynx. At this level the pre-epiglottic space is C shaped. The glossoepiglottic and pharyngoepiglottic folds are landmarks that signal the transition from the oropharynx above to the larynx and hypopharynx below.

(continued)

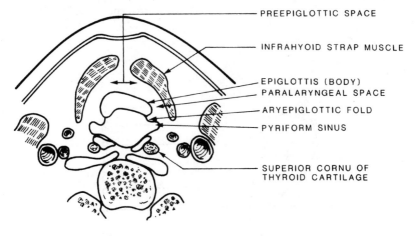

C   **HIGH SUPRAGLOTTIC LEVEL (2)**

PREEPIGLOTTIC SPACE

INFRAHYOID STRAP MUSCLE

EPIGLOTTIS (BODY)
PARALARYNGEAL SPACE
ARYEPIGLOTTIC FOLD
PYRIFORM SINUS

SUPERIOR CORNU OF
THYROID CARTILAGE

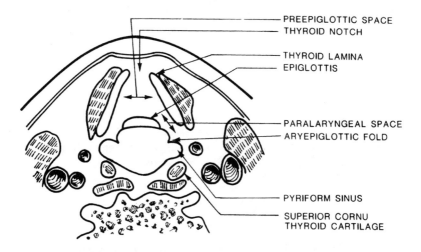

D   **HIGH SUPRAGLOTTIC LEVEL (3)**

PREEPIGLOTTIC SPACE
THYROID NOTCH

THYROID LAMINA
EPIGLOTTIS

PARALARYNGEAL SPACE
ARYEPIGLOTTIC FOLD

PYRIFORM SINUS

SUPERIOR CORNU
THYROID CARTILAGE

Fig. 11-4 *(continued)* **C,** Transaxial drawing through the high supraglottic level of the larynx again shows the C-shaped, pre-epiglottic space. The aryepiglottic folds are first seen at this level, separating the larynx from the pyriform sinus of the hypopharynx. **D,** Axial drawing, still in the high supraglottic level of the larynx, demonstrating the first evidence of the thyroid notch. Note that the anterior pre-epiglottic space now freely communicates with the posterolateral paralaryngeal space. No fascia separates these two endolaryngeal spaces. **E,** Transaxial drawing at the midsupraglottic level of the larynx revealing the hyoepiglottic ligament that now divides the lower pre-epiglottic space. The aryepiglottic folds are now defined more clearly as a sharp division between the endolarynx and the pyriform sinus of the hypopharynx. Tumor involving the aryepiglottic fold primarily is marginal supraglottic carcinoma. **F,** Axial drawing at the low supraglottic level of the larynx showing the thyroid notch to be closing. The paralaryngeal space represents the deep fatty space beneath the false vocal cords at this level.

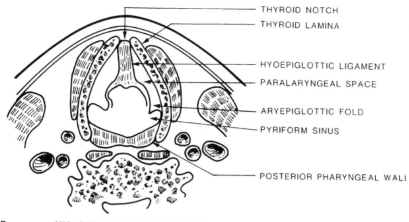

THYROID NOTCH
THYROID LAMINA

HYOEPIGLOTTIC LIGAMENT
PARALARYNGEAL SPACE

ARYEPIGLOTTIC FOLD
PYRIFORM SINUS

POSTERIOR PHARYNGEAL WALL

E   **MID-SUPRAGLOTTIC LEVEL (4)**

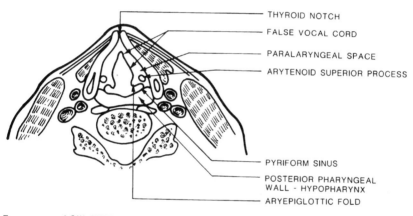

THYROID NOTCH
FALSE VOCAL CORD

PARALARYNGEAL SPACE
ARYTENOID SUPERIOR PROCESS

PYRIFORM SINUS

POSTERIOR PHARYNGEAL
WALL - HYPOPHARYNX
ARYEPIGLOTTIC FOLD

F   **LOW SUPRAGLOTTIC LEVEL (5)**

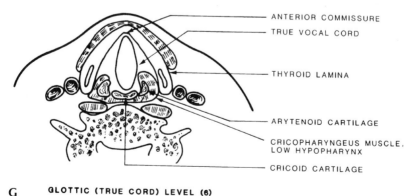

ANTERIOR COMMISSURE
TRUE VOCAL CORD

THYROID LAMINA

ARYTENOID CARTILAGE

CRICOPHARYNGEUS MUSCLE,
LOW HYPOPHARYNX
CRICOID CARTILAGE

G   **GLOTTIC (TRUE CORD) LEVEL (6)**

(continued)

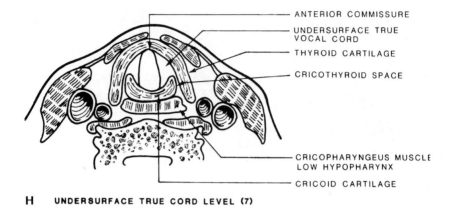

ANTERIOR COMMISSURE

UNDERSURFACE TRUE
VOCAL CORD

THYROID CARTILAGE

CRICOTHYROID SPACE

CRICOPHARYNGEUS MUSCLE
LOW HYPOPHARYNX

CRICOID CARTILAGE

H   UNDERSURFACE TRUE CORD LEVEL (7)

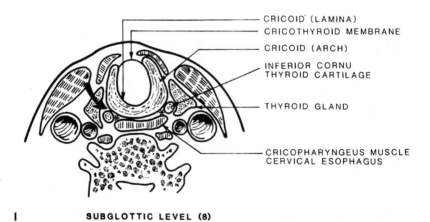

CRICOID (LAMINA)
CRICOTHYROID MEMBRANE

CRICOID (ARCH)

INFERIOR CORNU
THYROID CARTILAGE

THYROID GLAND

CRICOPHARYNGEUS MUSCLE
CERVICAL ESOPHAGUS

I   SUBGLOTTIC LEVEL (8)

Fig. 11-4   (*continued*)   **G**, Axial drawing through the glottic level (true vocal cord level) of the larynx demonstrates the thin (i.e., <1 mm) anterior commissure. The glottic level can be identified easily on axial images by the presence of cricoid and arytenoid cartilage on the same axial section. **H**, Axial drawing at the undersurface of the true vocal cord revealing the broad lamina of the cricoid cartilage posteriorly. The lack of arytenoid cartilage combined with a residual band of tissue where the true vocal cord is expected identifies this level as the undersurface of the true vocal cord. **I**, Transaxial drawing through the subglottic larynx shows the cricoid ring to be nearly complete. The cricothyroid joint (*curved arrow*) is immediately adjacent to the recurrent laryngeal nerve (*asterisk*) located in the tracheoesophageal groove. Dislocation of the cricothyroid joint often is associated with vocal cord paralysis secondary to recurrent laryngeal nerve injury.

    c. When the upper margin of the cricoid cartilage is imaged simultaneously with the arytenoid cartilage in the axial CT plane, the true vocal cord level is imaged (Fig. 11-4*G*).

8. Laryngeal compartments.

    a. The endolarynx can be subdivided into the supraglottis, glottis, and subglottis (Fig. 11-2, Table 11-1). The specific components of each area become important when staging SCCa.

    b. Supraglottis.

        1) The supraglottis extends from the tip of the epiglottis above to the laryngeal ventricles below.

        2) Components of the supraglottis include:

          a) Vestibule.

          b) Epiglottis.

          c) Pre-epiglottic space.

          d) Aryepiglottic folds.

          e) False vocal cords.

          f) Paraglottic (paralaryngeal) space.

          g) Arytenoid cartilages.

        3) A common error made in imaging this area is to include the components of the hypopharynx with those of the supraglottis. In particular, the pyriform sinus must be thought of as part of the

Table 11-1   Laryngeal and Hypopharyngeal Subdivisions

Larynx

Supraglottis
    Suprahyoid epiglottis (both lingual and laryngeal aspects)
    Infrahyoid epiglottis
    False vocal cords (ventricular bands)
    Aryepiglottic folds (laryngeal aspects)
    Arytenoid cartilages

Glottis
    True vocal cords, including anterior and posterior commissures

Subglottis
    Area from under surface of the true vocal cords to inferior surface of the cricoid cartilage

Hypopharynx

    Pyriform sinus
    Postcricoid area
    Posterior hypopharyngeal wall

hypopharynx and the epiglottis as part of the supraglottis (Table 11-1).

  a) These distinctions are important, because the behavior of primary SCCa is very different in these two areas.

4) Vestibule.

  a) The laryngeal vestibule is the air space within the supraglottic larynx.

5) Epiglottis.

  a) The epiglottis is a leaf-shaped cartilage that functions as a lid to the endolaryngeal "box."

  b) The "stem" of this leaf, which attaches the epiglottis to the thyroid lamina, is called the *petiole*. The petiole attaches to the thyroid cartilage via the thyroepiglottic ligament.

  c) The epiglottis is attached to the hyoid bone via the hyoepiglottic ligament. The ridge of mucous membrane over the hyoepiglottic ligament is called the *glossoepiglottic fold*. This fold sits in the midline between the valleculae (Figs. 11-1 and 11-4*A*).

  d) Some authors divide the epiglottis into suprahyoid and infrahyoid components. I find the terms *free margin* (i.e., suprahyoid) and *fixed portion* (i.e., infrahyoid) to be more useful.

6) False vocal cords.

  a) The false vocal cords represent the mucosal surfaces of the laryngeal vestibule of the supraglottis.

  b) Beneath the false vocal cords are the paired paraglottic spaces.

7) Arytenoid cartilage.

  a) The arytenoid cartilage spans the supraglottis and glottis, although most of the cartilage is in the supraglottis.

  b) The tissue projecting from the cephalad tip of the arytenoid cartilages to the inferolateral margin of the epiglottis is called the *aryepiglottic fold*. This fold represents the superolateral margin of the supraglottis, separating it from the pyriform sinus (i.e., hypopharynx).

Q#3

8) Paraglottic and pre-epiglottic spaces.

  a) These two fatty spaces of the supraglottis are critically important, because they serve as readily identifiable landmarks on CT and MRI scans. In addition, submucosal SCCa may lurk in these areas.

  b) The paraglottic spaces are paired, fatty regions beneath the false and true vocal cords. They terminate inferiorly at the level of the undersurface of the true vocal cords, and superiorly they merge into the pre-epiglottic space (Fig. 11-3). The surgical literature refers to the *paraglottic space*, while the radiologic literature describes the *paralaryngeal space*. These spaces are identical. In deference to our surgical colleague, this book uses the term *paraglottic space* preferentially.

c) The pre-epiglottic space is a C-shaped, fat-filled space set between the hyoid bone anteriorly and the epiglottis posteriorly. This space is halved by the hyoepiglottic ligament (Figs. 11-1 and 11-4*E*). The pre-epiglottic space, like the paraglottic space, is another important area where SCCa may lurk without clinical detection. Only imaging will tell the surgeon if tumor is present in either of these two fatty spaces.

Q#3

d) No fascia divides these two spaces. Consequently, SCCa can travel freely from one to the other.

c. Glottis.

1) The glottis includes the true vocal cords and both the anterior and posterior commissures.

2) True vocal cords.

a) True vocal cords are the only soft-tissue structures in the glottic region.

b) These cords extend in an oblique course from the vocal processes of the arytenoid cartilage posteriorly to the anterior commissure in the anterior midline. An axial image with the vocal process visible is by definition an image through the true vocal cord (i.e., glottic) level.

c) With quiet respiration the true vocal cords are in their relaxed, abducted (i.e., apart) state (Fig. 11-5*A*). Breath holding adducts (i.e., brings together) the vocal cords to an opposed, midline position (Fig. 11-5*B*).

3) Anterior commissure.

a) The anterior commissure represents the midline, anterior meeting point of the true vocal cords.

b) On axial CT or MRI scans, less than 1 mm of tissue should be discernible in this location (Figs. 11-4*G, H*). Even a small amount of soft-tissue thickening in the anterior commissure of patients with laryngeal SCCa indicates tumor in this location.

c) Only during quiet respiration is the anterior commissure adequately imaged in the axial plane.

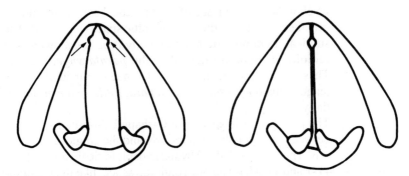

Fig. 11-5 Axial drawings of the normal true vocal cord level illustrating the cord in quiet respiration (*left*) and breath holding (*right*). *Left,* In quiet respiration the vocal cords are away from the midline with the vocalis processes pointing anteromedially. Note the small notch in the anterior aspect of the vocal cords (*arrow*). This represents the anterior–inferior outlet of the laryngeal ventricle. *Right,* With breath holding the vocal cords meet in the midline. The vocalis processes now point directly anteriorly.

      4) Posterior commissure.
         a) The posterior commissure is the mucosal surface on the anterior surface of the cricoid cartilage between the arytenoid cartilages.
         b) Soft tissues in the posterior commissure on quiet respiration should not exceed 1 mm.
   d. Subglottis.
      1) The subglottic area extends from the undersurface of the true vocal cords above to the inferior surface of the cricoid cartilage (Fig. 11-4*I*).
      2) Except for the immediate area of the undersurface of the true vocal cords, the mucosal surface of the subglottic area is closely applied to the cricoid cartilage.
         a) Any tissue seen on the airway side of the subglottic larynx should be viewed by the radiologist with great suspicion.
      3) The conus elasticus is a fibroelastic membrane that extends from the cricoid cartilage below to the medial margin of the true vocal cord above (Fig. 11-2). It forms the lateral wall of the subglottis.
         a) The conus elasticus tends to force SCCa to remain beneath the mucosal surface in the immediate subglottic area.
9. Laryngeal lymphatic drainage.
   a. The specific features of laryngeal lymphatic drainage are of more than academic interest to the radiologist imaging this region.

Depending on the location of the primary SCCa lesion within the larynx, the nodal metastases will vary considerably.

b. The glottis forms the embryologic barrier between superior and inferior lymphatic drainage of the larynx (Fig. 11-6).

1) A line drawn through the laryngeal ventricle just at the upper margin of the glottis defines the two embryologically separate pieces of the larynx.

2) The supraglottic larynx forms from the primitive buccopharyngeal anlage. This area has a lush lymphatic network that drains into the upper deep cervical nodal chain.

a) Supraglottic SCCa have a much higher incidence of nodal metastases at presentation compared with glottic and subglottic SCCa because of this rich lymphatic network.

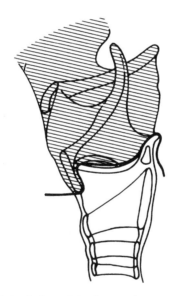

Fig. 11-6   Sagittal depiction of the larynx showing the two separate, embryologically defined regions of the larynx. A line drawn through the laryngeal ventricle just at the upper margin of the glottis defines the two pieces of the larynx. The upper area (*crosshatched*) has a lush lymphatic network that drains into the upper deep cervical nodal chain. Supraglottic squamous cell carcinoma has a much higher incidence of nodal metastases at presentation compared with glottic and subglottic tumors as a result of this rich lymphatic network. The inferior area (i.e., glottis and subglottis) is considerably less endowed with lymphatic channels. What lymphatic network exists drains into the low deep cervical nodal chain and the paratracheal nodal chain. It is not surprising given this separate embryologic derivation that both glottic and subglottic squamous cell carcinoma have low incidence of nodal metastases (i.e., <10%) at presentation.

b) It therefore is important to have the upper margin of the imaging scan begin at the mandibular fillings in the case of supraglottic SCCa to ensure a careful search for nodal metastatic disease at the same time as staging the primary tumor.

3) The glottic and subglottic larynx is formed from tracheobronchial buds. This area is considerably less endowed with lymphatic channels. What lymphatic network exists drains into the low deep cervical nodal chain and the paratracheal nodal chain.

    a) Glottic and subglottic SCCa have a low incidence of nodal metastases (i.e., <10%) at presentation because of this comparatively skimpy lymphatic drainage.

    b) Staging of glottic and subglottic SCCa can begin at the hyoid bone and extend to the level of the clavicle. Primary and nodal tumor are adequately staged by covering this area.

C. Laryngeal imaging.

1. Staging of squamous cell carcinoma.

    a. The goals of imaging the larynx when it is affected by SCCa are to stage both the primary tumor and nodal disease of the neck.

    b. Staging of primary tumor. Because the criteria for assigning a T stage to laryngeal carcinoma requires knowledge of movement of the true vocal cords and involvement of the anterior commissure, imaging is ideally performed with the cords adducted (i.e., breath-holding) and abducted (i.e., quiet respiration).

    c. Staging of nodal tumor. Intravenous contrast medium is necessary in the vascular phase to differentiate nodal disease from the normal vessels in the neck. This contrast medium also brings out the nodal inhomogeneities that help to mark a node as radiologically malignant (see Chapter 13).

    d. CT technique.

        1) Axial CT initially is completed with contiguous 5-mm scans from the lower mandibular margin to the clavicles, with bolus-drip infusion of intravenous contrast medium and quiet respiration. Angling the gantry angle parallel to the plane of the hyoid bone (i.e., approximately 10° toward the feet) will create scans parallel to the true vocal cords.

        a) This technique allows staging the nodes of the neck while simultaneously gaining a global perspective of the primary laryngeal tumor.

        b) During quiet respiration both vocal cords should be seen as displaced laterally from the midline (Fig. 11-5*A*). The anterior commissure is best seen with the cords in this position.

A cord that remains paramedian is either paralyzed or mechanically fixed (Fig. 11-7).

2) A second pass is then completed through the larynx with 3 × 3 mm contiguous scans and breath holding. No further contrast medium is necessary, because the natural fat of the paraglottic and pre-epiglottic spaces provides ample contrast.

    a) If spiral/helical CT is available and the patient is cooperative, a single breath-hold, dynamic acquisition is possible. Batched or single slice scanning with breath holding is alternatively employed.

    b) If a spiral/helical data set is acquired, coronal reconstructions are very informative about the cranial–caudal spread of the tumor.

    c) With breath holding the vocal cords oppose in the midline (Fig. 11-5*B*). A cord that remains paramedian is either paralyzed or mechanically fixed (Fig. 11-7).

    d) Cord motion can be assessed by comparing the initial, quiet respiration images with the subsequent breath holding images. Remember that cord motion is best assessed by the clinician during visualization, either indirectly or directly.

2. MRI technique.

  a. Only axial and coronal T1-weighted images are necessary for staging of the primary laryngeal tumor. Slice thickness must be 4 mm or less with interslice gap of 1 mm or less.

    1) Coronal T1-weighted images can greatly assist in the assessment of the transglottic nature of an individual tumor.

    2) Coronal images also help to differentiate subglottic tumor involvement from downward displacement of the true vocal cords by supraglottic tumor.

  b. Postcontrast, fat-saturated, T1-weighted imaging of the neck from the inferior angle of the mandible to the clavicles is then completed to stage the nodal neck disease. Postcontrast, T1-weighted axial images and axial T2- or T2*-weighted images are the most helpful in delineating cartilaginous invasion.

  c. MRI should not be attempted unless a neck surface coil is available and the radiologist has some experience with this tool. Attempts to image the larynx without the neck surface coil will result in a nondiagnostic study.

  d. Vocal cord motion cannot be assessed by current MRI techniques.

D. Squamous cell carcinoma of the larynx.

1. Both CT and MRI have had a major impact on the clinical staging of laryngeal SCCa. The submucosal information they provide about the

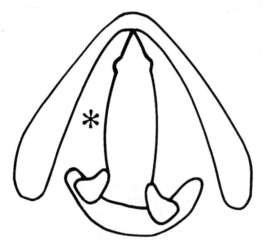

A

Fig. 11-7   Axial drawings at the level of the glottis showing vocal cord paralysis during quiet respiration (*A*), breath holding (*B*), and breath holding associated with a patulous laryngeal ventricle (*C*). **A,** A paralyzed right vocal cord (*asterisk*) in a paramedial location with the arytenoid process fixed in an anterior–medial position. The normal left vocal cord is off midline, as would be expected when seen during quiet respiration on a CT image. **B,** Paralyzed right vocal cord (*asterisk*) is displayed in the setting of breath holding. In such a case the axial CT image would show the normal left vocal cord "overcompensating" for the paralyzed right cord, actually crossing the midline (*arrow*) in an attempt to make contact with the paralyzed cord (i.e., close the glottis). **C,** Still another variation on the theme of paralyzed vocal cords. The right vocal cord is again the paralyzed cord. The patient is breath holding, with the opposite normal left vocal cord again seen to cross the midline in an attempt to close the glottis (*arrow*). The difference in this drawing is in the depiction of a patulous laryngeal ventricle (*asterisk*). The loss of tone from laryngeal muscles associated with vagus nerve injury at times may result in a patulous pyriform sinus and laryngeal ventricle. On axial CT images through the vocal cords, the paralyzed cord may be replaced by an air-filled laryngeal ventricle. Only the "fixed" arytenoid cartilage will remain as a clue to the side of the paralysis.

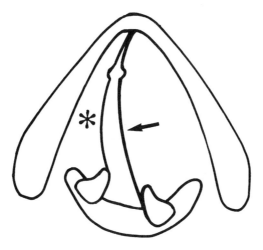

B

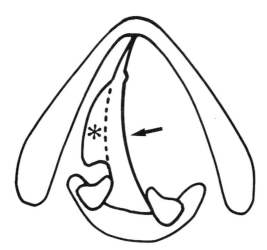

C

deep tissue activity and location of this malignant tumor cannot be gained by any other mechanism.

2. The overwhelming preponderance of malignant tumors of the larynx (i.e., 98%) are SCCa. Sarcoma, especially chondrosarcoma, is the rare exception.

3. Therapy for SCCa includes some combination of radiation therapy and conservative (i.e., partial laryngectomy) or radical (i.e., total laryngectomy) surgery. Smaller, endolaryngeal SCCa usually is not imaged and is treated with local radiation or laser surgery. Therapy for larger SCCa greatly benefits from precise pretreatment staging of the extent of tumor invasion. Deep tissue information from CT or MRI scans determines which treatment option will be undertaken.

   a. All conservative therapy aims to preserve a portion of the larynx and, therefore, some element of normal speech.

   b. The common speech-preserving partial laryngectomies are the vertical hemilaryngectomy and the supraglottic laryngectomy.

   c. Vertical hemilaryngectomy is used when the lesion involves the true vocal cord without fixation, there is little (1/3) involvement of the contralateral cord (i.e., <one third anteriorly), and less than 1 cm of subglottic extension, and the tumor remains inferior to the cephalad laryngeal ventricle and spares the thyroid cartilage. The goal is to preserve one intact vocal cord for speech and control of aspiration.

      1) The thyroid cartilage is incised near midline, and both the true and false vocal cords on one side are removed along with the ipsilateral thyroid ala (Fig. 11-8).

      2) Vocal cord SCCa actually can cross the midline at the anterior commissure and involve the anterior third of the opposite cord. In such cases the incision through the thyroid cartilage is moved more laterally to include a portion of the opposite thyroid cartilage.

      3) Contraindications to vertical hemilaryngectomy include significant subglottic extension (i.e., > 1 cm), involvement of the arytenoid cartilage, deep invasion at the anterior commissure, superior extension into the false vocal cord, and invasion of the thyroid cartilage.

   d. Horizontal (supraglottic) hemilaryngectomy is the treatment of choice for lesions that are isolated to the supraglottis above the laryngeal ventricle, spare the thyroid cartilage, and show no evidence for vocal cord fixation. The goal is to preserve both vocal cords for speech and control of aspiration.

      1) In this surgery the surgeon removes the upper half of the larynx, including part of the thyroid cartilage and often the hyoid bone (Fig. 11-9). The incision is directly through the ventricle, staying just above the level of the anterior commissure. The posterior

portion of the incision curves upward to spare the arytenoid cartilages and crosses the lower aryepiglottic fold.

2) Contraindications to horizontal hemilaryngectomy include tumor involvement of the glottis, subglottis, or tongue base. If the tumor crosses the laryngeal ventricle, this surgery is not feasible. Other findings that preclude this surgery are invaded cricoid or thyroid cartilage, vocal cord fixation, or involvement of both arytenoid cartilages.

4. Clinicoradiologic staging criteria for laryngeal carcinoma are presented in Table 11-2. Each of the three areas of the larynx (i.e., supraglottis, glottis, and subglottis) has its own criteria.

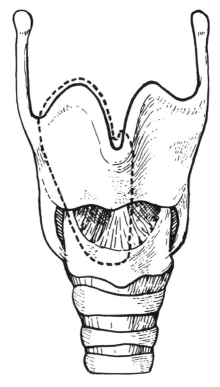

A

Fig. 11-8   Vertical hemilaryngectomy. **A**, Standard margins of vertical hemilaryngectomy (*dashed line*). This surgery generally is employed in the setting of glottic–supraglottic squamous cell carcinoma involving only one side of the larynx. The ipsilateral aryepiglottic fold as well as false and true vocal cords are removed along with the arytenoid cartilage and most of the ipsilateral thyroid cartilage.

(*continued*)

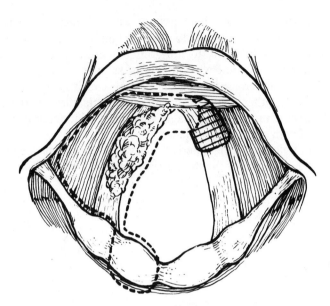

B

Fig. 11-8 (*continued*)   **B,** Axial drawing looking down on the vocal cords again showing the surgical margins (*dashed line*). Note that if the tumor crosses the anterior commissure to involve the anterior third of the contralateral vocal cord, an extended hemilaryngectomy may encompass this area as well (*crosshatched region*).

5. Supraglottic squamous cell carcinoma.
   a. Approximately 30% of all laryngeal carcinomas arise in the supra-glottis.
   b. Early nodal metastasis to the deep cervical nodal chain of the neck is common because of the lush lymphatic network within the supra-glottic larynx (Fig. 11-6).
      1) Regardless of their T stage, 55% of all patients with supraglottic carcinoma have nodal metastasis at presentation.
   c. Supraglottic carcinoma often is diagnosed late (e.g., stage T3 or T4), because there is no hoarseness until the vocal cord is involved.
   d. It is useful to divide the supraglottis into anterior (i.e., epiglottis) and posterolateral (i.e., aryepiglottic fold, false vocal cord, laryngeal ventricle) compartments when discussing tumor involvement, because routes of spread, surgical options, and general prognosis vary considerably between these areas.
      1) Anterior compartment (i.e., epiglottis) carcinoma tends to grow circumferentially. This relatively symmetrical growth allows epiglottic carcinoma to be missed easily on axial imaging.

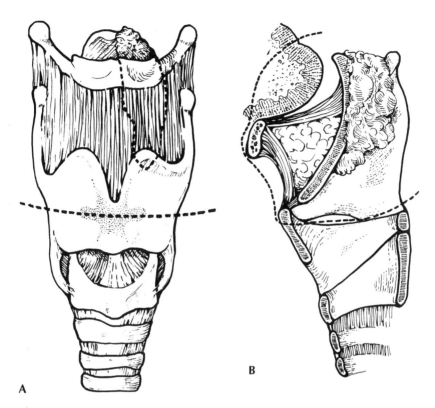

Fig. 11-9   Horizontal hemilaryngectomy. When the primary squamous cell carcinoma is truly supraglottic in origin and does not involve the glottis (i.e., ends at least 5 mm above the level of the true vocal cord), horizontal hemilaryngectomy is the conservative surgery used to preserve the speech and antiaspiration functions of both vocal cords acting in concert. **A,** Front view showing the horizontal surgical margin (*dashed line*). The upper half of the larynx, including part of the thyroid cartilage and often the hyoid bone, is removed in this surgery. **B,** Lateral perspective showing that the incision is carried directly through the ventricle, staying just above the level of the anterior commissure. The posterior portion of the incision curves upward to spare the arytenoid cartilages, crossing the lower aryepiglottic fold.

a)   This tumor initially spreads into the pre-epiglottic space. Only when tumor spread is more extensive are the tongue base above and the paraglottic space below accessed.

b)   Partial supraglottic laryngectomy is effective in less advanced epiglottic carcinoma. These lesions have a better prognosis than their posterolateral compartment counterparts.

Table 11-2 Staging Criteria for Laryngeal Squamous Cell Carcinoma

Supraglottis

T1: Tumor confined to site of origin with normal cord mobility

T2: Tumor involving adjacent supraglottic site or glottis without cord fixation

T3: Tumor limited to the larynx with cord fixation or extension to involve the postcricoid area, medial wall of pyriform sinus, or pre-epiglottic space

T4: Massive tumor extending beyond the larynx to involve the oropharynx (i.e., tongue base), soft tissues of the neck, or thyroid cartilage

Glottis

T1: Tumor confined to vocal cords with normal cord mobility (including involvement of the anterior or posterior commissures)

T2: Supraglottic or subglottic extension of tumor, or tumor extending to the posterior commissure with normal or impaired cord mobility

T3: Tumor confined to the larynx with cord fixation

T4: Massive tumor with destruction of thyroid cartilage or extension beyond the confines of the larynx (e.g., trachea, neck soft tissues such as thyroid)

Subglottis

T1: Tumor confined to the subglottic area

T2: Tumor extension to vocal cords with normal or impaired cord mobility

T3: Tumor confined to larynx with cord fixation

T4: Massive tumor with cartilage destruction or extension beyond the confines of the larynx or both

---

2) Posterolateral compartment (i.e., aryepiglottic fold, false vocal cord, laryngeal ventricle) carcinomas have two distinct patterns of spread.

   a) Early aryepiglottic fold carcinoma, also called *marginal supraglottic carcinoma*, is confined to the medial surface of the aryepiglottic fold. This lesion tends to grow exophytically, and as it enlarges it grows medially into the fixed portion of the epiglottis and inferiorly into the paraglottic space.

   b) False vocal cord and laryngeal ventricle carcinomas initially spread submucosally into the paraglottic space. More extensive tumor destroys thyroid cartilage and spreads transglottically across the laryngeal ventricle to involve the true vocal cords and subglottis below.

   c) Total laryngectomy with radiation therapy often is required for posterolateral compartment lesions. The prognosis for such lesions is poorer than for anterior compartment carcinomas.

  e. Radiologic staging issues for supraglottic carcinoma.

Q#4

1) The major clinical blind spots when staging supraglottic carcinoma are:
   a) Pre-epiglottic space and low tongue base.
   b) Paraglottic space.
   c) Thyroid cartilage involvement.

2) Both CT and MRI scans beautifully display involvement of the pre-epiglottic space, low tongue base and paraglottic space.

3) MRI is slightly better for detecting thyroid cartilage invasion, although neither technique detects the more subtle forms of this process.
   a) Variable ossification of the thyroid cartilage and microscopic invasion of this cartilage can make radiologic staging difficult.
   b) If the cartilage is ossified, a margin of cortical bone surrounds the normal fat–laden medullary cavity. In this case tumor within the medullary cavity is obvious on both CT and MRI scans.
   c) If the cartilage is not ossified, determining on CT scans if tumor is invading it may be impossible. The first- and second-echo T2-weighted MRI scans have the best chance of identifying tumor invasion of nonossified cartilage. On the longer-TR sequences the tumor remains high signal; the cartilage is seen as intermediate or low signal.
   d) Only when obvious fatty medullary invasion or tumor mass on the outer, extralaryngeal side of the thyroid cartilage is seen can cartilage invasion be diagnosed definitively using CT or MRI scans.
   e) If thyroid cartilage sclerosis is observed on CT scans, this means that the tumor is either abutting or invading the cartilage. Sclerosis alone does *not* indicate definite invasion.
   f) Comment. Because diagnosis of thyroid or cricoid cartilage invasion made radiologically is an indicator for total laryngectomy instead of conservative surgery or radiotherapy, this radiologic interpretation should be rendered only when no question exists about the finding. If questions remain despite adequate imaging, this should be conveyed to the surgeon.

4) Treatment is modified by radiologic findings as follows:
   a) Supraglottic laryngectomy is not undertaken unless more than 5 mm exists between the lower margin of the tumor and the vocal cord or anterior commissure. Axial CT therefore needs one normal slice between the vocal cord level and the inferior margin of the tumor. Coronal MRI will directly

image the relationship between the inferior margin of the tumor and the true vocal cord (i.e., thyroarytenoid muscle).

b) Supraglottic laryngectomy is not undertaken if cricoid or thyroid cartilage is invaded, a vocal cord is fixed, or both arytenoid cartilages are involved.

c) Involvement of the tongue base is a relative contraindication for partial laryngopharyngectomy or supraglottic laryngectomy.

d) Advanced supraglottic carcinoma generally is treated with total laryngectomy.

6. Glottic squamous cell carcinoma.

   a. Approximately 60% of laryngeal carcinomas occur at the glottic level. Because hoarseness is clinically obvious, these lesions usually are detected early in their natural history.

   b. Isolated glottic (i.e., true vocal cord) tumors rarely present with nodal metastasis, because the true vocal cord is relatively avascular and therefore alymphatic (Fig. 11-6). Only when the tumor has spread to the richer lymphatic bed of the supraglottis are associated malignant lymph nodes seen.

   c. In most cases stage T1 glottic carcinoma should not be imaged by either CT or MRI. These lesions respond well to radiation therapy or local surgical techniques, so radiologic evaluation adds little to their evaluation.

   d. Stage T2 to T4 lesions are imaged both to look at the deep tissue extent of tumor and to stage nodal disease in the neck.

   e. Glottic tumors show four distinct patterns of spread:

      1) Anterior to the anterior commissure.

      2) Posterior extension to the region of the arytenoid cartilage, cricoid cartilage, posterior commissure, and cricoarytenoid joint.

      3) Inferiorly into the subglottic region.

      4) Superiorly into the paraglottic space beneath the false vocal cord.

   f. Anterior spread of glottic carcinoma to involve the anterior commissure is readily detected with careful CT or MRI scans.

      1) More than 1 mm of tissue at the anterior commissure signals malignant invasion.

      2) The pre-epiglottic space above, subglottis below, and thyroid cartilage anteriorly are all at risk for carcinoma invasion once the tumor has spread to the anterior commissure.

      3) Carcinoma from one cord most commonly accesses the contralateral vocal cord across the anterior commissure.

         a) When both cords are involved symmetrically, thickening of the anterior commissure may be the only clue that both cords are infiltrated by tumor.

b) Involvement of more than the anterior third of the contralateral cord precludes partial hemilaryngectomy.

g. Posterior spread may be signaled by tissue in the posterior commissure, fixation of the arytenoid cartilage, widening of the cricothyroid space, or sclerosis of the arytenoid and/or cricoid cartilage.

1) If arytenoid or cricoid cartilage sclerosis is observed on CT images, the tumor is either abutting or invading the cartilage. Sclerosis alone does *not* indicate definite invasion.

h. Inferior extension into the subglottic region must be looked for carefully. If present, total laryngectomy is necessary.

7. Subglottic squamous cell carcinoma.

a. Subglottic carcinoma is the rarest form of laryngeal carcinoma, accounting for approximately 5% of all cases.

b. Total laryngectomy is usually required, because these lesions are detected late in their natural history.

c. The diagnosis of subglottic carcinoma is not hard to make radiologically, because the area below the undersurface of the true cord has no normal tissue between the mucosal surface and cricoid cartilage.

E. Chondroid tumors of the larynx.

1. Chondroma.

a. Rare, benign tumor of laryngeal cartilage.

b. CT scans may show the chondroid, mineralized matrix of an expansile lesion of the laryngeal cartilage.

c. The chondroma cannot be differentiated reliably from a smaller, low-grade chondrosarcoma.

2. Chondrosarcoma.

a. Rare, slow-growing malignancy of the laryngeal cartilages.

b. Primarily arises in the cricoid cartilage (i.e., 90% of cases) although rarely it may be centered in the thyroid cartilage.

c. CT scans show coarse or stippled calcification within the matrix of the tumor in virtually all cases. The lesion may remain endolaryngeal or more commonly extend into the immediate exolaryngeal soft tissues.

F. Laryngocele (Table 11-3).

1. Clinical presentation. Signs and symptoms resulting from laryngocele depend on its size and location. Internal laryngocele may cause hoarseness or stridor. Mixed laryngocele presents with an anterior neck mass just below the angle of the mandible.

2. Pathogenesis. When the laryngeal ventricle or its more distal sacculus (i.e., appendix) is functionally obstructed because of increased intraglottic pressure (e.g., from excessive coughing, playing a musical instrument, or blowing glass), laryngocele occurs (see Fig. 10-9, *right*).

Table 11-3   Types of Laryngocele

Internal laryngocele
Laryngocele confined to supraglottis, deep to the false vocal cord, in the paraglottic space

Mixed (external) laryngocele
Laryngocele with both internal and external components; lesion has herniated through the thyrohyoid membrane into the soft tissues of the anterior neck

Pyolaryngocele
Either internal or mixed laryngocele containing pus; superinfected

Secondary laryngocele
Internal or mixed laryngocele resulting from low supraglottic carcinoma obstructing the laryngeal ventricle

---

Obstruction of the proximal saccule by postinflammatory stenosis, trauma, or tumor is a less common cause. The cystic mass may be filled with air, fluid, or pus. With continued growth the laryngocele penetrates the thyrohyoid membrane and enters the neck in the lower submandibular space (see Fig. 10-9, *left*).

3. Radiologic features. (See Chapter 10 for details.)
   a. Internal laryngocele (see Fig. 10-10).
   b. Mixed (external) laryngocele (see Fig. 10-11).
   c. Secondary laryngocele (see Fig. 10-9, *left*).

G. Laryngeal trauma.

1. Imaging of the larynx is performed in two different trauma phases: the acute, and the chronic.
   a. Acute injuries to the larynx can be classified as iatrogenic, blunt, or penetrating trauma.
      1) Iatrogenic laryngeal injury refers to trauma that may occur inadvertently in the larynx at the time of an emergency or a planned intubation.
         a) Traumatic intubation usually is limited to bleeding from mucosal abrasions. Occasionally pharyngeal or laryngeal wall penetration occurs.
         b) When cartilaginous injury occurs during intubation, the most common form is dislocation of an arytenoid cartilage. The arytenoid cartilage typically is displaced anteriorly, forcing the vocal cord into a paramedial location. The cord will appear paretic both clinically and radiographically.

c) The radiologist must remember that a paramedial cord from vagus nerve injury may look very similar to a dislocated arytenoid cartilage. A clinical history of recent intubation is the key.

2) Blunt laryngeal trauma from athletic injuries, car accidents, and assault frequently causes symptoms suggestive of laryngeal injury (e.g., hoarseness, stridor). Although the clinician can assess clearly the mucosal surfaces for laceration and vocal cords for paralysis, assessing deep tissue injury or fracture of the cartilaginous laryngeal skeleton is difficult.

a) A blow to the larynx from the front of the neck tends to compress the cartilages against the bony cervical spine (Fig. 11-10).

b) The cricoid cartilage, like the pelvic bones, is a complete ring. It usually will fracture in two or more places. One of the more common forms is a vertical fracture through the posterior cricoid signet and bilateral fractures through the anterior cricoid ring (Fig. 11-10B). It is possible for severe, anterior neck trauma to cause such a fracture to the cricoid,

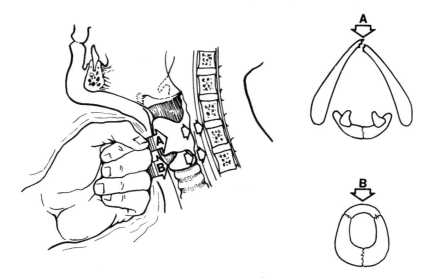

Fig. 11-10 Blunt trauma to the larynx. When a blunt object such as a fist strikes the anterior neck, the cartilaginous edifice of the larynx is compressed against the vertebral bodies of the cervical spine (*open arrows*). The thyroid cartilage most commonly will fracture along its anterior margin (*A*). The cricoid ring would be expected to break in at least two places; in this example the cricoid ring is fractured in three different locations.

with outward displacement of the cricoid fragments preserving an open airway.

c) An anterolateral blow to the larynx is the most common
mechanism of injury producing longitudinal fractures
through the thyroid cartilage ala. Such an injury may result
in folding of one thyroid ala inward on the other. Airway
compromise may or may not be associated. If no airway
compromise is present, the patient may not seek medical
attention. In such cases laryngeal distortion may be discovered only in the chronic phase of injury (discussed later).

d) In either form of injury to the larynx it is possible to have
associated arytenoid dislocation. Remember that arytenoid
dislocation usually occurs anteriorly and therefore can
mimic a paralyzed vocal cord on both physical examination
and CT images.

e) Abnormal loculations of submucosal air, often associated
with soft-tissue air in the neck (i.e., subcutaneous emphy-
sema), signal laryngeal mucosal laceration.

3) Penetrating laryngeal trauma may result in mucosal or cartilaginous injury. Direct surgical exploration is usually required.
Imaging of the larynx is only done when the acute phase has
passed and lingering clinical questions remain.

4) CT is the optimal imaging tool for evaluating significant injury
to the larynx. MRI has no role in this clinical setting.

b. Chronic laryngeal injury.

1) The most common presentation of chronic laryngeal injury, in
my experience, is seen in the patient with suspected anterior
neck mass where CT shows an infolded thyroid ala and tilted larynx (Fig. 11-11). The laryngeal deformity causes the clinician to
suspect a mass, and a history of previous neck injury almost
always can be elicited.

2) Head and neck surgeons can define a clinical syndrome signaling old trauma to the larynx. Such patients present with multiple
suggestive symptoms and signs, including a sensation of food
sticking in the throat, soreness in the throat brought on by a day
of talking, a bulging mass at the level of the false vocal cord with
intact mucosa, and laryngeal deformity on physical examination.
Again, inbuckling of thyroid alar cartilage at the site of old
injury seen on CT scans.

2. CT technique.

a. No intravenous contrast medium is necessary.

b. Angle the gantry parallel to the hyoid bone to make the scan plane
parallel to the true vocal cord.

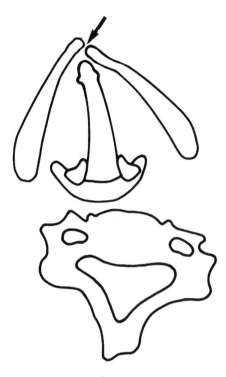

Fig. 11-11   Chronic posttraumatic larynx mimicking a neck mass. A patient sustaining blunt trauma to the larynx (Fig. 11-10) with thyroid cartilage fracture but no airway compromise may present months to years later during a physical examination of the neck as suspicious for a neck mass. This drawing illustrates what axial CT scans may show when a healed laryngeal fracture is found: an overlapping thyroid ala (*arrow*) associated with a larynx no longer centered in the midline of the neck. These findings are characteristic of old, healed laryngeal fracture. Questioning the patient will reveal a history of remote blunt trauma to the neck.

 c. Use contiguous, 3-mm slices. Scan from just above the hyoid bone to the first tracheal ring. Extend the scan as needed in either direction as dictated by the area containing the most severe injury.

 d. Photograph in the soft-tissue and bone windows to assess both the endolaryngeal soft tissue and cartilages.

 e. If spiral/helical technique is available, single breath holding acquisition is ideal. In the chronic phase of imaging this often is possible. In the acute phase it rarely is possible.

  1) Taking the 3-mm contiguous data set and reconstructing it into 1-mm contiguous images allows the radiologist to make exquis-

ite sagittal and coronal reconstructions. The relative positions of the cartilaginous edifice of the larynx can be displayed best with these reconstructions.

2) High detail, three-dimensional reconstructions now can be done with the spiral/helical data. In the past three-dimensional images were mostly cosmetic; however, these new images are now beginning to approach clinical usefulness.

3. CT findings.
   a. Supraglottic injuries.
      1) Acute findings.
         a) Hyoid bone fracture.
         b) Epiglottic laceration or avulsion.
         c) Thyroid cartilage transverse (adults) and vertical (children) fractures.
         d) Subcutaneous emphysema suggesting deep mucosal laceration.
         e) Aryepiglottic fold hematoma suggesting cricoarytenoid joint disruption.
      2) Chronic findings.
         a) Thyroid ala infolding is accompanied by tilting of the larynx relative to the vertebral body (Fig. 11-11). This configuration may be mistaken for a neck mass by an unsuspecting clinician with maladroit fingers.
   b. Glottic injuries.
      1) Acute findings.
         a) If the arytenoid cartilage is dislocated, it will move anteriorly, causing the vocal cord to look paretic (Fig. 11-12). CT scans can identify the anteriorly located arytenoid cartilage.
         b) If the cricothyroid joint is sprung, injury to the recurrent laryngeal nerve can cause vocal cord paralysis on the ipsilateral side.
         c) Avulsion and deep laceration of the vocal cord.
         d) Fixation of the arytenoid cartilage by hematoma.
   c. Subglottic injuries.
      1) Multiple cricoid ring fractures.
         a) Detection of cricoid ring fracture has great clinical significance, because if these fractures are not repaired, chronic stenosis and scarring of the larynx may result.
         b) The most common fracture of the cricoid ring is a posterior midline fracture associated with one or two anterolateral ring fractures (Fig. 11-10).
      2) Dislocation of the cricothyroid joint with widening of the cricothyroid space is seen on CT scans.

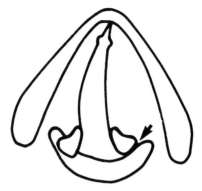

Fig. 11-12   Arytenoid cartilage dislocation. This axial drawing at the level of the true vocal cord during quiet respiration demonstrates left arytenoid dislocation. The arytenoid cartilage has "fallen off" its cricoid cartilage perch, now sitting ventral to the anterior cricoid margin (*arrow*). The vocal cord is paramedian or midline in arytenoid cartilage dislocation. A history of traumatic intubation and the anterior location of the arytenoid cartilage differentiate this appearance from simple vocal cord paralysis (compare with Fig. 11-7*B*).

> a) Recurrent laryngeal nerve injury often is associated with dislocation of the cricothyroid joint (Fig. 11-4, *I*).

HYPOPHARYNX

A. Introduction.

1. The hypopharynx is a distinct area of the upper aerodigestive tract and must be distinguished from the oropharynx above and the larynx below.
2. Because of the close association of the hypopharynx and larynx, surgery of hypopharyngeal tumors usually involves simultaneous surgery of the larynx.
3. Like the oropharynx and nasopharynx, the hypopharynx is a caudal continuation of the pharyngeal mucosal space.
   a. The mucosa, minor salivary glands, and inferior pharyngeal constrictor muscles are the only contents of the hypopharyngeal mucosal space.
   b. With such limited contents only SCCa and minor salivary gland benign and malignant tumors as well as retention cysts are included in the differential diagnosis for the hypopharyngeal mucosal space.
   c. The hypopharynx most often becomes an important focus to the imager when it is involved by SCCa.

B. Normal anatomy.

1. The three major subsites of the hypopharynx are:
   a. Pyriform sinus.
   b. Postcricoid area.
   c. Posterior hypopharyngeal wall.
2. Pyriform sinus.
   a. The pyriform sinus looks like two symmetric stalactites hanging from the hypopharynx behind the larynx.
      1) The inferior tip of the pyriform sinus is known as the *pyriform apex*. The apex reaches to the level of the cricoarytenoid joint (i.e., true vocal cord level).

Q#5

      2) The anteromedial margin of the pyriform sinus is the posterolateral wall of the aryepiglottic fold. The medial wall of the aryepiglottic fold is endolaryngeal (Fig. 11-4*C*, *D*, *E*, *F*).
         a) The aryepiglottic fold is considered to be part of the larynx. Tumors primary to the aryepiglottic fold are called *marginal supraglottic tumors*.
      3) The lateral wall of the pyriform sinus abuts the posterior thyroid cartilage ala.
      4) The posterior wall of the pyriform sinus actually is the most lateral aspect of the posterior hypopharyngeal wall.
   b. The landmarks used for resection of a pyriform sinus SCCa are closely related to those used for determining the feasibility of a supraglottic resection.
      1) A lesion located high in the pyriform sinus can be resected along with the supraglottic larynx.
      2) A lesion near the pyriform apex approaches the upper margin of the cricoid cartilage. When the SCCa is in the pyriform apex, it usually requires total laryngopharyngectomy.
3. Postcricoid area.
   a. The postcricoid area (pharyngeal–esophageal junction) extends from the level of the arytenoid cartilages and connecting folds to the inferior border of the cricoid cartilage. The postcricoid area is the anterior wall of the lower pharynx.
   b. This subsite of the hypopharynx is difficult to delineate clearly by either CT or MRI.
   c. A total laryngectomy is required for SCCa of the postcricoid area.
4. Posterior pharyngeal wall area.
   a. The posterior hypopharyngeal wall extends from the level of the valleculae to the level of the cricoarytenoid joints.

  b. This area consists of the mucosa and inferior pharyngeal constrictor muscles anterior to the middle layer of the deep cervical fascia.

C. Hypopharyngeal squamous cell carcinoma (Table 11-4).

1. Carcinomas of the hypopharynx are most common in the pyriform sinus (60% of cases), followed by the postcricoid area (25%) and the posterior pharyngeal wall (15%).
2. Because the hypopharynx is a "quiet" area regarding symptoms and signs, primary SCCa in this area usually is advanced (i.e., stage T3 or T4) at presentation.
   a. This tendency for primary tumor of the hypopharynx to be advanced at presentation is accompanied by a 50% incidence of nodal metastasis at diagnosis.
3. Clinical presentation.
   a. Early symptoms are often vague and include sore throat and intolerance to hot and cold liquids.
   b. The more common symptoms of advanced disease are dysphagia, weight loss, and cervical adenopathy.
   c. If ear pain is present initially, the tumor is usually large and has invaded the superior laryngeal nerve, causing referred pain via this root back through the vagus nerve.
   d. Virtually all patients with hypopharyngeal carcinoma are serious smokers and drinkers and usually are men.
       1) When hypopharyngeal carcinoma is detected in a woman, the diagnosis of Plummer-Vinson syndrome should be considered.
          a) Plummer-Vinson syndrome is characterized by atrophic mucosa, achlorhydria, and sideropenic anemia in women (90% of cases). Hypopharyngeal carcinoma is a complication of this syndrome.
4. Pyriform sinus carcinoma.
   a. Sixty percent of hypopharyngeal carcinomas are found in the pyriform sinus.

Table 11-4   Staging Criteria for Hypopharyngeal Carcinoma

T1: Tumor limited to one subsite* of the hypopharynx
T2: Tumor invades more than one subsite of the hypopharynx or an adjacent site *without* fixation of the hemilarynx
T3: Tumor invades more than one subsite of the hypopharynx or an adjacent site *with* fixation of the hemilarynx
T4: Tumor invades adjacent structures (e.g., thyroid or cricoid cartilages, soft tissues of the neck)

*Hypopharyngeal subsites are the pyriform sinus, postcricoid area (pharyngeal–esophageal junction), and posterior pharyngeal wall.

Q#6

b. Smaller lesions in the inferior reaches of the pyriform sinus may escape detection during clinical examination. When malignant adenopathy is the presenting symptom, the pyriform sinus is one of three major areas where the "unknown primary tumor" may hide.

1) The two other areas to examine in this circumstance are Waldeyer's lymphatic ring (i.e., lingual and faucial tonsil areas) and the nasopharynx.

c. Behavior of pyriform sinus carcinoma.

1) Pyriform sinus carcinoma is not confined by any cartilaginous boundary as endolaryngeal carcinoma is.

Q#7

2) The most common route of spread for pyriform sinus carcinoma is posterolaterally into the soft tissues of the neck. As the tumor spreads in this direction it often destroys the posterior margin of the ipsilateral thyroid cartilage ala.

3) Early invasion of soft tissue in the neck invasion, which is combined with nodal metastasis at presentation in 50% of patients, gives this tumor a particularly grim prognosis.

d. Radiologic staging.

1) In patients with malignant squamous adenopathy but no known primary tumor, carefully inspect the pyriform sinus for submucosal primary tumor.

2) Look for signs of invasion of the adjacent structures, especially the posterior aspect of the thyroid ala, cricothyroid space, soft tissues of the neck.

   a) Any of these findings stages the primary tumor as a T4 lesion.

3) Clinical staging relies heavily on "hemilarynx fixation" (Table 11-4). Although the vocal cords can be evaluated radiologically during breath holding and quiet respiration, visual inspection is faster and more accurate. The radiologic staging of pyriform sinus carcinoma should remain focused on deep tissue extent of the tumor.

5. Postcricoid carcinoma.

a. Accurate assessment of the extent of deep tissue tumor in the postcricoid area can be extremely difficult.

1) The normal soft tissue (i.e., a mixture of prevertebral muscles and inferior constrictor muscles) seen in the postcricoid area on CT or MRI scans varies in thickness.

2) Any radiologic assessment of postcricoid carcinoma must be done with a clear understanding of the endoscopic appearance of the mucosal extent of the tumor.

    b. Postcricoid carcinoma carries the worst prognosis of the three sub-
sites of the hypopharynx.

      1) Five-year survival rates are less than 25%.

6. Posterior pharyngeal-wall carcinoma.

    a. Posterior pharyngeal wall carcinomas generally are aggressive, infil-
trating tumors that invade the retropharyngeal space and run cephalad into the oropharynx and nasopharynx.

      1) Because of their posterior position these tumors often have
retropharyngeal adenopathy.

      2) Rather than examining only the anterior deep cervical nodal
chain for malignant adenopathy, it is important that the retropharyngeal nodes be scrutinized carefully in all cases of posterior
pharyngeal wall carcinoma.

      3) Retropharyngeal adenopathy is often subclinical. Discovering
adenopathy in this location may shift the patient from the
resectable to the unresectable group.

SUGGESTED READING

Archer CR, Sagel SS, Yeager VL, et al: Staging of carcinoma of the larynx: comparative accuracy of CT and laryngography. *Am J Roentgenol* 136:571–575, 1981.

Archer CR, Yeager VL, Herbold DR: Improved diagnostic accuracy in laryngeal
cancer using a new classification based on CT. *Cancer* 53:44–57, 1984.

Beahrs OH, Henson DE, Hutter RVP, Kennedy BJ (American Joint Committee on
Cancer): *Manual for staging of cancer*, ed. 4. Philadelphia, 1992, JB Lippincott.

Candela FC, Shah J, Jaques DP, et al: Patterns of cervical node metastases from
squamous carcinoma of the larynx. *Arch Otolaryngol Head Neck Surg*
116:432–435, 1990.

Castelijns GET, Gerritsen GJ, Kaiser MC, et al: Invasion of laryngeal cartilage by
cancer: comparison of CT and MR imaging. *Radiology* 166:199–206, 1987.

Castelijns JA, Doornbos J, Verbeeten B, et al: MR imaging of the normal larynx. *J
Comput Assist Tomogr* 9:919–925, 1985.

Castelijns JA, Golding RP, Schaik CV, et al: MR findings of cartilage invasion by
laryngeal cancer: value in prediction outcome of radiation therapy. *Radiology*
174:669–673, 1990.

Castelijns JA, Kaiser MC, Gerritsen GJ, et al: MR imaging of laryngeal cancer. *J
Comput Assist Tomogr* 11:134–140, 1987.

Cohn AM, Larson DL: Laryngeal injury: a critical review. *Arch Otolaryngol*
102:166–170, 1976.

Curtin HD: Imaging of the larynx: current concepts. *Radiology* 173:1–11, 1989.

DiSantis DJ, Balfe DM, Hayden RE, et al: The neck after total laryngectomy: CT
study. *Radiology* 153:713–717, 1984.

Hoover LA, Calcaterra TC, Walter GA, et al: Preoperative CT scan evaluation for
laryngeal carcinoma: correlation with pathological findings. *Laryngoscope*
94:310–315, 1984.

Horowitz BL, Woodson GE, Bryan RN: CT of laryngeal tumors. *Radiol Clin North Am* 22:265–279, 1984.

Lufkin RB, Hanafee WN: Application of surface coils to MR anatomy of the larynx. *AJNR* 6:491–497, 1985.

Lufkin RB, Hanafee WN, Wortham D, et al: Larynx and hypopharynx: MR imaging with surface coils. *Radiology* 158:747–754, 1986.

Mafee MF, Schild JA, Michael AS, et al: Cartilage involvement in laryngeal carcinoma: correlation of CT and pathologic macrosection studies. *J Comput Assist Tomogr* 8:969–973, 1984.

Mafee MF, Schild JA, Valvassori GE, et al: CT of the larynx: correlation of anatomic and pathologic studies in cases of laryngeal carcinoma. *Radiology* 147:123–128, 1983.

Mancuso AA, Hanafee WN: CT of the injured larynx. *Radiology* 133:139–144, 1979.

Mancuso AA, Hanafee WN, Juillard GJF: The role of CT in the management of cancer of the larynx. *Radiology* 124:243–244, 1979.

Mancuso AA, Tamakawa Y, Hanafee WN: CT of the fixed vocal cord. *Am J Roentgenol* 135:429–434, 1980.

McGravan MH, Bauer WFC, Ogura JH: The incidence of cervical lymph node metastases from epidermoid carcinoma of the larynx and their relationship to certain characteristics of the primary tumor. *Cancer* 14:55–66, 1981.

Melgin AJ, Biedlingmaier JF, Mirvis SE: 3D CT in the evaluation of laryngeal injury. *Laryngoscope* 101:202–207, 1991.

Munoz A, Ramos A, Ferrando J, et al: Laryngeal carcinoma: sclerotic appearance of cricoid and arytenoid cartilage. CT-pathologic correlation. *Radiology* 189:433–437, 1993.

Nathan MD, El Gammal T, Hudson JH: CT in the assessment of thyroid cartilage invasion by laryngeal carcinoma: a prospective study. *Otolaryngol Head Neck Surg* 88:726–733, 1980.

Reid MH: Laryngeal carcinoma: high-resolution CT and thick anatomic sections. *Radiology* 151:689–696, 1984.

Sagel SS, Aufderheide JF, Aronbert DJ, et al: High resolution CT in the staging of carcinoma of the larynx. *Laryngoscope* 91:292–300, 1981.

Sakai F, Gamsu F, Dillon WP, et al: MR imaging of the larynx at 1.5T. *J Comput Assist Tomogr* 14:60–72, 1990.

Saleh EM, Mancuso AA, Stringer SP: CT of submucosal and occult laryngeal masses. *J Comput Assist Tomogr* 16:87–93, 1992.

Schaefer SD. The acute management of external laryngeal trauma. A 27-year experience. *Arch Otolaryngol Head Neck Surg* 118:598–604, 1992.

Schaefer SD, Brown OE: Selective application of CT in the management of laryngeal trauma. *Laryngoscope* 93:1473–1475, 1983.

Silverman PM, Korobkin M: High resolution CT of the normal larynx. *Am J Roentgenol* 140:875–879, 1983.

Wippold FJ, Smirniotopoulos JG, Moran CJ, et al: Chondrosarcoma of the larynx: CT features. *AJNR* 14:453–459, 1993.

II

Imaging of Primary and Nodal Squamous Cell Carcinoma

12

Squamous Cell Carcinoma: Primary Tumor Staging and Follow-Up

CRITICAL IMAGING QUESTIONS: PRIMARY TUMOR STAGING AND FOLLOW-UP OF SQUAMOUS CELL CARCINOMA

1. If primary squamous cell carcinoma is staged with CT or MRI, in what percentage of cases will the stage be upgraded from the initial clinical stage?
2. For each of the major areas of the upper aerodigestive tract, name the major clinical blind spots where CT or MRI will detect tumor that the clinician cannot feel or see.
3. In the follow-up radiologic evaluation of squamous cell carcinoma, at what point in time should a new primary tumor be called a *second primary lesion* and not a *primary site recurrence*?
4. Name the four major sites in the extracranial head and neck where unknown primary lesions hide.

Answers to these questions are found in the text beside the question number (Q#) in the margin.

RADIOLOGIC EVALUATION OF SQUAMOUS CELL CARCINOMA

A. Imaging issues in the staging and follow-up of squamous cell carcinoma in the head and neck.

1. Pretherapy questions:
   a. Clinical/radiologic stage determination. What is the objective clinical/radiologic stage (i.e., primary [T] and nodal [N]) of the squamous cell carcinoma (SCCa) lesion?
   b. Unknown primary tumor search. If needle biopsy of a neck node reveals SCCa but clinical examination shows no primary tumor, is there an "occult" primary tumor in the submucosal area?
   c. Radiation therapy port planning. What are the best radiation port configurations based on the radiologic evaluation?
2. Post-therapy questions:
   a. Treatment assessment. After the tumor has been treated with radiation therapy and/or chemotherapy, how has it responded?
   b. Tumor recurrence. Now that treatment (surgery and/or radiation therapy) has made the neck difficult to examine, has the tumor recurred?

B. Objective primary (T) and nodal (N) squamous cell carcinoma determination.

1. This section focuses on the process of staging primary SCCa tumor. Nodal staging is presented in Chapter 13. The advantages and disadvantages of CT versus MRI are discussed at the end of this chapter.
2. Either CT or MRI (CT/MRI) can be used effectively to stage the primary tumor and nodal disease in patients with SCCa.
3. CT/MRI provides an objective determination of the deep tissue extent of primary tumor and nodal disease compared with the more subjective clinical examination.
   a. Clinical staging of the primary tumor is based on the clinician's visual and tactile observations.
   b. Clinical assessment of the mucosal involvement by the primary tumor far exceeds radiographic assessment.
   c. The radiographic estimate of the deep tissue extent of the primary tumor usually exceeds the clinical estimate in accuracy.
   d. The most accurate pretreatment stage comes when the clinical stage is matched with the radiologic stage.
      1) The radiologist should not read the radiologic examination on a patient with SCCa in the upper aerodigestive tract without knowledge of the clinical stage. If the imaging study is interpreted without clinical input, serious interpretive errors will lead the clinician to cease using cross-sectional imaging in the staging process.

Q#1

2) When clinical/radiologic stage is compared with the pathologic stage, CT/MRI will upstage approximately 25% of cases.

3) CT/MRI does not detect the majority of mucosal lesions. In such a case the radiologist sees no deep tissue tumor on the scan and can suggest to the referring clinician that the primary tumor "be staged by mucosal extent alone."

4. Staging of primary tumor is divided by the major areas of the upper aerodigestive tract. Each individual area has unique clinical staging criteria.

   a. These clinical criteria readily translate into radiologic staging criteria.

   b. The specific criteria for each main anatomic region can be found in the American Joint Committee on Cancer *Manual for Staging of Cancer*. Anyone involved in the use of CT/MRI in staging SCCa of the head and neck should have a copy of this manual available for quick reference during the final review of each case.

   c. This manual can be obtained by writing the following address:

   The Executive Office American Joint Committee on Cancer
   55 East Erie Street
   Chicago, Illinois 60611

   Ask for a copy of the manual entitled *Manual for Staging of Cancer* (4th ed, 1992), published by J.B. Lippincott. The 5th edition will be available in mid-1995.

   d. Table 12-1 provides an abbreviated version of these staging criteria by primary tumor site. Most of the clinical staging terminology can be translated directly into radiologic staging terminology.

   e. Table 12-2 defines what structures or subsites are included in each of the major SCCa-bearing areas of the extracranial head and neck.

5. Primary tumor staging issues by site.

   a. The important clinical deep tissue staging issues that may cause difficulty in arriving at a primary tumor stage are listed here for each major area of the upper aerodigestive tract. Imaging increases the overall accuracy of the pretreatment stage because of these relative clinical blind spots.

Q#2

   b. Nasopharynx SCCa.

   1) Clinical presentation.

      a) The ratio of men to women is 2:1.

      b) Unilateral middle-ear fluid in an adult should trigger the search for nasopharyngeal carcinoma.

      c) If deeply invasive, any mixture of cranial nerve IX, X, XI, and XII neuropathy may be seen.

Table 12-1 Staging Criteria for Primary Squamous Cell Carcinoma by Site

Nasopharynx

T1: Tumor confined to one subsite in nasopharynx or no visible tumor (biopsy positive only)

T2: Tumor invades more than one subsite* in the nasopharynx

T3: Tumor invades nasal cavity and/or oropharynx

T4: Tumor involves skull base, cranial nerves, or both

Oropharynx

T1: Tumor is 2 cm or less in its greatest dimension

T2: Tumor is more than 2 cm but not more than 4 cm in its greatest dimension

T3: Tumor is more than 4 cm in its greatest dimension

T4: Tumor invades adjacent structures, including bone (mandible or maxilla), soft tissues of the neck, or deep (extrinsic) muscles of the tongue

Hypopharynx

T1: Tumor limited to one subsite of the hypopharynx

T2: Tumor invades more than one hypopharyngeal subsite* or adjacent site without hemilarynx fixation

T3: Tumor invades more than one hypopharyngeal subsite or adjacent site with hemilarynx fixation

T4: Tumor invades adjacent structures; thyroid or cricoid cartilage, or soft tissues of the neck

Oral Cavity

T1: Tumor is 2 cm or less in its greatest dimension

T2: Tumor more than 2 cm but not more than 4 cm in its greatest dimension

T3: Tumor more than 4 cm in its greatest dimension

T4: Tumor invades adjacent structures, including mandible, maxilla, skin, extrinsic tongue muscles, and soft tissues of the neck

Larynx: Supraglottis

T1: Tumor limited to one subsite of the supraglottis with normal cord mobility

T2: Tumor invades more than one subsite* of supraglottis or glottis while preserving normal cord mobility

T3: Tumor limited to the larynx with fixation of the vocal cord, and/or invades the postcricoid area, medial wall of the pyriform sinus, or pre-epiglottic space

T4: Tumor extends beyond larynx to the oropharyngeal soft tissues of the neck and/or invades the thyroid cartilage

Larynx: Glottis

T1: Tumor limited to one or both vocal cords with normal mobility (may include involvement of the anterior or posterior commissures)

T2: Tumor extends into supraglottic and/or subglottic areas with normal or impaired vocal cord mobility

T3: Endolaryngeal tumor only with cord fixation

(continued)

Table 12-1 *(continued)*

T4: Tumor invades thyroid cartilage and/or into the adjacent soft tissues of the neck

Larynx: Subglottis
  T1: Tumor confined to the subglottis
  T2: Tumor invades one or both vocal cords with normal or impaired cord mobility
  T3: Endolaryngeal tumor only with cord fixation
  T4: Tumor invades thyroid or cricoid cartilage and/or extends to the soft tissues of the neck

Maxillary Sinus
  T1: Tumor limited to the antral mucosa with no erosion or destruction of bone
  T2: Tumor erodes or destroys antral infrastructure, including hard palate and/or middle nasal meatus
  T3: Tumor invades skin of cheek, posterior wall maxillary sinus, floor or medial wall orbit, or anterior ethmoid sinus
  T4: Tumor invades orbital contents and/or cribriform plate, ethmoid or sphenoid sinuses, nasopharynx, soft palate, pterygopalatine fossa or masticator space, or skull base

Adapted from American Joint Committee on Cancer: *Manual for staging of cancer, edn 4.* Philadelphia, 1992, JB Lippincott. Used with permission.

*Each of the major areas where squamous cell carcinoma is found in the extracranial head and neck has multiple subsites within it (as summarized in Table 12-2).

2) Nodal manifestations at presentation.
  a) Nodal metastases are present in 90%.
  b) When the nodal mass is present with normal mucosal surfaces, a submucosal "unknown" primary in the nasopharynx is the most common cause.
3) Clinical blind spots where radiologic staging may be helpful.
  a) CT/MRI is mandatory in all cases of nasopharyngeal carcinoma, because the area is so inaccessible to clinical examination.
  b) MRI is the better tool in this area because of its multiplanar capabilities and sensitivity to intracranial extension.
  c) Nasal cavity involvement (T3) or intracranial/skull base invasion (T4) may be discovered at the time of imaging even if there is no clinical suspicion.
4) Treatment options.
  a) Nasopharyngeal carcinoma is the "oat cell carcinoma" of the head and neck. Both radiotherapy and chemotherapy are used in the treatment of this tumor. Surgery usually is reserved only for diagnostic biopsy purposes.

Table 12-2   Subsites Included in Each Primary Squamous Cell Carcinoma Site

Nasopharynx
  Posterosuperior wall
  Lateral wall (fossa of Rosenmuller)
  Inferior (anterior) wall

Oropharynx
  Anterior wall (glossoepiglottic area)
    Tongue base (posterior one third of tongue)
    Vallecula
  Lateral wall
    Faucial tonsil
    Tonsillar fossa
    Glossotonsillar sulci
  Posterior wall
  Superior wall
    Inferior surface of the soft palate
    Uvula

Hypopharynx
  Pyriform sinus
  Postcricoid area
  Posterior pharyngeal wall

Oral cavity
  Lip
  Buccal mucosa
  Lower alveolar ridge
  Upper alveolar ridge
  Retromolar trigone (gingiva)
  Floor of mouth
  Hard palate
  Anterior two thirds of tongue (oral tongue)

Larynx: supraglottis
  False vocal cord
  Arytenoids
  Epiglottis (both lingual and laryngeal aspects)
    Suprahyoid epiglottis
    Infrahyoid epiglottis
  Aryepiglottic folds

Larynx: glottis
  True vocal cords
    Anterior commissure
    Posterior commissure   (*continued*)

Table 12-2   (*continued*)

Larynx: subglottis
Subglottis to the first tracheal ring

Maxillary sinus
Anteroinferior portion (infrastructure)
Superoposterior portion (suprastructure)

Adapted from American Joint Committee on Cancer: *Manual for staging of cancer*, edn 4. Philadelphia, 1992, JB Lippincott. Used with permission.

  b) Radiotherapy is the mainstay of treatment for nasopharyngeal SCCa. The sagittal and coronal images provided by MRI are very useful in planning the boost-field ports.
 c. Oropharyngeal SCCa.
   1) Clinical presentations.
     a) When combined, oropharyngeal and oral cavity SCCa form 5% of all malignant tumors in the United States.
     b) Presents initially as a painless, nonhealing ulcer on the mucosal surface of the oropharynx.
     c) With increasing size of the tumor, the patient complains of pain, induration, and infiltration of the underlying tissues and regional lymphadenopathy.
     d) Tumors of the tongue base (i.e., lingual tonsil) and faucial tonsil area cause early symptoms, including severe pain on swallowing, thick and indistinct speech, mucosal ulceration, and focal increase in the size of the tonsil. Referred pain to the ear (i.e., otalgia) may be part of the clinical presentation.
     e) In advanced cases (i.e., stage T4 lesions) trismus signals masticator space invasion, chin numbness signals mandibular invasion with inferior alveolar nerve injury, and tongue muscle fasciculations/atrophy signal injury to the neurovascular pedicle in the posterior sublingual space.
   2) Nodal manifestations at presentation.
     a) Sixty percent of patients have malignant adenopathy at presentation; 15% have bilateral nodes.
     b) First-order drainage is into the high deep cervical chain (i.e., jugulodigastric node). From there drainage usually is down the deep cervical chain, but it is possible for the spinal accessory chain to receive nodal spread with more posterior oropharyngeal tumors.
   3) Clinical blind spots where radiologic staging may be helpful.
     a) Objective size of primary tumor:
       i) T1. Two cm or less in its greatest dimension.

      ii) T2. More than 2 cm but not more than 4 cm in its greatest dimension.

      iii) T3. More than 4 cm in its greatest dimension.

  b) T4 is designated when the tumor invades the bone of the mandible or maxilla, soft tissue of the neck, or tongue root.

  c) Soft palate SCCa may spread perineurally along the greater palatine nerve to the pterygopalatine fossa (V_2 spread) and from there via the foramen rotundum intracranially.

  d) Faucial tonsillar SCCa may invade deeply into the adjacent masticator space, proceeding from there on the V_3 branches to the skull base, foramen ovale, and intracranially.

  e) Lingual tonsil SCCa may invade deeply into the back of the sublingual space of the oral tongue, involving the neurovascular pedicle (i.e., lingual artery, cranial nerves IX and XII, and lingual nerve).

  f) Posterior oropharyngeal wall SCCa may invade deeply to involve the retropharyngeal space either directly or via drainage to retropharyngeal lymph nodes. If invasion continues posteriorly, the prevertebral aspect of the perivertebral space is involved next.

4) Treatment options.

  a) Complete surgical excision combined with radiotherapy remains the mainstay of treatment for oropharyngeal SCCa. Soft-tissue defects often require flaps for reconstruction.

  b) Suprahyoid or complete ipsilateral neck dissection often accompanies surgery because of the high incidence of known nodal metastases.

  d. Hypopharyngeal SCCa.

  1) Clinical presentation.

    a) More than 40% of patients present because of lymph node metastases in the jugulodigastric region (i.e., angle of the mandible).

    b) Patients also may present with dysphagia and otalgia (i.e., pain radiating to the ear).

    c) In advanced cases hoarseness and difficulty breathing signal endolaryngeal invasion.

  2) Nodal manifestations at presentation.

    a) Fifty percent of patients present as T3N1–2 tumors.

    b) Adenopathy is unilateral when the primary is in the pyriform sinus. Adenopathy is more often bilateral when the primary is in the posterior hypopharyngeal wall or postcricoid in location.

  3) Clinical blind spots where radiologic staging may be helpful.

    a) Fixation of the hemilarynx by a large lesion obscuring endolarynx from direct view (i.e., stage T3).

    b) Invasion of bone or soft tissues of the neck (i.e., stage T4).

     4) Treatment options.

        a) Primary tumors are advanced at presentation, and nodal metastases are common.

        b) Surgery usually is extensive, requiring pharyngectomy or laryngopharyngectomy (if larynx is invaded). Musculocutaneous flaps from the neck or chest wall often are necessary.

        c) Unilateral or bilateral neck dissection usually is necessary depending on the clinical and radiologic evidence for nodal metastases.

        d) Radiotherapy before or after surgery is routine.

  e. Oral cavity SCCa.

     1) Clinical presentations. See Chapter 8.

     2) Nodal manifestations at presentation. See Chapter 8.

     3) Clinical blind spots where radiologic staging may be helpful.

        a) Objective size of primary tumor up to stage T3.

        b) Invasion of the maxillary antrum, pterygoid muscles, or tongue base with stage T4 primary tumor.

  f. Laryngeal SCCa.

     1) For details, see Chapter 11.

     2) Clinical blind spots where radiologic staging may be helpful.

        a) Supraglottic SCCa.

          i) Pre-epiglottic space tumor (stage T3).

          ii) Invasion of soft tissues of the neck (stage T4).

          iii) Thyroid cartilage destruction (stage T4).

        b) Glottic SCCa.

          i) Subglottic or supraglottic submucosal extension (stage T2).

          ii) Tumor extension outside the larynx (stage T4).

          iii) Thyroid cartilage destruction (stage T4).

        c) Subglottic SCCa.

          i) Tumor extension beyond laryngeal confines (stage T4).

          ii) Cartilage destruction: Cricoid or thyroid (stage T4).

  g. Maxillary sinus SCCa.

     1) Clinical presentation.

        a) Because the presenting signs and symptoms are similar to those of sinusitis (i.e., nasal obstruction, postobstructive sinusitis), these tumors often are diagnosed late, when the tumor has already infiltrated the adjacent deep tissues.

     2) Clinical blind spots where radiologic staging may be helpful.

        a) Infrastructure (stage T1) versus suprastructure (stage T2) involvement.

        b) Tumor invasion of cheek, orbit, anterior ethmoid sinuses, or pterygoid muscles (stage T3).

        c) Tumor invasion of cribriform plate, posterior ethmoid sinuses, or sphenoid sinus (stage T4).

6. Perineural tumor spread from SCCa primary tumor.
   a. Any malignancy can spread perineurally. SCCa is the most common tumor to spread in a perineural fashion, because it is by far the most common head and neck malignancy. Minor salivary gland malignancy (i.e., adenoid cystic carcinoma, mucoepidermoid carcinoma) and lymphoma, however, also undergo perineural spread in the extracranial head and neck.
   b. Because perineural spread is a direct extension of the tumor, its recognition is critical to the initial, complete resection of the primary tumor. Complete surgical resection remains the single best therapy for head and neck malignancy.
   c. The most commonly involved cranial nerves are the trigeminal (i.e., mandibular [V_3] and maxillary [V_2] divisions) and the facial nerve.
      1) When tumor involves the maxillary sinus, the pterygopalatine fossa and foramen rotundum need careful inspection. These are the major anatomic landmarks through which the maxillary division of the trigeminal nerve runs.
      2) Tumor located in the masticator space and spreading laterally from the nasopharyngeal and oropharyngeal mucosal space can access the foramen ovale via the mandibular division of the trigeminal nerve. Perimandibular lesions also may spread in a perineural fashion along cranial nerve V_3 by accessing the inferior alveolar nerve in the bony canal in the mandible.
      3) Parotid space tumors access the temporal bone along the facial nerve through the stylomastoid foramen.
   d. Thin-section, contrast-enhanced, fat-saturated, T1-weighted MRI scans in the axial and coronal planes best demonstrate perineural tumor. Perineural tumor is seen as perineural thickening and enhancement, with widening of the affected foramen.
   e. When the cavernous sinus is reached by the perineural tumor, MRI scans show a mass within the sinus, lateral bowing of the dura (which forms the wall), and/or narrowing or displacement of the cavernous carotid artery.
   f. It is important to identify perineural spread of tumor on the pretreatment radiologic examination. This tumor is contiguous to the primary tumor mass and must be resected during the initial surgical treatment for a surgical cure to be achieved.

C. Diagnosis of tumor recurrence with CT/MRI.

1. The radiated and/or operated neck resembles leather to the palpating hand. In 25% of cases, radiologic evaluation alone will be the only method of diagnosing tumor recurrence.

2. Submucosal tumor recurrence and some high nodal recurrences can be impossible to diagnose by clinical examination. This is especially true in more obese patients.
   a. Nodal recurrence in the retropharyngeal chain or beneath postradiated skin may be difficult to diagnose by palpation.
3. Both the primary site and nodal recurrence should be evaluated when imaging is used to search for recurrent SCCa.

Q#3

4. If it is over 2 years since the patient's initial tumor treatment, any lesion found should be staged as a second primary tumor, because the vast majority of SCCa lesions that recur do so within 2 years of their first diagnosis and therapy.
5. Patients at high risk for tumor recurrence based on the initial stage or poor surgical result may benefit from close radiologic follow-up in the first 2 years following treatment.
   a. Recommendation. Perform a baseline radiologic study 3 months after therapy. This information facilitates the diagnosis of recurrence if a growing mass is seen on follow-up examination.

D. Unknown primary tumor search.

1. "Unknown primary."
   a. Definition. Needle biopsy diagnosis of malignant SCCa in the neck nodes is made and no obvious primary SCCa can be seen on any mucosal surface of the upper aerodigestive tract.
   b. This patient subpopulation may benefit from imaging to search for a hidden or submucosal primary.
   c. Directed therapy to the primary site may be instituted if the primary is identified.

Q#4

2. Frequent sites of unknown primary.
   a. Nasopharynx, especially in the lateral pharyngeal recess.
   b. Pyriform sinus, most inferior aspect (i.e., apex).
   c. Faucial and lingual tonsillar crypts.
   d. A scan ordered to search for the unknown primary must include all of these areas. Because lymph nodes also should be staged during this examination, the imaging study must cover the entire neck from the skull base to the clavicles.
3. Why the clinician cannot see tumor in these locations.
   a. In the case of the nasopharynx 20% of the tumors found are submucosal. The natural undulations of the nasopharynx make identification of smaller mucosal lesions difficult.
   b. In the tongue base the SCCa spreads into the root of the tongue from the deeper crypts of the lingual tonsil. Faucial tonsillar crypts also

will hide primary tumors when the lesion dives into the adjacent deep tissues.

    c. Pyriform sinus tumor that is undetectable on the initial clinical examination usually lurks in the inferior recess of the pyriform sinus, beyond the sight of the inspecting eye.

4. The role of imaging in the setting of an "unknown primary" is to:

    a. Identify the primary tumor site.

    b. If none is found, suggest possible sites to biopsy (i.e., "suspicious" sites on CT/MRI scans).

    c. Stage the nodal disease in the neck.

E. Assessment with imaging of squamous cell carcinoma treatment.

1. Imaging is most helpful when the lesion under treatment is inaccessible to sight or touch.

2. Radiation therapy or chemotherapy response is easily evaluated by CT/MRI.

3. Early clinical trials suggest that MRI may be more sensitive than CT in evaluating tumor response to radiation therapy especially in nasopharyngeal carcinoma.

F. Radiation therapy port planning.

1. To date CT has functioned to help with planning radiation treatment. CT is limited compared with MRI in tumor versus normal tissue differentiation. CT also lacks MRI's multiplanar capabilities.

2. MRI provides excellent assistance here, in that its coronal and sagittal images can be translated directly onto anterior–posterior and lateral-simulation films.

3. Once the radiologist becomes familiar with the anatomy of the extracranial head and neck, especially near the skull base, he or she can greatly assist the radiation therapist by accurately depicting the tumor on simulation films.

G. CT vs. MRI in evaluating squamous cell carcinoma.

1. The choice of technology depends on the availability, expertise, and experience of the radiologist, and on the quality of the CT vs. MRI equipment available.

2. Either technology can objectively stage any T2 or greater SCCa of the upper aerodigestive tract.

3. Advantages of CT.

    a. Fast acquisition times (i.e., 1 sec/slice vs. spiral acquisition). Especially important in the case of bulky tumor that requires patient to swallow continually (too much motion for MRI). Patients with excessive respiratory motion secondary to accompanying lung disease also will benefit from CT.

      b. CT is a more "open system" with a lower rate of claustrophobia than MRI.

      c. CT is sensitive to bone destruction (e.g., mandible and skull base). As we become more familiar with MRI interpretation, however, we find much of this information also is present in the MRI scan.

      d. Nodal architecture. CT uses the low density within neck nodes as a malignant signature. MRI does not see an equivalent signature without the use of T1-weighted contrast-enhancement or T2-weighted images.

      e. CT is significantly less expensive than MRI, especially when contrast is used during MRI.

      f. Patients with absolute contraindications to MRI (e.g., cardiac pacemakers) can be imaged using CT.

4. Advantages of MRI.

      a. No iodinated contrast is necessary.

         1) Patients allergic to contrast or with renal failure can be imaged.

         2) There is limited risk of allergic reaction or renal damage from MRI contrast.

      b. No radiation is necessary.

         1) Patients who are pregnant will not have unnecessary exposure to radiation from MRI.

         2) Patients who will be imaged repeatedly will not accumulate a significant radiation dose from MRI.

      c. Multiplanar acquisition. Coronal and sagittal views can be obtained without patient discomfort. These images are more useful to the radiotherapist in port planning.

      d. Dental artifact. MRI is frequently unaffected by dental amalgam artifact in the oropharynx/oral cavity as compared with CT.

      e. Soft-tissue contrast. MRI is superior to CT is providing soft-tissue contrast, which provides greater lesion conspicuity and definition of tumor–normal soft tissue margins. This is especially true in the nasopharynx, oropharynx, and oral cavity. MRI "sees through" dental amalgam artifact in the oropharynx and oral cavity that may completely obscure the lesion on CT.

      f. MRI is a technology "on the move." With continued development of millisecond imaging techniques, spectroscopy, and node-seeking contrast agents, MR eventually may exceed all advantages of CT.

5. Appearance of SCCa primary tumor on CT/MRI.

      a. Tumor appearance by CT.

         1) SCCa primary tumor generally shows mild contrast enhancement during CT scanning.

         2) Tumor margins often are difficult to discern when the tumor abuts or invades adjacent muscle or lymphoid tissue in Waldeyer's ring.

3) Tumor margins usually are better defined on MRI scans because of the many different looks provided by this modality.
   a) T1-weighted, dual-echo T2-weighted, and contrast-enhanced fat-saturated images give the radiologist five different looks at the tumor margin.

b. Tumor appearance by MRI.
   1) SCCa generally is isointense to muscle and hypointense to fat on T1-weighted MRI, with mild to moderate hyperintensity observed on T2-weighted imaging.
   2) Some degree of enhancement usually is seen in primary SCCa when MRI contrast is employed with T1-weighted imaging. When combined with fat-saturation techniques, reregistration of the gray scale creates the appearance of significant tumor enhancement.
   3) Loss of tumor margins when adjacent to fatty areas in enhanced, T1-weighted images has been touted as a potential major imaging pitfall. In practice the combination of nonenhanced, T1-weighted images with dual-echo T2-weighted images fills in the needed information when the tumor margin abuts fat.

H. CT and MRI protocols for staging of SCCa.

1. CT imaging protocol in head and neck malignancy.
   a. CT protocols vary depending on the site of the primary tumor.
   b. In general the more inferior the primary tumor, the lower in the extracranial head and neck the scan can begin.
   1) Extent of CT scan.
      a) Primary tumor of the nasopharynx requires the most extensive scan extent. Axial images are obtained from the skull base to the clavicles.
      b) With oropharyngeal primary tumors the scan begins at the hard palate and extends to the clavicles. In a very rare circumstance a large, invasive primary oropharyngeal SCCa can spread uphill into the nasopharynx. This rare patient can be brought back for further imaging at a later time.
      c) Oral cavity tumors often are obscured at least in part by dental amalgam spray artifact. Begin the scan at the lower margin of the mandibular fillings seen on the preliminary scout scanogram, and continue it inferiorly to the clavicles.
      d) Hypopharyngeal laryngeal tumors also only require scanning the neck below the mandibular fillings. The inferior margin is to the clavicles.
      e) Thyroid malignancy, although not a SCCa, is mentioned here as a reminder that unlike staging SCCa, the inferior extent of

thyroid malignancy scanning is the aortic arch. Why? Because again unlike SCCa, thyroid malignancy spreads via the paratracheal chain directly into the superior mediastinum. SCCa never drains primarily into the mediastinum, so the CT scans can be terminated at the clavicles.

c. Both the primary tumor and nodal drainage of the tumor are imaged at the same sitting. This is so a radiographic primary tumor stage (T) and nodal stage (N) can be rendered in the report.

d. Routine factors for all primary sites include:
   1) kvp = 120.
   2) mAs ≥ 300 in all cases; higher through facial bones or in the cervical–thoracic junction.
   3) Slice thickness = 5-mm contiguous.
      a) When the lesion is small or margins indistinct, 3-mm, contiguous axial images through the tumor as a second pass may help to define tumor better.
      b) When the primary tumor is in the hypopharynx/larynx, 3-mm axial images are critical to obtain after the 5-mm images are taken. The 5-mm images are used to look for adenopathy, while the 3-mm images are used to stage the primary tumor. (See Chapter 11 for further technical details.)
   4) Contrast is used in all cases. Maximum intravascular contrast is sought by using an initial 50-mL bolus of 240 mg of iodinated contrast per milliliter, followed by rapid drip of another 100 mL of 240 mg of iodinated contrast per milliliter.
      a) If an injector is used along with dynamic or spiral imaging, the initial contrast bolus is given at 2 mL/sec for a total a 60 mL. A 30 second scan delay is employed to deliver the starting bolus. The remaining contrast is then delivered at 1 mL/sec up to a total of 90 mL.
      b) Either strategy allows the use of one 150-mL bottle only containing 240 mg of iodinated contrast per milliliter. This becomes very important if nonionic contrast is selected.
   5) Scan plane is axial in all cases.
      a) Coronal CT images are obtained only when the lesion is orbital, sinonasal, or nasopharyngeal.
      b) Axial images are angled around the fillings if this area is being scanned ("butterfly technique").
      c) When the primary is in the hypopharynx/larynx, the axial scan plane is parallel to the true vocal cords. Use the line of the hyoid bone if you are not comfortable with this concept. The gantry usually is angled approximately 10° to 15° toward the feet.

2. MRI protocol in head and neck malignancy.

    a. An anterior or anterior–posterior neck coil is essential to imaging the neck with MRI. The head coil is used only if the lesion is high in the oropharyngeal or in the nasopharynx proper. With oropharyngeal or nasopharyngeal primary tumors a neck coil is still needed to evaluate the cervical neck for malignant adenopathy.

    b. Routine use of water bags (or bags with Kaopectate in them) on the cervical neck creates a more uniform imaging volume at the junction of the chin and the cervical neck. This significantly reduces the bulk susceptibility artifacts that may lead to asymmetric fat-suppression in this area.

        1) The asymmetric fat-suppression artifact seen at the level of the hyoid bone results when no water bags are used during fat-suppression, postcontrast, T1-weighted imaging.

        2) Under these circumstances the volume change from tissue at the chin level and above and that below causes a change in the main magnetic field.

        3) These magnetic field inhomogeneities in turn cause water/fat frequency shifts within the imaging volume.

        4) As a result a presaturation, fat-selective radiofrequency pulse (fat sat) that overlies the fat frequency in one portion of the imaging volume may overlie the water frequency in a different portion of the imaging volume. It then becomes theoretically possible for a fat-saturated image to obscure a lesion through asymmetric suppression of the water signal in that lesion.

        5) Remember to remove the water bags for T2-weighted imaging; they will become very bright and cause gray-scale distortion. If commercially available bags or Kaopectate-filled bags are used, removal during T2-weighted imaging is not necessary.

    c. Patient instructions.

        1) Motion is the enemy of good head and neck imaging by MRI.

        2) Both the technologist and patient being aware of this fact goes a long way toward solving this problem.

        3) Specific instructions regarding quiet respiration, coughing, swallowing, tongue motion, and eye motion are necessary in all cases.

    d. Scan planes.

        1) Coronal, T1-weighted, localizing images recommended (TR/TE/NEX, 800/30/2; 4 mm with a 0.5-mm interslice gap). This coronal image is especially important in the case of lesions of the high oropharynx, nasopharynx, skull base, sinonasal area, orbit, and larynx (Use 3 mm with a 0.5-mm interslice gap in the larynx).

2) Axial T1-weighted, precontrast images (TR/TE/NEX, 800/30/2; 4 mm with a 0.5-mm skip slice) through lesion and first-order lymph nodes.

3) Axial T2-weighted (standard spin-echo sequence; TR/TE/NEX, 2500/30–90/2; 4 mm with a 0.1-mm skip slice or dual-echo, fast-spin echo) through primary lesion and nodal drainage. The technologist should match the T1- and T2-weighted axial images as closely as possible so that crosscomparison is easily accomplished.

4) Postcontrast, T1-weighted images in the axial and coronal planes with the same techniques as above and the addition of fat suppression in the axial plane.

   a) Routine use of contrast is controversial. When any question of perineural, intracranial, orbital, or extradural extension is present, contrast both with and without fat suppression is recommended.

   b) When postcontrast, fat-saturation, T1-weighted images are obtained, reregistration of the gray scale creates the appearance of significant tumor enhancement. This technique is at times very useful in defining the deep tissue extent of the tumor.

   c) Fat-saturated, postcontrast, T1-weighted images in the area of the orbit, nose, sinus, skull base, and temporal bone may be affected adversely by magnetic-susceptibility artifact produced at the air–bone interfaces. This "blooming" signal void may obscure both normal and diseased anatomy. Axial images generally are less affected than coronal images through these areas.

   d) Fat-saturated, postcontrast, T1-weighted images through the orbit often will display high signal in the area of intraconal fat. If dental amalgam is asymmetric, this signal may be very asymmetric in one orbit, simulating pathology. The high signal results from asymmetric fat suppression. The presaturation pulse misses the fat frequency in that area, resulting in a focal area where no fat suppression has occurred on the T1-weighted, fat-suppressed image (i.e., high-signal retroglobar area).

e. Additional imaging parameters to suppress image artifacts.

1) Flow compensation used in all sequences as possible.

2) Presaturation pulses (sat bands) placed as appropriate.

3) Phase-encoding gradients should be placed in the anterior–posterior direction. This puts the phase-encoding artifacts commonly seen in association with blood flow in vessels in the anterior–posterior direction and not across the tissues of the neck.

SUGGESTED READING

General References

Barakos J, Dillon WP, Chew WM: Orbit, skull base, and pharynx: contrast-enhanced fat suppression MR imaging. *Radiology* 179:191–198, 1991.

Beahrs OH, Henson DE, Hutter RVP, et al (American Joint Committee on Cancer), editors: *Manual for staging of cancer*, edn 4. Philadelphia, 1992, JB Lippincott.

Dillon WP, Harnsberger HR: The impact of radiologic imaging on staging of cancer of the head and neck. *Semin Oncol Hematol* 18:64–79, 1991.

Gatenby RA, Mulhern CB, Strawitz J, et al: Comparison of clinical and CT staging of head and neck tumors. *AJNR* 6:399–401, 1985.

Gussack GS, Hudgins PA: Imaging modalities in recurrent head and neck tumors. *Laryngoscope* 101:119–124, 1991.

Harnsberger HR, Dillon WP: The radiologic role in diagnosis, staging, and follow-up of neoplasia of the brain, spine, and head and neck. *Semin Ultrasound CT MR* 10:431–452, 1989.

Harnsberger HR, Mancuso AA, Muraki AS: The upper aerodigestive tract and neck: CT evaluation of recurrent tumors. *Radiology* 159:503–509, 1983.

Mancuso AA, Hanafee WN: Elusive head and neck carcinomas beneath intact mucosa. *Laryngoscope* 93:133–139, 1983.

Marchant FE, Lowry LD, Moffitt JJ, et al: Current national trends in post treatment follow-up of patients with squamous cell carcinoma of the head and neck. *Am J Otolaryngol* 14:88–93, 1993.

Parker GD, Harnsberger HR: Clinical-radiologic issues in perineural tumor spread of malignant diseases of the extracranial head and neck. *RadioGraphics* 11:383–399, 1991.

Schaefer SD, Merkel M, Burns DK, et al: CT of upper aerodigestive tract squamous cell carcinoma: assessment following induction chemotherapy. *Arch Otolaryngol* 110:236–240, 1984.

Tien RD, Hesselink JR, Chu PK, et al: Improved detection and delineation of head and neck lesions with fat suppression spin-echo MR imaging. *AJNR* 12:19–24, 1991.

Nasopharyngeal Carcinoma

Bass IS, Haller JO, Berdon WE: Nasopharyngeal carcinoma: clinical and radiographic findings in children. *Radiology* 156:651–654, 1985.

Dillon WP, Mills CM, Kjos B, et al: Magnetic resonance imaging of the nasopharynx. *Radiology* 152:731–738, 1984.

Hoover LA, Hanafee WN: Differential diagnosis of nasopharyngeal tumors by CT scanning. *Arch Otolaryngol* 109:43–47, 1983.

Hudgins PA, Gussack GS: MR imaging in the management of extracranial malignant tumors of the head and neck. *Am J Roentgenol* 159:161–169, 1992.

Mancuso AA, Bohman L, Hanafee W, et al: CT of the nasopharynx: normal and variants of normal. *Radiology* 137:113–121, 1980.

Moloy PJ, Chung YT, Krivitsky PB, et al: Squamous cell carcinoma of the nasopharynx. *West J Med* 143:66–69, 1985.

Silver AJ, Mawad ME, Hilal SK, et al: CT of the nasopharynx and related spaces. Part II: pathology. *Radiology* 147:733–738, 1983.

Teresi LM, Lufkin RB, Vinuela F, et al: MR imaging of the nasopharynx and floor of the middle cranial fossa. Part II. Malignant tumors. *Radiology* 164:817–821, 1987.

Vogl T, Dresel S, Bilaniuk LT, et al. Tumors of the nasopharynx and adjacent areas: MR imaging with Gd-DTPA. *AJNR* 11:187–194, 1990.

Oropharyngeal Carcinoma

Larson SG, Mancuso AA, Hanafee WN: CT of the tongue and floor of mouth. *Radiology* 143:493–500, 1992.

Muraki AS, Mancuso AA, Harnsberger HR, et al: CT of the oropharynx, tongue base, floor of mouth: normal anatomy and range of variations, and applications in staging carcinoma. *Radiology* 148:725–731, 1983.

Schaefer SD, Merkel M, Diehl J: CT assessment of squamous cell carcinoma of the oral and pharyngeal cavities. *Arch Otolaryngol* 108:688–692, 1982.

Oral-Cavity Carcinoma

Takashima S, Ikezoe J, Harada K, et al: Tongue cancer: correlation of MR imaging and sonography with pathology. *AJNR* 10:419–424, 1989.

Teichgraeber JF, Clairmont AA: The incidence of occult metastases for cancer of the oral tongue and floor of the mouth: treatment rationale. *Head Neck* 7:15–21, 1984.

Hypopharyngeal and Laryngeal Carcinoma

Archer CR, Yeager VL: CT of laryngeal carcinoma with histopathological correlation. *Laryngoscope* 92:1173–1180, 1982.

Archer CR, Yeager VL, Herbold DR: CT versus histology of laryngeal cancer: the value in predicting laryngeal cartilage invasion. *Laryngoscope* 93:140–147, 1983.

Archer CR, Yeager VL, Herbold DR: Improved diagnostic accuracy in the TNM staging of laryngeal carcinoma using a new definition of regions based upon CT. *J Comput Assist Tomogr* 7:610–617, 1983.

Castelijns JA, Doornbos JN, Verbeeten B: MR imaging of the normal larynx. *J Comput Assist Tomogr* 9:919–925, 1985.

Disantis DJ, Balfe DM, Hayden RE, et al: The neck after total laryngectomy: CT study. *Radiology* 153:713–717, 1984.

Hoover LA, Calcaterra TC, Walter GA, et al: Preoperative evaluation for laryngeal carcinoma: correlation with pathological findings. *Laryngoscope* 94:310–315, 1984.

Isaacs JJ, Mancuso AA, Mendenhall WM, et al: Deep spread patterns in CT staging of T2–4 squamous cell laryngeal carcinoma. *Otolaryngol Head Neck Surg* 99:455–464, 1988.

Larsson S, Mancuso AA, Hoover L, et al: Differentiation of pyriform sinus cancer from supraglottic laryngeal cancer by CT. *Radiology* 141:427–432, 1981.

Lufkin RB, Hanafee WN: Application of surface coils to MR anatomy of the larynx. *AJNR* 6:491–497, 1985.

Lufkin RB, Hanafee WN, Wortham D, et al: Larynx and hypopharynx: MR imaging with surface coils. *Radiology* 158:747–754, 1986.

Mafee MF, Schield JA, Michael AS, et al: Cartilage involvement in laryngeal carcinoma: correlation of CT and pathologic macro section studies. *J Comput Assist Tomogr* 8:969–973, 1984.

Mafee MF, Schield JA, Valvassori GE, et al: CT of the larynx: correlation with anatomic and pathologic studies in cases of laryngeal carcinoma. *Radiology* 147:123–128, 1983.

Mancuso AA, Hanafee WN, Julliard GF, et al: The role of CT in management of cancer of the larynx. *Radiology* 124:243–244, 1977.

Reid MH: Laryngeal carcinoma: high resolution CT and thick anatomic sections. *Radiology* 151:689–696, 1984.

Sagel SS, AufderHeide JF, Aronberg DJ, et al: High resolution CT in the staging of carcinoma of the larynx. *Laryngoscope* 91:292–300, 1981.

Saleh EM, Mancuso AA, Stringer SP: Relative roles of CT and endoscopy for determining the inferior extent of pyriform sinus carcinoma: correlative histopathologic study. *Head Neck* 15:44–52, 1993.

Scott M, Forsted DH, Rominger J, et al: CT evaluation of laryngeal neoplasms. *Radiology* 140:141–144, 1981.

Silverman PM, Bossen EH, Fisher SR, et al: Carcinoma of the larynx and hypopharynx: CT-histopathologic correlations. *Radiology* 151:697–702, 1984.

Sinonasal Malignancy

Gadeberg CC, Hjelm-Hansen M, Sogaard H, et al: Malignant tumours of the paranasal sinuses and nasal cavity. *Acta Radiologica Oncology* 23:181–187, 1984.

Hasso AN: CT of tumors and tumor-like conditions of the paranasal sinuses. *Radiol Clin North Am* 22:119–130, 1984.

Hesselink JR, New PFJ, Davis KR, et al: CT of the paranasal sinuses and face. Part II: pathological anatomy. *J Comput Assist Tomogr* 2:568–576, 1978.

Kondo M, Horiuchi M, Shiga H, et al: CT of malignant tumors of the nasal cavity and paranasal sinuses. *Cancer* 50:226–231, 1982.

Kondo M, Ogawa K, Inuyama Y, et al: Prognostic factors influencing relapse of squamous cell carcinoma of the maxillary sinus. *Cancer* 55:190–196, 1985.

Lanzieri CF, Shah M, Krauss D, et al: Use of gadolinium-enhanced MR imaging for differentiating mucoceles from neoplasms in the paranasal sinuses. *Radiology* 178:425–428, 1991.

Silver AJ, Baredes S, Bello JA, et al: The opacified maxillary sinus: CT findings in chronic sinusitis and malignant tumors. *Radiology* 163:205–210, 1987.

Som PM, Dillon WP, Sze G, et al: Benign and malignant sinonasal lesions with intracranial extension: differentiation with MR imaging. *Radiology* 172:763–766, 1989.

Som PM, Shapiro MD, Biller HF, et al: Sinonasal tumors and inflammatory tissues: differentiation with MR imaging. *Radiology* 167:803–808, 1988.

Som PM, Shugar JMA, Biller HF: The early detection of antral malignancy in the postmaxillectomy patient. *Radiology* 143:509–512, 1982.

Van Tassel P, Lee YY: Gd-DTPA enhanced MR for detecting intracranial extension of sinonasal malignancies. *J Comput Assist Tomogr* 15:387–392, 1991.

13

Squamous Cell Carcinoma: Nodal Staging

CRITICAL IMAGING QUESTIONS:
NODAL STAGING OF SQUAMOUS CELL CARCINOMA

1. Name the nodal groups of the extracranial head and neck that are important in the staging of squamous cell malignant adenopathy.
2. What are the imaging criteria for assigning a radiologic nodal stage (N) using CT or MRI?
3. When is it appropriate to diagnose extranodal tumor based radiologic appearance?

Answers to these questions are found in the text beside the question number (Q#) in the margin.

NODAL STAGING OF SQUAMOUS CELL CARCINOMA

A. Cervical nodal anatomy and nomenclature.

1. Chapter 12 discussed imaging issues surrounding the use of CT or MRI in the staging of primary squamous cell carcinoma (SCCa) of the head and neck. This chapter completes the discussion, with attention to the use of either of these imaging techniques in staging SCCa adenopathy.
2. Because malignant adenopathy frequently is present when the patient first is seen (Table 13-1) and its presence associated with a 50% reduction in the long-term survival rate, precise staging information before initial treatment is essential.
3. Before pursuing the radiologic issues of SCCa nodal staging with CT or MRI, the normal cervical nodal anatomy and nomenclature must be mastered.
4. Normal cervical nodal anatomy.
   a. Nodal groups of importance in the staging of SCCa are:

Q#1

    1) Deep lateral cervical group.
    2) Anterior cervical group.
    3) Submental–submandibular group.
    4) Parotid group.
    5) Retropharyngeal group.
   b. The standard locations and global drainage patterns of these nodal groups are illustrated in Figs. 13-1 and 13-2.
5. Deep lateral cervical nodal group.
   a. Nomenclature.
       1) This nodal group is divided into three subgroups:
         a) Deep cervical chain (i.e., jugular).
         b) Spinal accessory chain (i.e., posterior triangle).

Table 13-1 Incidence of Nodal Disease in Squamous Carcinoma of the Head and Neck

Primary tumor site	Incidence of nodes at presentation (%)
Nasopharynx	86–90
Oropharynx	50–71
Oral cavity	30–65
Hypopharynx	50–72
Supraglottic larynx	31–54
Glottic larynx	<10
Sinonasal	<10

Data from Som PM: Lymph nodes of the neck. *Radiology* 165:593–600, 1987.

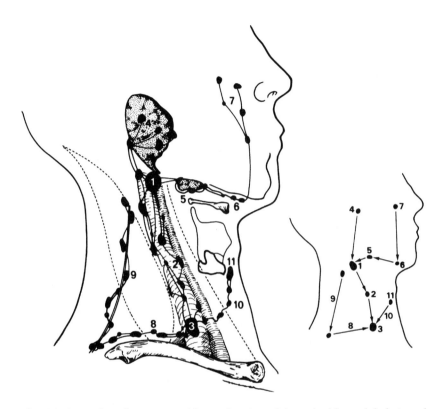

Fig. 13-1   *Left,* Right anterior oblique drawing of the palpable nodal chains of the neck. The retropharyngeal nodes of the deep oropharynx and nasopharynx are not included. *Right,* The *arrows* are vectors displaying the usual directions of lymphatic drainage in the head and neck region. Numbers for both panels represent:

Common Nodal Terms	Alternate Nodal Terms
1. Jugulodigastric node	"Sentinel" (highest) node of internal jugular chain
2. Internal jugular nodal chain	Deep cervical chain
3. Virchow's node	"Signal" (lowest) node of the internal jugular chain
4. Parotid nodal group	—
5. Submandibular nodal group	—
6. Submental nodal group	—
7. Facial nodal group	—
8. Transverse cervical nodal chain	Supraclavicular nodal chain
9. Spinal accessory nodal chain	Posterior triangle nodal chain
10. Anterior cervical nodal chain	Includes prelaryngeal, pretracheal, paratracheal nodal groups
11. Pretracheal nodal group	Delphian nodes

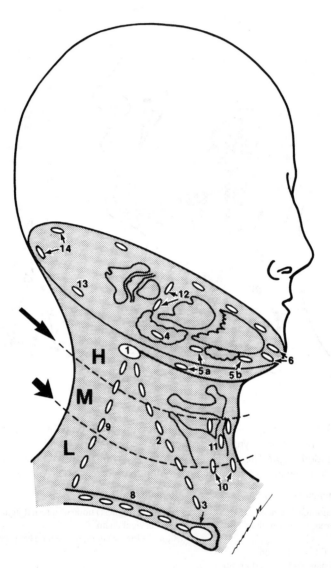

Fig. 13-2   The major nodal groups, including the retropharyngeal chain (*12*). The major nodal chains (i.e., internal jugular [*2*] and spinal accessory [*9*]) are subdivided into high (*H*), middle (*M*), and low (*L*) subgroups by a line drawn along the undersurface of the hyoid bone (*long, skinny arrow*) and a line drawn at the level of the cricoid cartilage (*short, fat arrow*).

(*continued*)

Fig. 13-2 *(continued)*

Common Nodal Terms	Alternate Nodal Terms
1. Jugulodigastric node	"Sentinel" (highest) node of internal jugular chain
2. Internal jugular nodal chain	Deep cervical chain
3. Virchow's node	"Signal" (lowest) node of the internal jugular chain
4. Parotid nodal group	—
5. Submandibular nodal group	*5a,* Posterior to submandibular gland
	5b, Anterior to submandibular gland
6. Submental nodal group	—
8. Transverse cervical nodal chain	Supraclavicular nodal chain
9. Spinal accessory nodal chain	Posterior triangle nodal chain
10. Anterior cervical nodal chain	Includes prelaryngeal, pretracheal, paratracheal nodal groups
11. Pretracheal nodal group	Delphian nodes
12. Retropharyngeal nodal group	Lateral group are nodes of Rouviere
13. Mastoid nodal group	—
14. Occipital nodal group	—

    c) Transverse cervical chain (i.e., supraclavicular).

  b. Deep cervical chain (i.e., jugular chain).

    1) Location. Found along the length of the internal jugular vein, often within the fascial layers of the carotid sheath.

    2) Important nodes found within this chain include:

      a) Jugulodigastric node. "Sentinel" (i.e., highest) node, found at the apex of the deep cervical chain at the angle of the mandible.

      b) Virchow's node. "Signal" (i.e., lowest) node, among the most inferior nodes of the deep cervical chain (Fig. 13-1).

        i) When this node is involved in the absence of upper neck nodes, primary tumor should be sought in the chest or abdomen.

    3) To provide direct clinicoradiologic correlation, the deep cervical chain is subdivided into three nodal regions: the high, middle, and low deep cervical chains (Fig. 13-2).

      a) The high deep cervical nodes are found above the level of the hyoid bone.

      b) The middle deep cervical group is found between the hyoid bone and the cricoid cartilage.

      c) The low deep cervical group is associated with the carotid space below the level of the cricoid cartilage.

      d) The hyoid bone and cricoid cartilage are easily seen on both CT and MRI scans. As radiologic landmarks they allow the radiologist to assign the abnormal node to the high, middle, or low deep cervical chain in a way that will correlate well with clinical or surgical assessment.

4) Drainage pattern. The deep cervical nodal group receives lymphatic drainage from the parotid, retropharyngeal, and submandibular nodes. They in turn form the jugular lymphatic trunks and empty into the subclavian or the internal jugular vein. At times this trunk empties directly into the lymphatic duct on the right and the thoracic duct on the left.

   a) Because this distal termination is into the venous system, SCCa lymph nodes are not found in the upper mediastinum.

   b) Consequently, imaging of lymph node disease can be terminated at the level of the clavicles. There is no need to worry about the upper mediastinum when staging SCCa nodes.

   c) The upper mediastinal nodes are important when thyroid carcinoma is imaged, because this tumor may drain via the paratracheal chain into the mediastinum.

5) Malignant nodes most frequently are located in the deep cervical chain, because it serves a final common pathway for all lymphatics of the upper aerodigestive tract and neck.

c. Spinal accessory chain.

   1) Location. This nodal chain follows the course of the spinal accessory nerve (i.e., cranial nerve XI) in the posterior cervical space (i.e., posterior triangle) of the neck. The chain courses downward in an oblique, posterolateral direction (Fig. 13-1).

   2) Nodes of the spinal accessory chain merge at its apex with nodes of the deep cervical chain, making them indistinguishable on CT or MRI scans.

   3) Drainage pattern. The spinal accessory chain receives lymphatic drainage from the occipital and mastoid nodes, parietal scalp, and lateral neck and shoulder lymphatics. Principal drainage from the spinal accessory chain is into the transverse cervical nodal chain (Fig. 13-1, *right*).

   4) Comment. When a malignant node appears in the spinal accessory chain without a clinically apparent primary site, the occult primary tumor most frequently is found in the nasopharynx.

d. Transverse cervical chain.

   1) Location. These nodes run in a transverse direction parallel to the clavicles (Fig. 13-1).

   2) Drainage pattern. The transverse cervical chain receives drainage from the spinal accessory chain, deep cervical chain, subclavicular nodes, upper anterior chest wall, and skin of the anterolateral neck. Drainage from the transverse cervical chain is the same as for the deep cervical chain.

6. Anterior cervical nodal group.
    a. Nomenclature.
        1) This nodal group is divided into three subgroups:
            a) Pretracheal chain.
            b) Prelaryngeal chain.
            c) Paratracheal chain.
    b. Pretracheal nodal chain.
        1) Location. The nodes in the anterior jugular chain follow the course of the external jugular vein, lying in the superficial fascia of the neck external to the strap muscles.
        2) Drainage pattern. This nodal chain drains the lymph of the skin and muscles of the anterior neck. It then drains into the thoracic duct or anterior mediastinal nodes on the left and into the lowest deep cervical chain or highest intrathoracic node on the right.
    c. Prelaryngeal nodal chain.
        1) The Delphian node is an important midline superficial lymph node found at the upper end of the prelaryngeal chain.
            a) When this node is involved in the setting of laryngeal SCCa, it signals definite subglottic involvement that should be searched for and identified on radiologic examination.
    d. Paratracheal nodal chain.
        1) Location. Found within the visceral space of the infrahyoid neck. In most cases just lateral to the trachea and posterior to the thyroid in the tracheoesophageal groove.
        2) Drainage pattern. Receives lymph drainage from the supraglottic and subglottic larynx, pyriform sinuses, thyroid gland, trachea, and esophagus. It then drains as described for the pretracheal nodal chain.
        3) Comment. The majority of paratracheal nodes are seen in the tracheoesophageal grooves. The most cephalad of these nodes sits behind the superior pole of the thyroid gland and therefore can be mistaken for a parathyroid adenoma on either CT or MRI scans.
7. Submental–submandibular chain.
    a. Nomenclature.
        1) This group is subdivided by anatomic location into two groups:
            a) Submental nodes.
            b) Submandibular nodes.
        2) The two groups are discussed together because of their common drainage pattern.
    b. Submental nodes.
        1) Location. Found in the anterior submandibular space between the anterior belly of the two digastric muscles.

    2) Drainage pattern. Receives lymph drainage from the chin, lips, cheeks, floor of the mouth, and anterior tongue. They in turn drain into the submandibular nodes and then the high deep cervical chain.

  c. Submandibular nodes.

    1) Location. Located in the more posterolateral aspect of the submandibular space, in the vicinity of the submandibular gland. These nodes are strictly extraglandular, because the submandibular gland undergoes *early encapsulation* during embryogenesis, thereby excluding lymph nodes from the substance of the gland (compare with parotid nodal chain).

    2) Drainage pattern (Fig. 13-1, *right*). Both the submental and submandibular nodal groups drain the anterior facial structures and skin as well as the floor of mouth and anterior oral cavity contents.

    3) In describing submandibular nodes, use the submandibular gland as a reference point, and comment on whether the node seen is anterior, lateral, or posterior to the gland.

8. Parotid nodes.

  a. Nomenclature.

    1) Nodes of the parotid space can be either inside or outside of the gland. For this reason they are referred to as *intraglandular* or *extraglandular*.

    2) The parotid gland undergoes *late encapsulation* during embryogenesis, incorporating lymph tissue within the gland as it does so. This phenomenon explains the existence of intraglandular parotid nodes.

  b. Parotid nodes.

    1) Location. Found inside or outside of the parotid gland, but all are present within the parotid space.

    2) Drainage pattern. These nodes receive lymph from the external auditory canal, eustachian tube, skin of the forehead and temporal region, posterior cheek, gums, and buccal mucous membrane. They in turn drain into the high deep cervical chain.

  c. Comments.

    1) The principal area drained by the parotid nodes is the skin.

    2) As expected, the most common tumors to metastasize to these nodes are invasive skin SCCa and melanoma.

    3) Because the parotid space is not commonly thought of as a nodal station, patients with invasive skin malignancy both in and around the ear have received neck dissection of malignant nodes in the deep cervical chain without undergoing parotidectomy as part of the dissection. These patients are at great risk for devel-

oping nodal malignancy within the parotid gland with resultant facial nerve paralysis.

9. Retropharyngeal nodes.

   a. Nomenclature.

      1) The retropharyngeal nodes are found in two locations in the retropharyngeal space: medial, and lateral.

      2) Consequently, this nodal group is divided into two groups: the medial and lateral retropharyngeal nodes.

   b. Medial retropharyngeal nodes.

      1) Location. Medial nodes lie near the midline in the retropharyngeal space at the nasopharyngeal and oropharyngeal levels.

      2) Drainage pattern. These nodes drain lymph primarily from the nasopharynx and oropharynx. From there this lymph drains into the high deep cervical nodal chain.

   c. Lateral retropharyngeal nodes (nodes of Rouviere).

      1) Location. Found in the lateral aspect of nasopharyngeal and oropharyngeal retropharyngeal space, just lateral to the longus colli and capitus muscles and just medial to the internal carotid artery.

      2) Drainage pattern. Same as for medial retropharyngeal nodes.

   d. Comments.

      1) The lateral nodal group often is normally seen in the nasopharynx in younger patients, especially during MRI examination of the area. With increasing age of the patient (i.e., > 40 years), retropharyngeal nodes must be viewed with suspicion.

      2) Awareness of this nodal group is extremely important when staging SCCa, because these nodes often are clinically occult.

      3) The lateral retropharyngeal nodal mass may be difficult to distinguish from carotid space mass on axial images. See Chapter 1 for more details.

B. Lymph node division by levels.

1. New American Joint Committee on Cancer guidelines.

   a. The American Joint Committee on Cancer (AJCC) guidelines for nodal staging currently in use are discussed in Sections C and D in this chapter. For now (1994) the terminology presented here will suffice. A new "level terminology," however, is coming into use and is present briefly in this section.

   b. This scheme subdivides the lymph nodes of the neck into specific anatomic subsites, then groups them into seven levels for simplicity and ease of description.

   c. This level concept is driven by the fact that the extent and level of cervical nodal involvement by metastatic tumor is prognostically important.

2. Lymph nodes by level (Fig. 13-3).
   a. Level I nodes.
      1) Submental nodes.
      2) Submandibular nodes.
   b. Level II nodes.
      1) Upper deep cervical chain nodes.
   c. Level III nodes.
      1) Middle deep cervical chain nodes.
   d. Level IV nodes.
      1) Lower deep cervical chain nodes.
   e. Level V nodes.
      1) Spinal accessory nodes.
      2) Transverse cervical chain nodes.

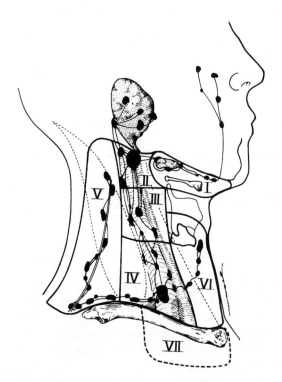

Fig. 13-3   Lymph node levels. This drawing shows the general anatomic locations for the different levels of lymph nodes in the neck. Level I nodes are submental and submandibular nodes; level II nodes, upper deep cervical nodes; level III nodes, middle deep cervical nodes; level IV nodes, lower deep cervical nodes; level V nodes, spinal accessory and transverse cervical nodes; level VI nodes, pretracheal, prelaryngeal, and paratracheal nodes; level VII nodes, upper mediastinal nodes.

    f. Level VI nodes.
      1) Pretracheal nodes.
      2) Prelaryngeal nodes.
      3) Paratracheal nodes.
    g. Level VII nodes.
      1) Upper mediastinal nodes.
3. Important nodes not yet incorporated into this scheme include the retropharyngeal and parotid groups.

C. Clinical issues in staging nodal squamous cell carcinoma.

1. When a patient has a history of smoking as well as a mass that appeared insidiously and is firm, painless, nontender, and at times fixed, SCCa adenopathy heads the list of differential diagnosis.
    a. In most cases the neck mass is seen along with a known primary SCCa that has been seen on a mucosal surface of the upper aerodigestive tract. In this case the nodal disease is staged both clinically and radiologically at the same time as the primary tumor.
    b. In the unusual circumstance where no associated primary SCCa is seen, radiologic staging of the SCCa nodal mass is done in conjunction with searching the head and neck area for the clinically occult or "unknown" primary tumor. (See Chapter 12.)
2. Once needle biopsy of the mass or identification of a primary tumor is completed, five specific questions regarding this nodal deposit arise.
    a. What is the size of the nodal mass?
    b. What side of the neck is the nodal mass on relative to the primary tumor?
    c. How many nodes are felt?
    d. Is there extracapsular spread?
    e. Is there carotid fixation?
    f. Although each of these questions can be answered by physical examination alone, CT or MRI can further define the nodal stage.
3. Information derived from the clinical examination is applied to the AJCC criteria for assigning a nodal stage (N) to the specific tumor (Table 13-2).
4. Multiple pitfalls in the clinical staging of SCCa adenopathy include:
    a. Approximately 10% of malignant nodes are clinically occult because of their deep location (too deep to palpate) in areas such as the retropharyngeal nodal chain and high deep cervical chain. Because even a single malignant node in the ipsilateral neck decreases the survival rate by 50%, detection of any nodal disease is extremely important.
    b. Nodal conglomerates may feel like a single node and therefore be staged as N1 rather than N2b.

Table 13-2   Criteria for Clinical Nodal Staging

NX: Nodes cannot be assessed
NO: No clinically positive nodes
N1: Single clinically positive ipsilateral node ≤ 3 cm
N2: Single clinically positive ipsilateral node >3 cm but not >6 cm, or multiple ipsilateral nodes not >6 cm in diameter
  N2a: Single clinically positive ipsilateral node >3 cm but not >6 cm in diameter
  N2b: Multiple clinically positive ipsilateral nodes not >6 cm in diameter
N3: Massive ipsilateral node or nodes, bilateral nodes, or contralateral node or nodes
  N3a: Ipsilateral node or nodes >6 cm in diameter
  N3b: Bilateral clinically positive nodes
  N3c: Contralateral node or nodes only

Modified from Beahrs OH, Henson DE, Hutter RVP, Kennedy BJ (American Joint Committee on Cancer), editors: *Manual for staging of cancer*, edn 4. Philadelphia, 1992, JB Lippincott. Used with permission.

c. No allowance is made in this system for extracapsular tumor, even though it is well known from the pathologic literature that extracapsular (extranodal) tumor decreases the patient survival rate by 50% and is the single best prognosticator of local treatment failure.

5. A more complete and objective staging approach would provide vital pretreatment information and help to direct therapeutic decisions. CT or MRI, if focused to this problem with definitive radiologic staging criteria, can serve this function.

D. Radiologic issues in staging nodal squamous cell carcinoma.

1. Either contrast-enhanced CT or MRI can be used to stage radiologically the nodes of the neck.
2. The following rules are useful for staging neck nodes with CT or MRI:
    a. Nodal staging should be done simultaneously with primary tumor staging.
    b. Nodal staging should not add to the overall cost of the examination.
    c. At the very least the first- and second-order drainage nodes of the primary tumor should be imaged. If there is doubt about what this constitutes, the entire neck to the clavicles must be scanned.
    d. Once a CT or MRI protocol is established to scan the required neck area in contiguous slices, do not deviate from it so as to establish a reliable, reproducible set of images.
3. CT or MRI criteria for malignant nodes.

Q#2

a. A node ≥ 1.5 cm in maximum diameter in the deep cervical chain, spinal accessory, or submental–submandibular nodal group.

1) Some argue that sensitivity is more important than specificity in this discussion. They recommend use of a 1.0-cm maximum diameter as a cutoff, because they feel limited neck dissections of suspicious nodes is a better approach to this problem.

2) If your institution has a high-quality radiology–pathology team that can needle biopsy suspicious nodes with ultrasonic guidance and interpret the specimen with a high degree of accuracy, this technique makes the absolute size issue less important.

b. A node ≥ 1.0 cm in maximum diameter in the parotid or retropharyngeal nodal groups.

c. A node of any size with central low density (on CT scans) or central low intensity (on contrast-enhanced fat-suppressed MRI scans).

1) The presence of central nodal necrosis is directly related to nodal size. The larger the node, the more likely it will demonstrate central nodal necrosis.

d. These criteria only apply to enhanced CT and T1-weighted, contrast-enhanced MRI scans. In the absence of contrast-enhanced T1-weighted MRI, T2-weighted images may provide information about internal nodal architecture. Size criteria alone, however, must be relied on.

e. Pitfalls in the use of these radiologic nodal staging criteria are rare.

1) Postinflammatory fatty infiltration of nodes can occur and appears as central low density on CT scans. In most cases the node remains oval, and the fat is not centrally located.

2) Suppurative adenopathy from fulminant infection in the head and neck region can "necrose" the center of adjacent nodes and in all respects mimic the radiologic appearance of a malignant node. Consequently, in the unusual circumstance where SCCa and abscess coexist, care must be exercised to avoid erroneously diagnosing malignant adenopathy.

4. Once the CT or MRI scans of the neck nodes are obtained and the described criteria applied, information about nodal size, side, and number of nodes should be compared with modified AJCC nodal staging guidelines (Table 13-3).

Q#3

5. Extranodal disease is diagnosed radiologically by the following observations:

a. Extranodal radiologic criteria.

1) The lymph node will appear to have amorphous, spiculated margins.

Table 13-3   Modified American Joint Committee on Cancer Radiologic Nodal Staging Guidelines

NO: All nodes <1.5 cm in diameter with no central low density (on CT scans) or central low intensity (on MRI scans)

N1: Single ipsilateral node 15 to 29 mm in diameter, or single ipsilateral node <15 mm with central low density (CT) or central inhomogeneous intensity (MRI)

N2: Single ipsilateral node 3 to 6 cm in diameter, or multiple ipsilateral nodes all <6 cm
    N2a: Single ipsilateral node 3 to 6 cm in diameter
    N2b: Multiple ipsilateral nodes all <6 cm

N3: Massive ipsilateral node or nodes, one or more >6 cm in diameter
    N3a: Ipsilateral node or nodes, at least one >6 cm
    N3b: Bilateral malignant nodes
    N3c: Contralateral malignant nodes only
    (N3d):   Extranodal malignant nodes (see text for radiologic criteria used to make this diagnosis)

Adapted from Stevens MH, Harnsberger HR, Mancuso AA: Computed tomography of cervical lymph nodes: staging and management of head and neck cancer. *Arch Otolaryngol* 11:735–739, 1985. Used with permission.

    2) Its contents appear to spill into the adjacent fatty spaces of the neck.

    3) Nodal contents "encase" the adjacent vessels and muscles. When the nodal contents completely surround the carotid artery, this form of extranodal tumor is termed *carotid fixation*. This radiologic diagnosis is made cautiously, because most surgeons will not operate on a neck with suspected carotid fixation and surgery still offers the best chance for cure of head and neck cancer.

  b. Note that the (N3d) classification (Table 13-3) does not have formal approval of the AJCC at this time. It is included, however, to remind the radiologist how important the diagnosis of extranodal tumor is to treatment and overall prognosis.

6. The accuracy of CT nodal staging is approximately 90% to 95%, compared with 75% to 80% for clinical nodal staging.

7. The initial study done by Yousem et al (1992) regarding the accuracy of MRI in the staging neck nodes shows similar accuracy statistics if compulsive imaging techniques and strict criteria for malignant adenopathy are maintained.

  a. In that study it was found that CT was slightly more accurate than MRI in identifying central nodal necrosis and extranodal spread.

8. CT or MRI can have a profound impact on the process of nodal staging by providing objective nodal staging information not necessarily available from clinical examination alone.

SUGGESTED READING

Bataskis JG: *Tumors of the head and neck: clinical and pathological considerations*, edn 2. Baltimore, 1979, Williams & Wilkins.

Beahrs OH, Henson DE, Hutter RVP, Kennedy BJ (American Joint Committee on Cancer), editors: *Manual for staging of cancer*, edn 4. Philadelphia, 1992, JB Lippincott.

Dooms GC, Hricak H, Crooks LE, et al: Magnetic resonance imaging of the lymph nodes: comparison with CT. *Radiology* 153:719–728, 1984.

Friedman M, Roberts N, Kirshenbaum GL, et al: Nodal size of metastatic squamous cell carcinoma of the neck. *Laryngoscope* 103:854–856, 1993.

Friedman M, Shelton V, Mafee M, et al: Metastatic neck diseases: evaluation by computed tomography. *Arch Otolaryngol* 110:443–447, 1984.

Glazer HS, Niemeyer JH, Balfe DM, et al: Neck neoplasms: MR imaging. I: initial evaluation. *Radiology* 160:343–348, 1986.

Last RJ: *Anatomy: regional and applied*, edn 6. New York, 1978, Churchill-Livingstone.

Lindberg R: Distribution of cervical lymph node mestastases from squamous cell carcinoma of the upper respiratory and digestive tracts. *Cancer* 29:1446–1449, 1972.

Mancuso AA, Harnsberger HR, Muraki AS, et al: Computed tomography of cervical and retropharyngeal lymph nodes: normal anatomy, variants of normal, and application in staging head and neck cancer. I: normal anatomy. *Radiology* 148:709–714, 1983.

Mancuso AA, Harnsberger HR, Muraki AS, et al: Computed tomography of cervical and retropharyngeal lymph nodes: normal anatomy, variants of normal, and application in staging head and neck cancer. II: pathology. *Radiology* 148:715–723, 1983.

Mancuso AA, Maceri D, Rice D, et al: CT of cervical lymph node cancer. *Am J Roentgenol* 136:381–385, 1981.

Reede DL, Bergeron RT, Whelan MA, et al: Computed tomography of cervical lymph nodes. *RadioGraphics* 3:339–351, 1983.

Rouviere H: *Lymphatic system of the head and neck*. In Tobias MJ, editor: *Anatomy of the human lymphatic system*. Ann Arbor, 1938, Edwards Brothers.

Sako K, Pradier RN, Marchetta FC, et al: Fallibility of palpation in the diagnosis of metastasis to cervical nodes. *Surg Gynecol Obstet* 118:989–990, 1964.

Snyderman NL, Johnson JT, Schramm VL, et al: Extracapsular spread of carcinoma in cervical lymph nodes: impact upon survival in patients with carcinoma of the supraglottic larynx. *Cancer* 56: 1597–1599, 1985.

Som PM: Detection of metastasis in cervical lymph nodes: CT and MR criteria and differential diagnosis. *Am J Roentgenol* 158:961–969, 1992.

Som PM: Lymph nodes of the neck. *Radiology* 165:593–600, 1987.

Steinbrich W, Beyer D, Modder U: Malignant lymph nodes disease: diagnosis with MRI in comparison with other imaging modalities. *Radiology* 25:199–205, 1985.

Stevens MH, Harnsberger HR, Mancuso AA: Computed tomography of cervical lymph nodes: staging and management of head and neck cancer. *Arch Otolaryngol* 11:735–739, 1985.

Tart RP, Mukherji SK, Avino AJ, et al: Facial lymph nodes: normal and abnormal CT appearance. *Radiology* 188:695–700, 1993.

Van den Brekel MWM, Castelijns JA, Stel HV, et al: Modern imaging techniques and ultrasound-guided aspiration cytology for the assessment of neck node metastases: a prospective comparative study. *Eur Arch Otorhinolaryngol* 250:11–17, 1993.

Yousem DM, Som PM, Hackney DB, et al: Central nodal necrosis and extracapsular neoplastic spread in cervical lymph nodes: MR imaging versus CT. *Radiology* 182:753–759, 1992.

III

Imaging of the Face

14

The Normal and Diseased Orbit

CRITICAL IMAGING QUESTIONS: THE ORBIT

1. What four major anatomic areas are used to subdivide the orbit when constructing a differential diagnosis?
2. Along what scan plane is the orbit best imaged in the axial direction by CT or MRI? Why?
3. The superior orbital fissure has what bone (or bones) as its lateral and medial borders? Is the optic strut a piece of the greater or lesser wing of the sphenoid bone?
4. What is Zinn's ligament, or the "ring of Zinn?" What structures pass through it?
5. What is the most common pediatric malignancy of the globe? How often is it unilateral? How often is it bilateral? What is the CT signature of this lesion?
6. What are the two common tumors of the optic nerve/sheath complex? Describe the differences in clinical presentation and radiologic appearance of these two lesions.
7. What is the most common cause of an intraorbital mass lesion in an adult? What are the two most common intraorbital structures involved by orbital pseudotumor?

Answers to these questions are found in the text beside the question number (Q#) in the margin.

THE ORBIT

A. Introduction.

1. The orbit and its contents have come into better focus as CT and MRI have been tailored to answer the ophthalmologic questions of the region.
2. As with all confined areas of the body, the problem of interpreting images of lesions in the orbit is one of creating a rational method that allows the radiologist to subdivide the anatomic region, reducing the number of possible diagnoses.

Q#1

3. In the orbit this is done by dividing the area into its major anatomic components:
   a. Globe.
   b. Optic nerve and sheath.
   c. Conal–intraconal area.
   d. Extraconal area.
4. From the differential diagnosis for each of these anatomic components the general category of congenital–pediatric lesions can be extracted. Thus there are differential diagnoses for five groups of lesions:
   a. Congenital-pediatric orbital lesions (Table 14-1).
   b. Globe lesions (Table 14-2).

Table 14-1   Differential Diagnosis of Congenital and Pediatric Lesions of the Orbit

Congenital Lesions
  Neurofibromatosis type I*
    Optic nerve glioma
    Optic nerve sheath meningioma
    Optic nerve hemangioblastoma
    Optic nerve sheath schwannoma
    Plexiform neurofibroma
    Sphenoid wing dysplasia
  Septooptic dysplasia
    Optic nerve hypoplasia
  Coloboma
  Orbit or globe hypoplasia or aplasia
  Fibrous dysplasia
    Bony orbit enlargement
  Congenital glaucoma
    Globe enlargement (buphthalmos)
  Frontolateral meningocele or encephalocele

(continued)

Table 14-1   *(continued)*

Globe lesions
Retinoblastoma*
Medulloepithelioma
Coats' disease
Persistent hyperplastic primary vitreous
Retrolental fibroplasia
Sclerosing endophthalmitis (*Toxocara canis*)

Inflammatory and Infectious Diseases
Optic neuritis (without multiple sclerosis)
Orbital cellulitis (usually from ethmoids, with or without subperiosteal abscess)
Orbital pseudotumor

Tumors
Rhabdomyosarcoma*
Capillary hemangioma*
Lymphangioma
Optic nerve glioma
Dermoid or epidermoid
Non-Hodgkin lymphoma, leukemia
Secondary tumor
    Neuroblastoma, Ewing sarcoma

Vascular Lesions
Arteriovenous malformation
Carotid–cavernous fistula
Venous varix

Trauma
Foreign body*
Penetrating injury*

*These are more common lesions.

    c. Optic nerve sheath lesions (Table 14-3).
    d. Conal–intraconal lesions (Table 14-4).
    e. Extraconal lesions (Table 14-5).
5. Once a lesion is identified on CT or MRI scans as primary to one of these anatomic sites, the imaging features of the specific lesion (e.g., lesion morphology, contrast enhancement) are matched with the relevant differential diagnosis to further shorten the list of possibilities.

Table 14-2   Differential Diagnosis of Lesions of the Globe

Congenital
Persistent hyperplastic primary vitreous
Coats' disease
Coloboma
Globe hypoplasia or aplasia

Degenerative
Optic nerve drusen (hyaline bodies)
Phthisis bulbi (end-stage injured eye)

Trauma
Vitreous hemorrhage*
Choroidal hematoma*
Choroidal effusion
Foreign body

Inflammatory
Orbital pseudotumor (uveal or scleral thickening)*
Sclerosing endophthalmitis (*Toxocara canis*)

Ocular Tumor
Uveal melanoma (adults)*
Retinoblastoma (children)*
Ocular metastasis
Choroidal hemangioma
Medulloepithelioma

*These are more common lesions.

    a. This approach to orbital lesions is somewhat artificial. Many lesions are seen in more than one general category (e.g., pseudotumor) or may cross between anatomic sites (e.g., rhabdomyosarcoma).

    b. When the lesion is in its early phase of growth, it will be confined to one anatomic area. When the lesion is larger and has transgressed the bounds of a distinct anatomic site, it still often will be centered in one of the areas defined previously.

    c. In any event one can use this approach to analyzing orbital lesions as a starting point both for the study of the anatomy of the area and for assigning an initial differential diagnosis. Obviously, this construct will be enriched by one's individual experiences with lesions of the orbit.

6. This chapter first considers the ideal technical approach to the orbit using CT and MRI. Orbital anatomy is then considered. Finally, lesions of the orbit, including the congenital–pediatric group, are discussed by major anatomic area.

Table 14-3   Differential Diagnosis of Optic Nerve Sheath Lesions

Tumor
  Optic nerve glioma*
  Meningioma*
  Optic nerve sheath neurofibroma or schwannoma
  Lymphoma or leukemia
  Metastasis
    Direct extension of retinoblastoma or uveal melanoma
    Distant metastasis from lung or breast carcinoma
  Hemangioblastoma
  Hemangiopericytoma

Inflammatory
  Optic neuritis (with or without multiple sclerosis)
  Idiopathic orbital pseudotumor
  Sarcoidosis
  Toxoplasmosis
  Tuberculosis
  Syphilis

Trauma
  Contusion*
  Hematoma*
  Optic nerve avulsion

Vascular
  Central retinal vein occlusion

Endocrine
  Graves' disease

Miscellaneous
  Increased intracranial pressure*
  Optic hydrops

*These are more common lesions.

  a. Specific lesions found in multiple anatomic areas are discussed under the category where they are seen most frequently in vivo.

B. Technical imaging considerations.

1. The orbit is one area of the body where MRI has not completely supplanted CT as the clear choice for diagnostic imaging.
   a. Two important reasons for this are:

Table 14-4   Differential Diagnosis of Conal and Intraconal Lesions

Tumor
  Cavernous hemangioma (adults)*
  Capillary hemangioma (children)*
  Lymphangioma*
  Lymphoma*
  Metastasis (breast, lung, thyroid gland; melanoma)*
  Rhabdomyosarcoma (children)
  Hemangiopericytoma
  Neurofibroma/schwannoma (III, IV, V1)
  Ectopic meningioma

Inflammatory
  Pseudotumor*
  Cellulitis*
  Abscess
  Granulomatous disease (sarcoid, Wegener's syndrome)

Vascular
  Carotid–cavernous fistula with large superior orbital vein*
  Venous varix*
  Superior ophthalmic vein thrombosis*
  Venous angioma
  Arteriovenous malformation

Trauma
  Hematoma*
  Foreign body*

Endocrine
  Graves' disease*

*These are more common lesions.

  1) The presence of a superb natural contrast provided by retrobulbar fat, bony orbit, sinus air, and any lesion that may be present.
  2) The inherent sensitivity of MRI to globe and lid motion.
2. The continuing development of MRI techniques and technology make the role of MRI in orbital imaging subject to constant reappraisal. Fat suppression and faster scan techniques more recently have overcome most of these MRI limitations.
  a. In my imaging center MRI has become the initial imaging sequence of choice for the orbit and cranial nerve II.
    1) The main reason for this shift is MRI's ability to see intraaxial lesions (e.g., multiple sclerosis plaques), sella and parasellar lesions, and intraorbital lesions with equal clarity.

Table 14-5   Differential Diagnosis of Extraconal Lesions

Congenital/Development
Cephalocele

Trauma
Medial blowout fracture
Hematoma

Inflammatory
Subperiosteal cellulitis or abscess secondary to ethmoid or sphenoid sinusitis
Pseudotumor

Lacrimal gland
Congenital
  Dermoid
Tumor
  Benign mixed tumor
  Adenoid cystic carcinoma
  Non-Hodgkin lymphoma (bilateral)
Inflammatory
  Postviral syndrome
  Sjögren's syndrome
  Mikulicz's syndrome

Tumor
Metastasis*
Maxillary sinus malignancy
  Squamous cell carcinoma*
Nasal malignancy

*These are more common lesions.

    2) If the patient can cooperate with the demands of MRI, this modality is the more sensitive tool to the clinical–radiologic questions concerning the orbit and the optic nerve.
  b. CT is used as an adjunctive imaging tool when movement, clips, or some metallic foreign body compromises the MRI scans.
    1) In my experience only smaller, "tram-track" meningioma may be missed by MRI. Fat-saturated, T1-weighted axial images along the plane of the intraorbital optic nerve usually will allow identification of this lesion, but the smaller, mostly calcified lesions may be detected only by CT.
    2) A second clinical setting where CT is preferred is the infant with suspected retinoblastoma. With CT the question of calcification within a mass in the globe can be answered readily.

3. The MRI contrast agent gadolinium has not been a panacea for orbital MRI, because when used with T1-weighted imaging, it may make a lesion disappear into the orbital fat if it enhances intensely.

 a. Chemical fat-suppression techniques combined with gadolinium have now developed sufficiently to solve this problem most of the time.

 b. Fat-suppression artifacts at times still render these MRI scans non-diagnostic. Newer autoshimming equipment now makes fat-saturation artifacts less of a problem.

4. CT technique.

Q#2

 a. Contiguous, 3- × 3-mm images are obtained along the anthropologic baseline or infraorbitomeatal line (i.e., −10° to the orbitomeatal baseline). Some authors argue that 1.5-mm contiguous sections are necessary for orbital imaging.

Q#2

 1) A plane of section along the anthropologic baseline is chosen, because imaging in this plane closely parallels the orbital axis, permitting visualization of the optic nerve and horizontal eye muscles along their entire orbital course.

 2) Using this plane also minimizes the low-density, beam-hardening artifacts from the temporal bone seen with more positive angulation.

 b. A bolus-drip, intravenous contrast technique with an injector is used to maximize contrast in the vascular structures both in and around the orbit. When lesions extend outside the orbit, contrast often is a great help in identifying the extraorbital aspect of the lesion.

 c. Both soft-tissue and bony reconstructions should be performed, with subsequent photography to emphasize soft-tissue contrast (window width, 150–400 HU) and bone detail (window width, 2000 to 3000 HU).

 d. Coronal images are not acquired routinely. When a lesion affects either the superior or inferior wall of the orbit, coronal images definitively elucidate wall destruction and craniocaudal spread.

 e. If the lesion involves the orbital apex or intracranial compartment, MRI can be a great help in determining the true extent of the lesion and its involvement with the optic nerve and chiasm.

5. MRI technique.

 a. Coil selection.

 1) In most circumstances the standard head coil is well suited to image the orbit and surrounding structures.

 2) Special orbital surface coils provide even higher anatomic detail of the orbital contents (i.e., increased signal-to-noise ratio).

a) The globe and other anterior orbital structures benefit most from these special orbital surface coils.

b) The limitation of orbital surface coils becomes apparent when the lesion penetrates intracranially and surface coil–related signal falloff degrades the image to a nondiagnostic level.

b. Limiting motion artifacts from globe and lid motion.

1) Instruct the patient to fix his or her gaze on a point with both eyes open.

2) Keep imaging times to a minimum by limiting the repetition time (TR), number of excitations (NEX), and matrix size.

Q#2

c. Use T1-weighted (short TR) semiaxial (i.e., along the course of the optic nerve) and coronal imaging sequences as the initial screening MRI examination.

1) T2-weighted (long TR) sequences are used only if a lesion is seen and further characterization is required.

a) Fast spin echo has supplanted conventional spin echo in T2-weighted imaging both in and around the orbit. This allows more rapid imaging and is not affected significantly by the interface susceptibility artifacts commonly encountered in this area.

2) Limited flip-angle (i.e., gradient echo) scanning is of limited use in the orbit, because it often is badly affected by the blooming artifacts secondary to interface susceptibility phenomenon.

d. Slice thickness in orbital MRI should not exceed 4 mm in most situations. Contiguous sections are ideal.

e. Photography of orbital MRI scans requires some degree of initial physician supervision so that subtle lesions are not masked by inadequate photography.

C. Normal anatomy of the orbit.

1. Bony orbit.

a. Orbital roof.

1) The main portion of the triangular orbital roof is comprised of the frontal bone, with the frontal sinus within (Figs. 14-1 and 14-2).

2) Anteriorly the orbital roof is thin. In its more posterior aspect it becomes thick.

3) The anterolateral part of the orbital roof forms a shallow fossa for the lacrimal gland (Fig. 14-1).

4) The orbital roof can be imaged completely only in the coronal plane.

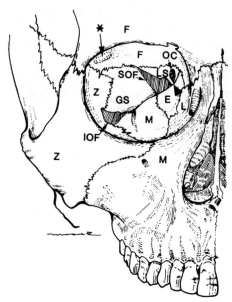

Fig. 14-1   Bony orbit from a frontal view. Six bones contribute to the bony walls of the orbit: the frontal (*F*), sphenoid (*S*), ethmoid (*E*), maxillary (*M*), lacrimal (*L*), and zygomatic (*Z*). The superior orbital fissure (*SOF*) is bordered by the greater wing of the sphenoid bone (*GS*) laterally and the lesser wing of the sphenoid bone (*LS*) medially. The optic canal (*OC*) is bordered inferiorly by the optic strut (*arrowhead*), which is a spike of bone from the LS. *Asterisk*, Lacrimal gland fossa; IOF, inferior orbital fissure.

    b. Orbital floor.
       1) The floor of the orbit is triangular.
       2) The floor is formed by the orbital plate of the maxilla (Figs. 14-1 and 14-2), the orbital process of the palatine bone, and the orbital surface of the zygomatic bone.
       3) Because the orbital plate of the maxilla is quite thin, inferior blowout fractures usually occur in this area.
       4) Like the orbital roof the orbital floor is studied completely only from the coronal perspective.
    c. Medial orbital wall.
       1) The medial orbital wall is a flat rectangular structure (Figs. 14-1 and 14-2).
       2) The anterior aspect is formed by the frontal process of the maxillary bone.
         a) Together with the lacrimal bone the frontal process of the maxillary bone forms the lacrimal fossa (Fig. 14-2). The lacrimal sac fossa contains the lacrimal sac.

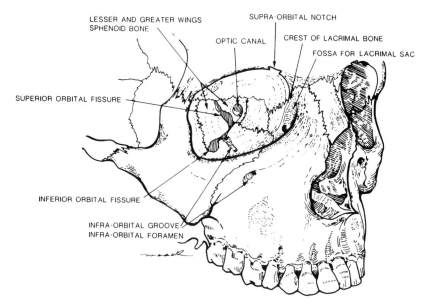

Fig. 14-2   Oblique view of the orbital cavity. The optic canal is situated at the apex of the conical orbital cavity between the two bony spikes of the lesser wing of the sphenoid bone. The infraorbital groove and foramen contain the infraorbital nerve (i.e., cranial nerve V$_2$ branch).

     3) The lamina papyracea (Latin for "paper plate") of the ethmoidal air cells forms the midportion of the medial orbital wall.

       a) For obvious reasons this very thin bony wall is the site of medial blowout fractures.

       b) Spontaneous dehiscence of orbital fat also may occur through the lamina papyracea into the ethmoid sinus, mimicking "occult medial blowout fracture" on CT or MRI scans.

     4) A small portion of the sphenoid bone forms the posterior portion of the medial orbital wall.

   d. Lateral orbital wall.

     1) The anterior portion of the lateral orbital wall is formed by the orbital surface of the zygomatic bone.

   e. Superior orbital fissure.

     1) The superior orbital fissure sits at the margin between the lateral wall and the orbital roof.

Q#3

     2) This bony fissure is surrounded by the sphenoid bone. The greater wing of the sphenoid bone forms its lateral boundary and the lesser wing its medial boundary (Figs. 14-2 and 14-3).

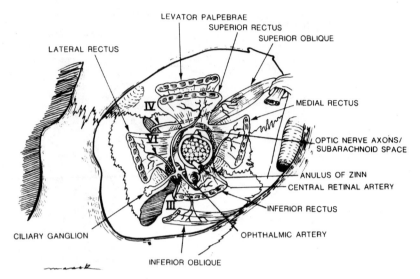

LEVATOR PALPEBRAE
SUPERIOR RECTUS
SUPERIOR OBLIQUE
LATERAL RECTUS
MEDIAL RECTUS
IV
VI
OPTIC NERVE AXONS/
SUBARACHNOID SPACE
ANULUS OF ZINN
CENTRAL RETINAL ARTERY
III
INFERIOR RECTUS
CILIARY GANGLION
OPHTHALMIC ARTERY
INFERIOR OBLIQUE

Fig. 14-3 Frontal (coronal) view of posterior muscle cone with associated nerves and arteries. The optic nerve axons are wrapped within its pial, arachnoid, and dural sheaths. A fibrous cuff is formed by the four rectus muscles and called the *annulus of Zinn*. Through the gap in the cuff come the optic nerve/sheath complex, ophthalmic artery, and cranial nerves III and VI.

Q#3

    3) The medial tip of the superior orbital fissure lies beneath the optic canal (Fig. 14-2). It is separated from the canal by the optic strut, which is a bridge of bone formed by the lesser wing of the sphenoid bone.

    4) Contents.

        a) Superior ophthalmic vein.

        b) Oculomotor (III), trochlear (IV), abducens (VI) nerves.

        c) Ophthalmic division of trigeminal nerve (V_1).

    5) As the largest communication between the orbit and intracranial area, the superior orbital fissure may be a conduit for inflammatory or neoplastic disease between the orbital apex and the cavernous sinus.

  f. Inferior orbital fissure.

    1) The inferior orbital fissure is found between the floor and the lateral wall of the orbit.

    2) This bony fissure connects with the pterygopalatine fossa and the nasopharyngeal masticator space (i.e., infratemporal fossa) inferolaterally.

3) Inflammatory and neoplastic lesions of the deep face can gain access to the orbital apex via the inferior orbital fissure.

4) Contents.

a) Infraorbital and zygomatic nerves.

b) Nerve branches from pterygopalatine ganglion.

c) Venous connections between inferior ophthalmic vein and pterygoid plexus.

g. Optic canal.

1) The optic canal is completely formed by the lesser wing of the sphenoid bone.

2) The canal contains the optic nerve and the ophthalmic artery, both of which are contained in a dural sheath.

3) The canal courses from its origin in the suprasellar cistern in an anterior, inferolateral direction. Its most intracranial portion has no bony roof.

2. Soft-tissue structures of the orbit.

a. Spatial subdivisions of the orbit.

1) The orbit can be divided into four distinct anatomic areas for creating limited differential diagnoses by region (Fig. 14-4):

a) Globe.

b) Optic nerve and sheath.

c) Conal–intraconal area.

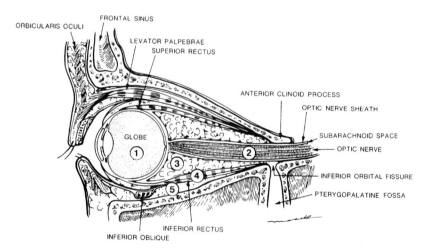

Fig. 14-4   Large (sagittal) view of the orbit, which best delineates its five anatomic areas: globe (*1*), optic nerve/sheath complex (*2*), intraconal area (*3*), conus (*4*), and extraconal area (*5*). Observe the potential pathway for infection or neoplasia into the orbit through the pterygopalatine fossa into the inferior orbital fissure, then on to the orbital apex.

    d) Extraconal area.
  b. Globe.
    1) The sphere of the globe is divided into anterior and posterior segments by the lens.
    2) The layers of the globe wall normally cannot be visualized by either CT or MRI.
    3) The optic nerve head, where the nerve fibers of the retinal ganglion cells accumulate in front of the lamina cribrosa, appears as a slight prominence approximately 3-mm nasal to the posterior pole of the globe.
  c. Optic nerve and sheath.
    1) The optic nerve is best thought of as containing three segments: orbital, canalicular, and intracranial.
    2) In all the optic nerve is approximately 4.5 cm in length, with the orbital segment making up the majority.
    3) The orbital segment follows a tortuous course from the optic canal to its insertion onto the back of the globe. It is a nearly round collection of axons surrounded by the same meningeal sheaths as the brain.
    4) MRI sections parallel to the intraorbital optic nerve can be designed from sagittal, T1-weighted, localizing images. Some centers do their high-resolution, T1-weighted imaging in the coronal plane.
  d. Conal–intraconal area.
    1) Extraocular muscles.
      a) The extraocular muscles of the orbital cone originate from a common, tendinous ring in the orbital apex, and they insert on the globe a few millimeters behind the corneoscleral border.
      b) The four rectus muscles and the fibrous septa webbed between them make up the muscle cone, which is filled with orbital fat. The intraconal area also contains orbital vessels, sensory and motor nerves to the extraocular muscles, and the optic nerve/sheath complex.
      c) Although in the intraconal area, the optic nerve/sheath complex is discussed separately, because lesions primary to these structures are somewhat unique.
      d) The seven extraocular muscles are the superior, inferior, lateral, and medial recti; the superior and inferior oblique muscles; and the levator palpebrae (Figs. 14-5 and 14-6).

Q#4

      e) The four recti, superior oblique, and levator palpebrae muscles originate from the common annulus tendineus communis (i.e., Zinn's ligamentous ring). This tendinous ring encloses the central portion of the superior orbital fissure and the optic foramen. The optic nerve/sheath complex, ophthalmic artery, and distal aspects of cranial nerves III and VI all pass through the annulus (Fig. 14-3).

  f) Coronal imaging provides the best routine imaging plane when assessing the size of extraocular muscles.

2) Orbital vessels.

  a) The superior ophthalmic vein is visualized routinely by both CT and MRI as it courses in the superior aspect of the orbit and passes out of the orbit through the superior orbital fissure (Figs. 14-5*A* and 14-6*A,B*).

  b) The ophthalmic artery comes through the optic canal with the optic nerve. Most commonly it then leaves the dural sheath beneath the nerve to cross over the nerve and run upward and medially within the muscle cone (Figs. 14-3, 14-5*A*, and 14-6*A,B*).

3) Orbital nerves.

  a) The orbital nerves include the optic nerve (i.e., cranial nerve II); cranial nerve III, IV, and VI branches; and cranial nerve V_1.

  b) See Chapter 18 for discussion of their locations and functions.

e. Extraconal area.

1) The extraconal area is the region between the muscle cone and bony orbit (Fig. 14-4).

2) This area contains only fat and the lacrimal gland.

3) Lacrimal gland.

  a) The lacrimal gland (Fig. 14-5*A*) is a lens-shaped organ located in the anterior orbit superolateral to the globe.

  b) The gland appears on routine CT and MRI scans as a mass in the upper temporal extraconal area.

  c) On coronal images the upper margin of the gland should be convex and the lower margin concave. The lower margin lies on the levator palpebrae and the lateral rectus muscles.

D. Lesions of the globe.

1. Most lesions of the globe can be diagnosed by the ophthalmologist without using CT or MRI.
2. CT, and sometimes MRI, are used to image globe lesions when:
   a. A child has leukokoria (Table 14-6) and the possibility of retinoblastoma with extraocular extension.
   b. A patient has opacity of the cornea, lens, or vitreous, precluding adequate ophthalmologic examination.
   c. An older patient has unilateral lens opacity secondary to trauma or malignant tumor.

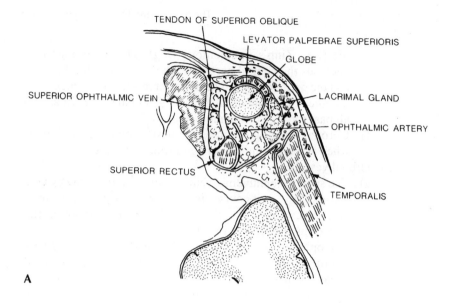

TENDON OF SUPERIOR OBLIQUE

LEVATOR PALPEBRAE SUPERIORIS

GLOBE

SUPERIOR OPHTHALMIC VEIN

LACRIMAL GLAND

OPHTHALMIC ARTERY

SUPERIOR RECTUS

TEMPORALIS

A

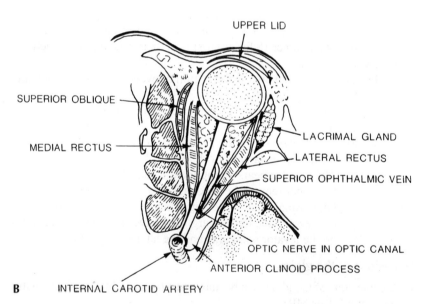

UPPER LID

SUPERIOR OBLIQUE

MEDIAL RECTUS

LACRIMAL GLAND

LATERAL RECTUS

SUPERIOR OPHTHALMIC VEIN

OPTIC NERVE IN OPTIC CANAL

ANTERIOR CLINOID PROCESS

B   INTERNAL CAROTID ARTERY

Fig. 14-5 Axial drawings along the infraorbitomeatal line from the top of the orbit (*A*) to the bottom (*D*). **A,** Most cephalad axial drawing along the plane of the ophthalmic artery and the superior ophthalmic vein. The lacrimal gland is seen in the anterior temporal recess of the orbital cavity in the extraconal area. **B,** Axial drawing through the plane of the optic nerve/sheath complex. Imaging along the infraorbitomeatal line often allows visualization of the entire intraorbital optic nerve from the optic canal to its attachment to the globe. The bellies of the lateral

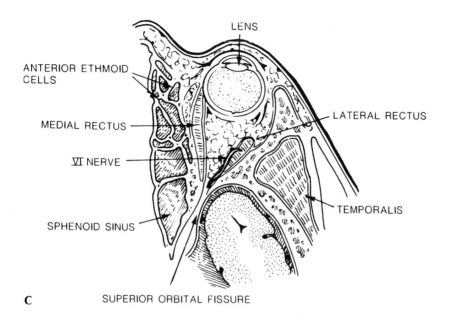

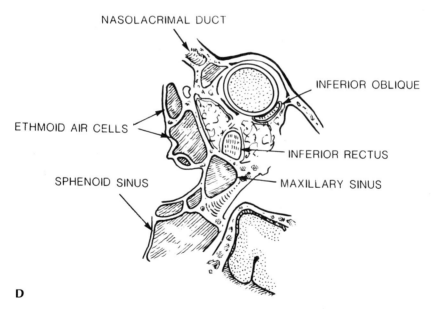

and medial rectus muscles are largest at this level. **C,** Axial drawing just below the plane of the optic nerve. Note the proximity of the ethmoid and sphenoid sinuses to the medial extraconal area. Infection of these two sinuses can lead to subperiosteal abscess in this area. **D,** Axial drawing through the lower orbit showing the belly of the inferior rectus muscle at its largest.

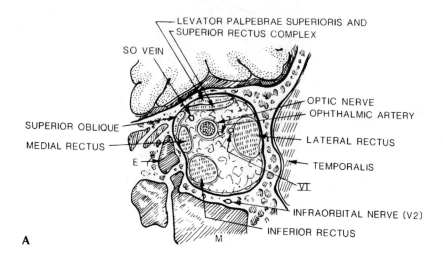

A

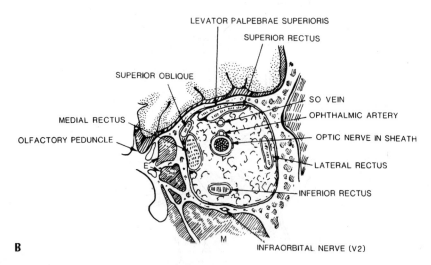

B

Fig. 14-6   Coronal drawings from the back of the orbit to the front. **A**, Just anterior to the muscle cone in the back of the orbit, revealing the ophthalmic artery to be inferolateral to the optic nerve and the superior ophthalmic nerve superomedial the optic nerve. The size of the extraocular muscles is evaluated much more easily in the coronal plane. **B**, The midorbit, showing that the ophthalmic artery

(continued)

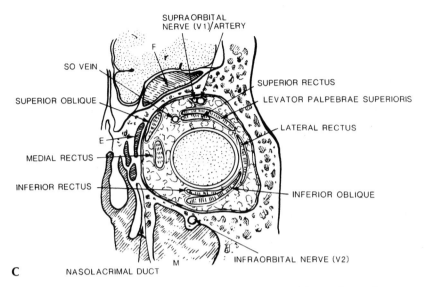

SUPRAORBITAL
NERVE (V1)/ARTERY

SO VEIN

SUPERIOR OBLIQUE

MEDIAL RECTUS

INFERIOR RECTUS

SUPERIOR RECTUS

LEVATOR PALPEBRAE SUPERIORIS

LATERAL RECTUS

INFERIOR OBLIQUE

INFRAORBITAL NERVE (V2)

C   NASOLACRIMAL DUCT

Fig. 14-6 (*continued*) has rotated to a position superior to the optic nerve. The superior ophthalmic vein remains above the optic nerve. **C**, Most anterior view, showing the supraorbital nerve (i.e., cranial nerve V_1 branch) in the extraconal area above and the infraorbital nerve (i.e., cranial nerve V_2 branch) below. *E*, Ethmoid bone; *F*, frontal sinus; *M*, maxillary bone; *SO*, superior ophthalmic vein.

   d. A patient has a known mass of the globe, and radiologic examination is requested to evaluate its extraocular extent.
3. Developmental lesions.
   a. Microphthalmia.
      1) Definition. Microphthalmia is a congenital underdevelopment or acquired diminution in the size of the globe.
      2) Bilateral microphthalmia and cataract are seen with congenital rubella, persistent hyperplastic vitreous, retinopathy of prematurity, retinal folds, and Lowe syndrome.
      3) In older patients microphthalmia results from trauma, surgery, or inflammation with disorganization of the eye (i.e., phthisis bulbi).
      4) Radiologic characteristics.
         a) Congenital microphthalmia is seen on CT or MRI scans as a small globe associated with a small, poorly developed bony orbit.
         b) In acquired microphthalmia CT scans show a shrunken, calcified globe.

Table 14-6   Common Causes of Leukokoria (White Pupil)

Developmental
  Coats' disease
  Persistent hyperplastic primary vitreous
  Retina dysplasia
  Congenital retinal fold

Tumor
  Retinoblastoma
  Medulloepithelioma

Inflammatory
  Sclerosing endophthalmitis

Degenerative
  Cataract
  Retrolental fibroplasia

Trauma
  Organized vitreous hemorrhage
  Long-standing retinal detachment

---

    b. Macrophthalmia.
       1) Definition. Enlargement of the globe.
       2) Macrophthalmia most commonly results from juvenile glaucoma or myopia. Its most severe form, buphthalmos, is caused by juvenile-onset glaucoma.
    c. Coloboma.
       1) Definition. Congenital defect in the globe, usually at the point of insertion of the optic nerve.
       2) Pathologic features. Coloboma represents a defect in the fusion of the fetal optic fissure. It presents as a localized defect in the sclera, uvea, and retina.
       3) Radiologic characteristics.
          a) CT or MRI scans usually show a small globe with a cystic outpouching of vitreous at the site of attachment of the optic nerve to the globe.
          b) A retroocular cyst may be associated.
    d. Persistent hyperplastic primary vitreous.
       1) Clinical presentation. Unilateral leukokoria (Table 14-6) in male infants, which may simulate retinoblastoma.
       2) Pathologic features.
          a) Persistence of the primary vascular vitreous, which normally undergoes involution by the sixth embryonic month.

b) Hyperplasia of the residual embryonic connective tissue occurs after involution.
3) Radiologic characteristics.
   a) Microphthalmic globe with enhancing, increased density in the vitreous humor.
   b) Unilateral or bilateral. A tissue density band may extend from the back of the lens to the posterior inner surface of the globe (following Cloquet's canal).
  e. Retinopathy of prematurity (retrolental fibroplasia).
1) Clinical presentation. Premature baby requiring long-term ventilator support with high concentrations of oxygen.
2) Pathologic features. Abnormal proliferation of the retinal vascular buds, often associated with use of high concentrations of oxygen for premature infants in neonatal intensive care units.
3) Radiologic characteristics.
   a) CT scans show increased density in the vitreous bilaterally.
   b) Calcification is not typical.
  f. Coats' disease.
1) Clinical presentation. Leukokoria unilaterally in a 6- to 8-year-old boy. Symptoms develop when the retina detaches, with loss of central vision.
2) Pathologic features.
   a) Coats' disease is a congenital vascular malformation of the retina characterized by multiple telangiectatic vessels.
   b) Leakage of serous and lipoproteinaceous exudate from these vessels leads to retinal detachment.
3) Radiologic characteristics.
   a) CT scans show increased density in part or all of the vitreous of the globe.
   b) Normal globe size and lack of calcification are part of the radiologic picture.
   c) Can appear identical to persistent hyperplastic vitreous or retinopathy of prematurity.
4. Ocular inflammatory lesions.
  a. Scleritis.
1) Clinical presentation.
   a) Anterior scleritis presents with pain, erythema, photophobia, and tenderness.
   b) Posterior scleritis presents without pain and may mimic uveal melanoma.
2) Pathologic features.
   a) Idiopathic scleral inflammation or associated with systemic disease.

b) Inflammation may be unilateral or bilateral; commonly affects women.

   3) Radiologic characteristics. Thickened, enhancing sclera is seen on enhanced CT or MRI scans. Choroidal detachment may be associated.

b. Sclerosing endophthalmitis or larval granulomatosis.

   1) Clinical presentation.

      a) Typically a 2- to 8-year-old child infected by playing in soil contaminated by dog excrement.

      b) Unilateral, localized granuloma may simulate retinoblastoma or endophthalmitis and may involve the entire vitreous.

   2) Pathologic features. Ingestion of the ova of the nematode *Toxocara canis* results in uveitis or more generalized endophthalmitis.

   3) Radiologic characteristics.

      a) Dense vitreous without a discrete mass usually is seen on CT or MRI scans.

      b) Calcification is not present, making differentiation from retinoblastoma possible when the localized granulomatous form occurs.

5. Ocular tumors.

a. Retinoblastoma.

   1) Clinical presentation.

      a) Child younger than 3 years of age (98%) with leukokoria (abnormal pupillary reflex known as *white pupil*) (Table 14-6).

      b) Less common presentations include strabismus, decreased visual acuity, positive family history, eye pain, or proptosis.

Q#5

   2) Pathologic features.

      a) Retinoblastoma is the most common tumor of the globe during childhood.

      b) This tumor is believed to arise from either primitive photoreceptor or neuronal retinal cells.

Q#5

      c) Of all retinoblastomas, 75% are unilateral and 25% bilateral.

   3) Radiologic characteristics.

      a) CT is the preferred method for evaluating leukokoria because of its sensitivity to calcification. MRI serves an adjunctive role only when further delineation of the extraocular extent of tumor is required.

Q#5

    b) When CT scans show an intraocular mass with calcification in a child younger than 3 years of age, the lesion should be considered a retinoblastoma. Calcifications can be clumped or punctate. When the tumors are small, calcification may be difficult to identify.

    c) CT scans also may show extraocular tumor spread along the optic nerve to the orbital apex and intracranial area. When a pinealoma is seen in concert with bilateral retinoblastoma, the term *trilateral retinoblastoma* is applied.

    d) The major differential diagnostic considerations in a child with leukokoria are toxocara endophthalmitis, persistent hyperplastic vitreous, retinopathy of prematurity, and Coats' disease. Calcification in these lesions is rare and, if present, late in the course of disease.

  b. Uveal melanoma.

    1) Clinical presentation.

      a) Adults (i.e., those 50 to 70 years of age) with a unilateral ocular complaint.

      b) Diagnosis is confidently made with combined ophthalmoscopic and ultrasound examinations. The diagnostic error rate ranges from 1% to 3%.

    2) Pathologic features.

      a) Uveal melanoma is the most common primary intraocular malignancy in adults.

      b) The tumor is unilateral, with 85% arising from the choroid, 9% from the ciliary body, and 6% from the iris.

    3) Radiologic characteristics.

      a) Because the clinical–ultrasonic diagnosis of uveal melanoma is made so confidently, neither CT nor MRI is used routinely in the work-up of this tumor.

      b) CT or MRI is used for diagnosis when opaque ocular media prevent a clear view, or when ophthalmoscopic visualization is suboptimal because of vitreous opacification or large amounts of subretinal effusion.

      c) CT features. CT scans show a soft-tissue mass adjacent to the outer layer of the globe that bulges inward toward the vitreous. When the soft-tissue mass is large and breaks through Bruch's membrane, it has a characteristic "mushroom cloud" appearance. When the lesion is small and flat, it may be difficult to see or to differentiate from metastatic tumor to the globe.

      d) MRI features. MRI scans demonstrate an elevated, sharply circumscribed lesion with high signal on T1-weighted images because of the paramagnetic properties of melanin and/or associated hemorrhage.

    e) Care must be taken to differentiate retinal detachment from uveal melanoma when seen together.

  c. Ocular metastasis.

    1) Clinical presentation. Only 50% of patients with ocular metastasis have a known primary tumor.

    2) Pathologic features.

      a) Metastatic tumor to the globe most commonly involves the uveal tract (i.e., vascular layer between the retina and the sclera).

      b) Lung and breast carcinomas are the most common primary lesions that metastasize to the globe.

    3) Radiologic characteristics.

      a) CT scans show ocular metastases as thickened areas of increased density. The lesions usually are small, multiple, and associated with subretinal fluid.

      b) Bilateral ocular lesions, especially in the posterior temporal portion of the uveal tract near the macula (an area of rich vascular supply), should suggest the diagnosis of ocular metastasis rather than choroidal hemangioma, uveal melanoma, or atypical nevi, all of which may mimic this lesion.

  d. Choroidal hemangioma.

    1) Clinical presentation.

      a) The lesion may be isolated or occur in association with Sturge-Weber syndrome.

      b) Sturge-Weber syndrome includes a mixture of the following features: "port-wine" vascular nevus flammeus in cranial nerve V distribution (part or all of the face, may involve sclera), leptomeningeal venous angiomatosis, seizures, dementia, mental retardation, hemiparesis, hemianopia, congenital glaucoma, buphthalmos (i.e., "cow eye"), and visceral angiomas.

    2) Pathologic features. Choroidal hemangioma is a benign vascular lesion that can mimic more ominous intraocular masses.

    3) Radiologic characteristics. CT scans show a lenticular to flat, intensely enhancing ocular wall mass.

  e. Astrocytic hamartoma, retinal angioma, choroidal osteoma, and medulloepithelioma are extremely rare intraocular tumors.

6. Ocular degenerative changes.

  a. Cataract.

  b. Retinal detachment.

  c. Disc drusen.

    1) Clinical presentation. Headache. Visual field defects. Pseudopapilledema. May be asymptomatic.

2) Pathologic features. Disc drusen is a cellular accretion of hyaline-like material on the surface of the optic disc.
3) Radiologic characteristics.
    a) CT scans show a globe with discrete, flat calcification of the optic nerve disc.
    b) Bilateral in 75% of cases.
    c) Most commonly encountered incidentally on head CT scans for other clinical indications.

E. Optic nerve–sheath lesions.

1. Thickening of the optic nerve/sheath complex has been described as tubular, fusiform, and excrescent.
   a. Tubular thickening refers to uniform enlargement of the nerve sheath complex. It is the most common type of thickening seen. This pattern can be seen in both neoplastic and nonneoplastic disorders, making it a nonspecific radiologic finding.
   b. Fusiform thickening describes a nerve/sheath complex that is lens shaped, tapering at either end.
   c. Excrescent thickening refers to a lesion of the optic nerve/sheath with single or multiple focal nodules along the complex.
      1) Fusiform and excrescent thickening of the optic nerve/sheath complex are significantly more specific findings for tumor.
2. Developmental lesions.
   a. Hypoplasia of the optic nerve.
      1) Hypoplasia may be an isolated congenital anomaly or be associated with other ocular, cranial, facial, or systemic abnormalities.
      2) When the ophthalmologist notes hypoplasia of the optic nerve, CT or MRI is ordered to exclude the possibility of an intraorbital or intracranial lesion affecting the visual pathway.
      3) Septooptic dysplasia.
         a) Septooptic dysplasia is one of many conditions associated with optic nerve hypoplasia.
         b) This syndrome consists of bilateral or unilateral optic nerve hypoplasia, with absence of the septum pellucidum, and dysplasia of the third ventricle, hypothalamic hypopituitarism, and growth-hormone deficiency.
         c) MRI scans show small optic nerves, absence of a septum pellucidum, and pointing of the frontal horns inferiorly.
3. Inflammatory lesions.
   a. Optic neuritis.
      1) Clinical presentation.
         a) Decreased visual acuity or visual field defects occurring over hours to days.

b) Pain on eye movement and tenderness when pressure is applied to the globe are other clinical symptoms that may be present.
2) Optic neuritis in adults may be sporadic or a harbinger of multiple sclerosis.
   a) Approximately 50% of patients with idiopathic optic neuritis develop multiple sclerosis.
   b) If optic neuritis is discovered on fat-suppressed, T1-weighted, enhanced MRI scans, a T2-weighted, whole-brain sequence should be performed to search for other radiologic stigmata of multiple sclerosis.
3) Other, less common causes of optic neuritis include pseudotumor, sarcoidosis, radiation therapy, viral, tuberculous, or syphilitic neuritis.
4) The role of MRI in patients with suspected optic neuritis is:
   a) To document the presence of an enhancing optic nerve (fat-saturated, T1-weighted, contrasted images).
   b) To search for multiple sclerosis plaques within the brain (T2-weighted, whole brain sequence).
   c) To exclude tumor or other compressive causes of visual impairment.
4. Tumors.

Q#6

a. The two major optic nerve/sheath tumors (i.e., optic nerve glioma, and optic nerve/sheath meningioma) do not ordinarily cause diagnostic problems because of their very different clinical settings. Even in a child with neurofibromatosis, differentiation of these two lesions usually can be accomplished radiologically.
b. Optic nerve glioma.
   1) Clinical presentation.
      a) Optic nerve glioma is a childhood disease presenting within the first 10 years of life in 75% of cases.
      b) The initial symptom is decreased vision in the affected eye with minimal axial proptosis.
      c) Hypothalamic disorder and obstructive hydrocephalus signal the presence of a larger tumor with intracranial extension.
   2) Pathologic features.
      a) Optic nerve glioma accounts for 80% of primary tumors of the optic nerve.
      b) One third of patients have neurofibromatosis type I. Conversely, 15% of patients with neurofibromatosis type I have optic nerve or optic chiasm glioma.

c) Histologically, childhood optic nerve glioma is most commonly a low-grade malignancy of the pilocytic astrocytoma variety.
d) The much more rare adult optic nerve glioma tends to be glioblastoma, with much more aggressive behavior.
3) Radiologic characteristics.
   a) On CT or MRI scans, optic nerve glioma may appear tubular, fusiform, or excrescent. The tubular configuration is the most common shape seen.
   b) Approximately 50% of optic nerve gliomas demonstrate contrast enhancement, but calcification is rare.
   c) A search for intracranial optic pathway involvement is an integral part of the radiologic examination. T2-weighted and gadolinium-enhanced MRI are significantly more sensitive than CT to more central spread of tumor.
   d) Spread of optic nerve glioma intracranially along the optic pathway helps to differentiate this lesion from optic nerve sheath meningioma. A complete comparison of the clinical and radiologic features of optic nerve glioma and optic nerve sheath meningioma is presented in Table 14-7.

Q#6
c. Optic nerve sheath meningioma.
1) Clinical presentation.
   a) A tumor of middle-aged women in most instances.
   b) Rarely seen in children with neurofibromatosis type II.
   c) Insidious onset, with progressive visual loss over months.
2) Pathologic features.

Table 14-7   Clinical and Radiological Features of Optic Nerve Glioma and Optic Nerve Sheath Meningioma

	Optic Nerve Glioma	Optic Nerve Sheath Meningioma
Age	Children: 33% have neurofibromatosis type I	Middle-aged women; children with neurofibromatosis type II
CT	Enlargement of optic nerve/sheath complex; usually fusiform or excrescent; no calcification	Enlargement of optic nerve–sheath complex; usually tubular calcification; "tram track" enhancement seen
MRI	Extension of tumor extensively along optic pathway intracranially	Minimal extension of tumor through optic canal only into prechiasmatic optic nerve

       a) Second most common primary neoplasm of the optic nerve/ sheath complex.

       b) Tumors arise from the meningoendothelial cells of the arachnoid layer. Because the optic nerve carries all three leptomeningeal layers with it to the globe, optic nerve sheath meningioma can occur anywhere along this tract.

   3) Radiologic characteristics.

       a) Most commonly causes tubular thickening of the optic nerve/sheath complex, but growth can be fusiform or excrescent as well.

       b) Marked contrast enhancement of the tumor is characteristic on CT examination.

       c) Enhancing tumor around the nonenhancing optic nerve results in a "tram track" appearance on axial images. When the tumor is still small, it may be difficult to differentiate from optic neuritis or a normal variant.

       d) Calcification is common. Hyperostosis also may be seen in the enlarged, remodeled optic canal, which is commonly involved.

       e) Although intracranial extension may occur, it is clearly contiguous with the intraorbital meningioma, and it extends only a short distance along the prechiasmatic optic nerve sheath. This feature often helps to differentiate optic nerve sheath meningioma from optic nerve glioma (Table 14-7).

       f) Careful MRI and inspection are required to avoid missing the more subtle, early, optic nerve sheath meningioma. Linear calcifications that may be readily apparent on CT may be invisible on MRI scans. Only the fat-saturated, T1-weighted, axial enhanced images along the course of the nerve may demonstrate early meningioma. If fat-saturation artifacts obscure this imaging sequence, it is possible to miss this lesion. Use CT in equivocal cases.

  e. Other tumors of the optic nerve sheath.

   1) Other tumors primary to the optic nerve/sheath complex are extremely rare.

   2) Distant metastasis or local spread of retinoblastoma or uveal melanoma can occur.

   3) When lymphoma or leukemic infiltrates involve the optic nerve/ sheath complex, they usually do so as part of a systemic disease.

   4) Plexiform neurofibroma or schwannoma also are rarely seen along the course of the optic nerve/sheath complex.

5. Increased intracranial pressure.

  a. Elevation of the intracranial cerebrospinal fluid pressure, transmitted to the perioptic nerve subarachnoid space, results in distention of the optic sheath.

1) . In older patients it is possible to see an enlarged cerebrospinal fluid space around the optic nerve without this necessarily meaning that hydrocephalus is present.

b. CT or MRI scans show a bilateral, tortuous, enlarged, optic nerve/sheath complex. Enhanced thin-section CT or T2-weighted MR scans show the cause of this enlargement to be a swollen perioptic-nerve subarachnoid space.

   1) Careful examination may reveal the cause of the increased intracranial pressure.

      a) Increased intracranial pressure with secondary enlargement of the perioptic nerve subarachnoid space may result from intracranial mass lesions, hydrocephalus, malignant hypertension, diffuse cerebral edema, increased venous pressure, elevated cerebrospinal fluid protein levels, and pseudotumor cerebri among other disorders.

   2) Although clinical examination shows papilledema, the degree of distention of the perioptic nerve subarachnoid space does not correlate with the severity of the papilledema.

F. Conal and intraconal lesions.

1. Either singly or together, the conal muscles and intraconal fat are affected by the same group of diseases. For this reason the two areas are combined for construction of an orbital differential diagnosis for the conal–intraconal area.

2. Inflammatory lesions.

   a. Idiopathic inflammatory pseudotumor.

      1) Clinical presentation.

         a) Rapidly developing, unilateral, painful ophthalmoplegia; proptosis; or chemosis (i.e., edema of the ocular conjunctiva) with a rapid and lasting response to steroid therapy in an otherwise healthy patient is highly suggestive of orbital pseudotumor.

Q#7

         b) Pseudotumor is the most common cause of intraorbital mass lesion in adults.

      2) Pathologic features.

         a) Biopsy of the involved orbital area reveals a lymphocytic infiltrate that may have a variable histologic appearance. Early in the disease process an "inflammatory infiltrate" is seen. Later in the disease fibrosis and collagen fibers appear in the pathologic specimen.

         b) Pseudotumor may be seen in association with Wegener's granulomatosis, fibrosing mediastinitis, thyroiditis, or cholangitis.

      3) Radiologic characteristics.

a) Orbital pseudotumor can involve many of the structures within the orbit, including:

Q#7

1) Retrobulbar fat (76%).
2) Extraocular muscle or muscles (57%).
3) Optic nerve (38%).
4) Uveal–scleral area (33%).
5) Lacrimal gland (5%).
   b) The two principal pseudotumor types are tumefactive (i.e., diffuse involvement of conal and intraconal structures) and myositic (i.e., involving the extraocular muscles).
   c) The tumefactive type must be differentiated from true orbital tumor. Clinical presentation and response to steroids dictate the need for biopsy.
   d) The myositic type must be differentiated from thyroid ophthalmopathy. Unilateral involvement of a single extraocular muscle, including the tendinous insertions, is highly suggestive of pseudotumor.
   e) CT manifestations. Unilateral, enhancing mass (95% of cases) primarily conal and intraconal (i.e., tumefactive type) or involving a single extraocular muscle, including the tendinous insertions (i.e., myositic type).
   f) MRI manifestations. The morphologic features of pseudotumor are the same on CT and MRI scans. An additional feature supporting the diagnosis of pseudotumor on MRI scans is its tendency to produce signal that is hypo- or isointense to fat on T2-weighted images. Orbital tumors usually are hyperintense on T2-weighted images compared with orbital fat.
3. Endocrine lesions.
   a. Thyroid ophthalmopathy.
      1) Clinical presentation.
         a) Thyroid ophthalmopathy is the most common cause of unilateral or bilateral exophthalmos in adults.
         b) Most patients with thyroid ophthalmopathy have symptoms of hyperthyroidism. A history of gradually progressive, painless ocular prominence and proptosis often is associated with lid lag.
         c) In 70% of these patients levels of thyroxine (T4), triiodothyronine (T3), T3 resin uptake, or the free T4 index is elevated.
         d) Ten percent of patients with thyroid ophthalmopathy are free of clinical or laboratory evidence of thyroid dysfunction or "euthyroid ophthalmopathy."

2) Pathologic features. Biopsy of the affected extraocular muscles or retroorbital fat reveals deposition of hygroscopic mucopolysaccharides and infiltration of lymphocytes and plasma cells.
3) Radiologic characteristics.
   a) Characteristic findings on CT or MRI scans of thyroid ophthalmopathy are enlargement of extraocular muscles with sparing of the tendinous attachments to the globe. Compare this with the tendency of pseudotumor to involve the attachments.
   b) In descending order of frequency, the inferior, medial, lateral, and superior rectus muscles are involved.
   c) Eighty percent of patients have bilateral muscle involvement.
   d) In 10% of patients, one isolated muscle belly is involved.
   e) Enhanced images reveal moderate to prominent extraocular muscle belly enhancement.
   f) Retroglobar fat volume may be increased.
   g) If isolated lateral rectus muscle enlargement is seen on CT or MRI scans, causes other than thyroid ophthalmopathy should be sought.
4) Treatment options.
   a) When loss of vision accompanies thyroid ophthalmopathy, CT or MRI are used to evaluate the orbit in preparation for decompressive surgery or radiotherapy.
   b) Visual loss from compressive optic neuropathy results from increased extraocular muscle size and often massive increases in orbital fat.

4. Vascular lesions.
   a. Carotid–cavernous fistula.
   1) Clinical presentation.
      a) A spontaneous or posttraumatic communication between the cavernous carotid artery and cavernous sinus causes suffusion of the globe and orbit, pulsating exophthalmos, and a bruit on auscultation.
      b) Visual loss is present in the larger fistulous communications in 50% of cases.
   2) Radiologic characteristics.
      a) CT or MRI scans reveal enlargement (i.e., engorgement) of the superior ophthalmic vein and extraocular muscles.
      b) In addition, MRI scans show signal void in the ipsilateral cavernous sinus and enlarged superior ophthalmic vein because of the arterial flow within each.
      c) MRA reveals the enlarged superior ophthalmic vein. Phase-contrast MRA with directional emphasis can show the reversal of normal flow in this vessel.

  b. Venous varix.
   1) Pathologic features.
    a) Venous varix is an enormously dilated vein of either congenital or acquired origin.
    b) The lesion may occur as a congenital venous malformation or a venous wall weakness. Alternatively, the lesion may occur in association with either intraorbital or intracranial arteriovenous malformation.
   2) Radiologic characteristics.
    a) Contrast-enhanced CT scans show the varix as a lobulated, densely enhancing, intraconal structure that enlarges with Valsalva maneuver. Phleboliths may be seen.
    b) MRI permits documentation of the blood flow characteristics within the lesion. When the flow is rapid, flow void will be seen; slow flow may be visualized as flow-related enhancement. Because spontaneous thrombosis of a venous varix is common, variable signal intensity from a clot may be seen.
  c. Superior ophthalmic vein thrombosis.
   1) Clinical presentation.
    a) Superior ophthalmic vein thrombosis often occurs in conjunction with cavernous sinus thrombosis.
    b) Subsequent dysfunction of cranial nerves III, IV, and VI as well as associated ophthalmoplegia are seen.
   2) Radiologic characteristics.
    a) CT scans show an enlarged superior ophthalmic vein with an enhancing rim and low-density central clot. The ipsilateral cavernous sinus usually also is enlarged.
    b) MRI scans show an enlarged superior ophthalmic vein without central flow void. Central clot will vary in signal intensity depending on its age.
    c) Phase-contrast MRA with velocity encoding will prove there is no flow in the vessel when the intraluminal clot has confusing signal intensities.
5. Tumors.
  a. Cavernous hemangioma.
   1) Clinical presentation.
    a) Cavernous hemangioma occurs in early to middle adult life (i.e., 20 to 40 years of age).
    b) It presents as unilateral proptosis with diplopia and diminution of vision resulting from optic nerve compression by tumor.
   2) Pathologic features.

      a) Cavernous hemangioma is the most common orbital tumor.

      b) It is composed of a large, vascular space without recognizable feeder vessels. It has a dense, fibrous pseudocapsule.

      c) When isolated from the systemic circulation, it will thrombose, with subsequent phlebolith formation and hemosiderin deposition.

   3) Radiologic characteristics.

      a) CT scans show cavernous hemangioma as an intraconal, sharply circumscribed, rounded, dense mass that often spares the orbital apex. Uniform enhancement is the rule. Deformity of the bony orbit because of erosion is common, but bone destruction never occurs.

      b) MRI better delineates the relationship of the cavernous hemangioma to the optic nerve and extraocular muscles.

b. Capillary hemangioma.

   1) Clinical presentation. Infant patient (i.e., <1 year of age) with proptosis as well as eyelid and conjunctiva swelling that increases with crying or Valsalva maneuver.

   2) Pathologic features.

      a) Proliferation of endothelial cells with multiple capillaries.

      b) These lesions tend to regress spontaneously in the first few years of life.

   3) Radiologic features.

      a) Enhanced CT scans reveal an enhancing mass spanning the conal–intraconal the extraconal areas.

      b) The mass usually is not well marginated and may have irregular margins, suggesting a malignant cause.

c. Lymphangioma.

   1) Clinical presentation. Infant or young child with proptosis, often with associated periorbital swelling.

   2) Pathologic features.

      a) Histologic examination reveals that these lesions are comprised of dilated, thin, endothelium-lined vascular channels containing a variable amount of lymphocytic infiltration.

      b) Unlike capillary hemangioma, lymphangioma does not involute but continues to grow.

   3) Radiologic characteristics.

      a) Enhanced CT scans reveal a multiloculated, lobular, rim-enhancing mass that may be intraconal, conal, or extraconal.

      b) MRI scans may reveal hematoma of various duration within the lesion. Fluid-fluid levels may be present.

d. Lymphoma.

   1) Clinical presentation.

a) Orbital lymphoma presents in middle-aged patients (average age, 50 years) with painless swelling of the eyelids.
b) Exophthalmos occurs later in the course of the disease. If the primary area of involvement is the muscle cone, motion of the extraocular muscles is limited.
c) Orbital lymphoma usually presents without evidence of systemic disease. A majority of patients subsequently develop systemic lymphoma.

2) Pathologic features.
a) Orbital lymphoma is the third most common cause of proptosis after orbital pseudotumor and cavernous hemangioma.
b) The orbital lymphomas are B-cell (non-Hodgkin) lymphoma. Hodgkin lymphoma rarely involves the orbit.

3) Radiologic characteristics.
a) Orbital lymphoma may involve any area of the orbit. In descending order of frequency involvement is seen in the lacrimal gland (i.e., extraconal area), conal–intraconal area, and optic nerve/sheath complex.
b) Enhanced CT scans show orbital lymphoma as a spectrum of findings ranging from a well-defined, high-density mass to diffuse infiltration of the intraconal area. Bilateral orbital masses suggest the diagnosis of orbital lymphoma.

G. Extraconal lesions.

1. Strictly speaking, the extraconal area contains only the lacrimal gland and fat. Primary lesions of this area consequently are limited to lesions of the lacrimal gland; however, the extraconal area is the first part of the orbit into which surrounding infection and tumor invade on their way to deeper orbital structures.
2. Lesions of the lacrimal gland.
   a. Enlargement of the lacrimal gland is a nonspecific finding that can be caused by inflammation or neoplasm.
   b. Lacrimal gland inflammatory lesions.
      1) Most acute, inflammatory enlargement of the lacrimal gland in younger patients results from postviral syndrome. Chronic lacrimal gland inflammation is secondary to Sjögren's syndrome, Mikulicz's syndrome, or sarcoidosis.
      2) Sjögren's syndrome.
         a) Lymphocytic infiltration of the lacrimal and salivary glands causes decreased lacrimation and xerostomia.
         b) Many patients have associated rheumatoid arthritis, systemic lupus erythematosus, scleroderma, or polymyositis.

         3) Mikulicz's syndrome.
            a) Mikulicz's syndrome represents a nonspecific enlargement of the lacrimal and salivary glands associated with sarcoidosis, lymphoma, or leukemia.
    c. Tumors of the lacrimal gland.
         1) Tumors of the lacrimal gland may be epithelial, lymphoid, or metastatic.
         2) Benign mixed tumor and adenoid cystic carcinoma. These two epithelial tumors account for 50% of all lacrimal gland tumors.
         3) Lymphoma. Non-Hodgkin lymphoma of the orbit most frequently is found in the lacrimal gland.
         4) Metastasis. Metastasis to the lacrimal gland is rare.
3. Inflammatory lesions.
    a. See Chapter 15.
    b. Sinus infection with secondary subperiosteal abscess.
    c. Mucocele.
4. Tumors.
    a. Epidermoid and dermoid tumors.
         1) Orbital epidermoid or dermoid tumors usually arise anteriorly, between the globe and the orbital periosteum in the extraconal area. (See Chapter 15.)
         2) These lesions are well-circumscribed cystic masses. Containing only squamous debris and cholesterol, epidermoid tumors are fluid density on CT; dermoid tumors, which in addition may contain fat, sebaceous glands, teeth, and hair, usually are fat density on CT.
    b. Meningioma.
         1) Meningioma may involve the extraconal area from above or either side.
         2) The most common meningioma in the extraconal area is the sphenoid wing meningioma.
    c. Paranasal sinus malignancy.
         1) See Chapter 15.
         2) Squamous cell carcinoma of the maxillary or ethmoid sinus where CT or MRI scans have shown spread into the orbit requires orbital exenteration at the time of surgical treatment.
         3) Malignancy accesses the orbit through the weaker inferior and lateral walls in most cases. If the tumor breaks through the posterior maxillary sinus wall, it also may gain access to the orbital apex through the pterygopalatine fossa–infraorbital fissure.
5. Developmental lesions.
    a. See Chapter 16.
    b. Fibrous dysplasia.

1) Orbital involvement with fibrous dysplasia may be focal or diffuse.
2) Symptoms of diplopia and proptosis usually result from displacement of the globe by bony overgrowth. Late in the disease process the optic nerve atrophies because of optic canal impingement.
3) CT scans show thickened bone with coarsened trabeculae. Cystic areas may be present in the active phase of the disease, representing replacement of normal bone with fibrous tissue.
4) The differential diagnosis for this lesion includes en plaque meningioma, aneurysmal bone cyst, and Paget disease.

c. Paget disease.
1) Involvement of the bony orbit by Paget disease is infrequent, only occurring late in the disease process.
2) When involved, the roof and lateral orbital walls are the most frequently diseased areas.
3) CT scans show thickened bone with both lytic and sclerotic areas.

d. Neurofibromatosis type I.
1) The manifestations of neurofibromatosis are protean.
2) Orbital involvement is seen as optic nerve glioma, optic nerve sheath meningioma, plexiform neurofibroma, and dysplasia of the sphenoid bone portion of the posterior orbital wall.
3) Sphenoid wing dysplasia.
   a) Partial absence of the sphenoid wing results in enlargement of the superior orbital fissure and middle cranial fossa.
   b) At times the temporal lobe herniates through the enlarged superior orbital fissure, forming a meningioencephalocele with subsequent pulsatile exophthalmos.
   c) Although CT better delineates the bony abnormality of the sphenoid wing dysplasia, use of MRI to evaluate tissues in the cephalocele and to examine the rest of the brain and cisterns is strongly recommended.

SUGGESTED READING

Albert A, Lee BC, Saint-Louis, et al: MRI of the optic chiasm and the optic pathways. *AJNR* 7:255–258, 1986.

Armington WG, Bilaniuk LT: The radiologic evaluation of the orbit: conal and intraconal lesions. *Semin Ultrasound CT MR* 9:455–473, 1988.

Atlas SW, Grossman RI, Savino PJ, et al: Surface coil MR of orbital pseudotumor. *AJNR* 8:141–146, 1987.

Azar-Kia B, Mafee MF, Horowitz SW, et al: CT and MRI of the optic nerve and sheath. *Semin Ultrasound CT MR* 9:443–454, 1988.

Bencherif B, Zouaoui A, Chedid G, et al: Intracranial extension of an idiopathic orbital inflammatory pseudotumor. *AJNR* 14:181–184, 1993.

Bilaniuk LT, Schenck HF, Zimmerman RA, et al: Ocular and orbital lesions: surface coil MR imaging. *Radiology* 156:669–674, 1985.

Char DH, Unsold R, Sobel DF, et al: *Ocular and orbital pathology.* In Newton TH, Hasso AN, Dillon WP, editors: *Computed tomography of the head and neck,* ed 1. New York, 1988, Raven Press.

Cohn EM: Optic nerve sheath meningioma: neuroradiologic findings. *J Clin Neurol Ophthalmol* 3:85–89, 1983.

Enzmann D, Donaldson SS, Kriss JP: Appearance of Graves' disease on orbital CT. *J Comput Assist Tomogr* 3:815–819, 1979.

Enzmann D, Donaldson SS, Marshall WH, et al: CT in orbital psuedotumor (idiopathic orbital inflammation). *Radiology* 120:597–601, 1976.

Flanders AE, Mafee MF, Rao VM, et al: CT characteristics of orbital pseudotumors and other orbital inflammatory processes. *J Comput Assist Tomogr* 13:40–47, 1989.

Graeb DA, Rootman J, Robertson WD, et al: Orbital lymphangiomas: clinical, radiologic, and pathologic characteristics. *Radiology* 175:417–421, 1990.

Hiak BG, Saint-Louis L, Smith ME, et al: Magnetic resonance imaging in the evaluation of leukocoria. *Ophthalmology* 92:1143–1152, 1985.

Harnsberger HR: State of the art orbital imaging. *Semin Ultrasound CT MR* 9:379–483, 1988.

Hedges TR, Possi-Mucelli R, Char DH, et al: CT demonstration of ocular calcification: correlations with clinical and pathological findings. *Neuroradiology* 23:15–21, 1982.

Hesselink JR, Davis KR, Dallow RL, et al: CT of masses of the lacrimal gland region. *Radiology* 131:143–147, 1979.

Hilborn MD, Munk PL, Lin DTC, et al: Sonography of ocular choroidal melanomas. *Am J Roentgenol* 161:1253–1257, 1993.

Holman RE, Grimson BS, Drayer BP, et al: MRI of optic gliomas. *Am J Ophthalmol* 100:596–601, 1985.

Hopper KD, Sherman JL, Boal DK, Eggli KD: CT and MR imaging of the pediatric orbit. *RadioGraphics* 12:485–503, 1992.

Hosten N, Sander B, Cordes M, et al: Graves ophthalmolopathy: MR imaging of the orbits. *Radiology* 172:759–762, 1989.

Johns TT, Citin CM, Black J, et al: CT evaluation of perineural orbital lesions: evaluation of the "tram-track" sign. *AJNR* 5:587–590, 1984.

Just M, Kahaly G, Higer HP, et al: Graves opthalmology: role of MR imaging in radiation therapy. *Radiology* 179:187–190, 1991.

Levine HL, Ferris EJ: The neuroradiologic evaluation of "optic neuritis." *Am J Roentgenol* 125:702–716, 1975.

Lloyd GA: Lacrimal gland tumours: the role of CT and conventional radiology. *Br J Radiol* 54:1034–1038, 1981.

Mafee MF, Goldberg MF, Greenwold MJ, et al: Retinoblastoma and simulating lesions: role of CT and MR imaging. *Radiol Clin North Am* 25:667–682, 1987.

Mafee MF, Goldberg MF, Valvassori GE, et al: CT in the evaluation of patients with persistent hyperplastic primary vitreous (PHPV). *Radiology* 145:713–717, 1982.

Mafee MF, Peyman GA, Grisolano JE, et al: Malignant uveal melanomas and simulating lesions: MR imaging evaluation. *Radiology* 160:773–780, 1986.

Mafee MF, Peyman GA, McKusick MA: Malignant uveal melanoma and similar lesions studied by CT. *Radiology* 156:403–408, 1985.

Mihara F, Gupta KL, Murayama S, et al: MR imaging of malignant uveal melanoma: role of pulse sequence and contrast agent. *AJNR* 12:991–996, 1991.

Nugent RA, Belkin RI, Neigel JM, et al: Graves orbitopathy: correlation of CT and clinical findings. *Radiology* 177:675–682, 1990.

Peyster RG, Augsberger JJ, Shields JA, et al: Choroidal melanoma: comparison of CT, fundoscopy, and US. *Radiology* 156:675–680, 1985.

Peyster RG, Hoover ED, Hershey BL, et al: High resolution CT of lesions of the optic nerve. *Am J Roentgenol* 140:869–874, 1983.

Price HI, Batnitzky S, Danziger A, et al: The neuroradiology of retinoblastoma. *RadioGraphics* 2:7–23, 1982.

Ramirez H, Blatt ES, Hibri NS: CT identification of calcified optic nerve drusen. *Radiology* 148:137–139, 1983.

Rothfus WE, Curtin HD: Extraocular muscle enlargement: a CT review. *Radiology* 151:677–681, 1984.

Sandberg-Wollheim M, Bynke H, Cronqvist S, et al: A long term prospective study of optic neuritis: evaluation of risk factors. *Ann Neurol* 27:386–393, 1990.

Sherman JL, McLean IW, Brallier DR: Coats disease: CT-pathologic correlations in two cases. *Radiology* 146:77–78, 1983.

Shnier R, Parker GD, Hallinan JM, et al: Orbital varices: a new technique for non-invasive diagnosis. *AJNR* 12:717–718, 1991.

Skedros DG, Haddad J Jr, Bluestone CD, Curtin HD: Subperiosteal orbital abscess in children: diagnosis, microbiology, and management. *Laryngoscope* 103:28–32, 1993.

Swenson SA, Forbes GS: Radiologic evaluation of tumors of the optic nerve. *AJNR* 3:319–326, 1982.

Tien RD, Chu PK, Hesselink JR, Szumowski J: Intra- and paraorbital lesions: value of fat-suppression MR imaging with paramagnetic contrast enhancement. *AJNR* 12:245–253, 1991.

Tong KA, Osborn AG, Mamalis N, et al: Radiologic-pathologic correlation: occular melanoma. *AJNR* 14:1359–1366, 1993.

Turner RM, Gutman I, Hilal SK, et al: CT of drusen bodies and other calcific lesions of the optic nerve: case report and differential diagnosis. *AJNR* 4:175–178, 1983.

Unsold R, de Groot J: *Normal anatomy of the orbit*. In Newton TH, Hasson AN, Dillon WP, editors: *Computed tomography of the head and neck*, ed 1. New York, 1988, Raven Press.

Wells RG, Sty JR, Gonnering RS: Imaging of the pediatric eye and orbit. *RadioGraphics* 9:1023–1044, 1989.

Yousem DM, Atlas SA, Grossman RI, et al: MR imaging of Tolosa-Hunt syndrome. *AJNR* 10:1181–1184, 1989.

15

Sinonasal Imaging:
Imaging Issues in Sinusitis

CRITICAL IMAGING QUESTIONS:
SINONASAL IMAGING

1. Describe the normal drainage of each paranasal sinus. What is the name of the primary passage through which each sinus drains?
2. What are the three parts of the hard portion of the nasal septum?
3. What are the principal components of the ostiomeatal unit? In what plane is this unit best displayed?
4. What normal structures link the pterygopalatine fossa to the nasopharyngeal masticator space, nose, orbit, middle cranial fossa, and oral cavity?
5. In what order do the four paranasal sinuses aerate? Approximately when would you see each sinus aerated on plain-film radiographs of the sinuses?
6. What four nonmalignant diseases of the sinonasal region can mimic radiologically malignant squamous cell carcinoma?

Answers to these questions are found in the text beside the question number (Q#) in margin.

SINONASAL IMAGING: EMPHASIZING IMAGING ISSUES IN SINUSITIS

A. Normal Anatomy of the Paranasal Sinuses and Nose.

1. General remarks.
   a. The paranasal sinuses and nose are intimately associated in their development. An understanding of the anatomy of one without that of the other precludes one from grasping the complete picture of the normal and diseased sinonasal region.
   b. The key to normal anatomy of the paranasal sinuses lies in a clear understanding of the structures of the lateral wall of the nose, into which the paranasal sinuses drain (Figs. 15-1 through 15-4).
   c. The anatomy of the sinuses is relatively simple, whereas that of the lateral wall of the nose is complex.
   d. The anatomy of the pterygopalatine fossa and the sphenopalatine foramen is discussed in this chapter because of the interaction of these normal anatomic structures in the spread of sinonasal disease.
2. Anatomy of the paranasal sinuses.
   a. Specific anatomic considerations of the paranasal sinuses are best discussed with reference to the four sinus groups.
   b. Maxillary sinuses.
      1) Bone of origin. Paired air cells in the maxillary bone.
      2) Maxillary sinus walls. The roof of the maxillary sinus is the floor of the orbit. The medial wall is a portion of the lateral wall of the nose. The posterior wall abuts the retromaxillary fat pad and pterygopalatine fossa.

Q#1

      3) Drainage. Maxillary sinus drainage is primarily via the maxillary ostium into the infundibulum, which in turn empties into the posterior aspect of the hiatus semilunaris of the middle meatus (Figs. 15-3 and 15-4).
   c. Ethmoid sinuses.
      1) Bone of origin. Ethmoid bone.
         a) The ethmoid bone consists of four parts: the horizontal lamina above, called the *cribriform plate*; a perpendicular plate; and two lateral masses, called the *ethmoid labyrinths*.
         b) The roof of the ethmoid labyrinth is called the *fovea ethmoidalis*.
      2) The number of air cells per side varies from three to 18. Anterior, middle, and posterior groups generally can be identified.
         a) When describing a lesion within the ethmoid sinuses, localize it to one of these three areas (i.e., anterior, middle, posterior).

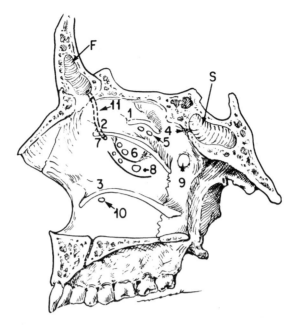

Fig. 15-1 Simplified drawing of the normal lateral wall apertures of the nose. The superior (*1*), middle (*2*), and inferior (*3*) turbinates have been pruned to display critical ostia of the nasal lateral wall. From front to back, the frontal sinus (*F*) drains through the nasofrontal duct (*11*) into the most anterior aspect of the hiatus semilunaris of the middle meatus. Anterior ethmoid air cells drain into the anterior hiatus semilunaris/cephalad maxillary infundibulum area (*7*). Middle ethmoid air cells drain through the ethmoid bulla (*6*) into the middle portion of the hiatus semilunaris of the middle meatus. The maxillary sinus empties through its ostia (*8*) into the posterior–inferior hiatus semilunaris. Posterior ethmoid air cells (*5*) initially drain into the superior meatus, while the sphenoid sinus (*S*) empties through the sphenoid ostia (*4*) into the adjacent sphenoethmoidal recess. *9*, Sphenopalatine foramen; *10*, nasolacrimal duct ostia in the anterior aspect of the inferior meatus. (From Harnsberger HR, Osborn AG, Smoker WRK: CT in the evaluation of the normal and diseased paranasal sinuses. *Semin Ultrasound CT MR* 7:68–90, 1986. Used with permission.)

    b) Identification of which area one is looking at on coronal sinus CT images may be difficult at first. If definite identification of the specific cells affected is necessary for treatment, axial CT images will provide this information.

    c) The middle ethmoid air cells can be identified on coronal sinus CT images as the ethmoid air cells superior and lateral to the ethmoid bulla. Once the middle air cells are identified

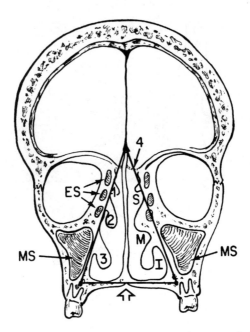

Fig. 15-2 Normal coronal scheme of the nose and paranasal sinuses. The nose is a triangular structure when viewed from the front and is divided down the middle by the septum (*open arrow*). At the apex of the triangle is the cribriform plate of the ethmoid bone (*4*). The base of the triangle is the hard and soft palates, and the sides are comprised of the lateral nasal walls. The coronal view best demonstrates the major relationships of the nasal and paranasal sinus structures. The lateral wall of the nose is dominated by the superior (*1*), middle (*2*), and inferior (*3*) turbinate bones. The areas lateral and inferior to each turbinate represent the meati of the nose; the major paranasal sinuses drain into these regions. *ES*, Ethmoid sinus; *I*, inferior meatus; *M*, middle meatus; *MS*, maxillary sinus; *S*, superior meatus. (From Harnsberger HR, Osborn AG, Smoker WRK: CT in the evaluation of the normal and diseased paranasal sinuses. *Semin Ultrasound CT MR* 7:68–90, 1986. Used with permission).

by this landmark, anterior and posterior ethmoid air cells can be identified.

3) Ethmoid sinus walls.
   a) The thin, lateral wall separating the ethmoid air cells from the orbit is called the *lamina papyracea*.
   b) The medial wall is shared with the nose.
   c) The roof of the ethmoid air cells (i.e., fovea ethmoidalis) also is the floor of the anterior cranial fossa.

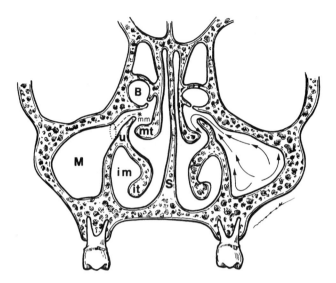

Fig. 15-3   Coronal drawing of the normal ostiomeatal unit. *Left,* Normal structures of the ostiomeatal unit, maxillary ostium (*dotted circle*), maxillary infundibulum (*dashed straight line*), uncinate process (*u*), hiatus semilunaris (*asterisk*), and
ethmoid bulla (*B*). *Right,* Normal mucociliary drainage of the maxillary sinus
(*arrows*). The mucus normally flows from the sinus proper, through the maxillary
ostium, up the maxillary infundibulum, and through the hiatus semilunaris into the
middle meatus. *im,* Inferior meatus; *it,* inferior turbinate bone; *M,* maxillary sinus;
mm, middle meatus; *mt,* middle turbinate bone; *S,* nasal septum. (From Pollei SR,
Harnsberger HR: The radiologic evaluation of the sinonasal region. *Postgrad
Radiol* 8:242–265, 1989. Used with permission.)

Q#1

 4) Drainage. Drainage of the ethmoid air cells is complex.
   a) Anterior ethmoid air cells empty into the anterior aspect of
       the hiatus semilunaris.
   b) Middle ethmoid air cells empty through the ethmoid bulla
       into the middle meatus.
   c) Posterior ethmoid air cells empty into the superior meatus,
       then into the sphenoethmoidal recess (Figs. 15-1 and
       15-4).
 5) Other special ethmoid sinus features are:
   a) Agger nasi air cells. These are defined as the anterior–infe-
       rior, most extramural ethmoid air cells. The term *extramural*
       is used when the air cell is not confined within the parent
       bone (in this case, the ethmoid bone).

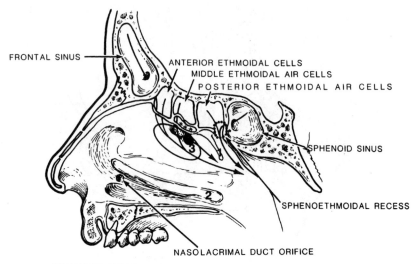

FRONTAL SINUS

ANTERIOR ETHMOIDAL CELLS
MIDDLE ETHMOIDAL AIR CELLS
POSTERIOR ETHMOIDAL AIR CELLS

SPHENOID SINUS

SPHENOETHMOIDAL RECESS

NASOLACRIMAL DUCT ORIFICE

✳✳✳: ETHMOIDAL BULLA
1: CUT MIDDLE TURBINATE
2: CUT INFERIOR TURBINATE
3: MAXILLARY SINUS OSTIUM

Fig. 15-4   Mucociliary drainage patterns of the individual sinus groups on the lateral wall of the nose. Frontal sinus drainage is via the nasofrontal canal into the anterior recess of the middle meatus. The anterior ethmoid complex drains into the anterior middle meatus area (*solid circled region*). The middle ethmoid complex drains through the ethmoid bulla (*asterisks*) into the cephalad portion of the ethmoid infundibulum, then into the middle part of the middle meatus. The posterior ethmoid air cells drain into the superior meatus, then into the sphenoethmoidal recess (*dotted circle*). The sphenoethmoidal recess also directly receives the drainage of the sphenoid sinus. (Adapted from Pollei SR, Harnsberger HR: The radiologic evaluation of the sinonasal region. *Postgrad Radiol* 9:242–265, 1989. Used with permission.)

      b) Haller's cells. These are defined as the extramural ethmoidal air cells extending along the medial floor of the orbit (i.e., infraorbital air cells).

      c) Ethmoid bulla (bulla ethmoidalis). This is defined as the convex, inferomedial bony wall overlying the middle ethmoid air cells. The ethmoid bulla protrudes inferomedially into the middle meatus.

   d. Sphenoid sinuses.

      1) Bone of origin. Sphenoid bone. Aeration usually is within the medial portion of the sphenoid bone. Less commonly, aeration spreads inferiorly into the pterygoid plates.

2) Sphenoid sinus walls. The roof of the sphenoid sinus is the sella turcica. The anterior wall is shared with the ethmoid sinuses. The posterior wall is the clivus, and the inferior wall is the roof of the nasopharynx.

Q#1

3) Drainage. The sphenoid sinuses drain into the sphenoethmoidal recess just posterior and medial to the superior meatus (Figs. 15-1 and 15-4).

e. Frontal sinuses.
1) Bone of origin. The paired, normally asymmetric frontal sinuses are located in the frontal bone.
2) Frontal sinus walls. The inferior wall of the frontal sinuses also is the anterior portion of the orbital roof. The posterior wall directly abuts the anterior cranial fossa.
   a) When a question regarding the integrity of the posterior wall of the frontal sinus (e.g., fracture, focal dehiscence from tumor or infection), axial CT is recommended in addition to coronal sinus CT.

Q#1

3) Drainage. The frontal sinuses most frequently drain via the nasofrontal duct through or adjacent to the anterior ethmoid air cells, then into the frontal recess of the middle meatus of the nose (Fig. 15-1).
   a) Communication between the frontal sinus and nasal cavity is not strictly a duct. Rather, it is an internal channel between the sinus and the frontal recess of the middle meatus.

3. Normal anatomy of the nose.
   a. General comments.
      1) The nose is a triangular structure when viewed from the front and is divided down the middle by the septum (Fig. 15-2). At the apex of the triangle is the cribriform plate of the ethmoid bone. The base of the triangle is the hard and soft palates, and the sides are comprised of the lateral nasal walls.
      2) The lateral wall of the nasal cavity contains the passages from the paranasal sinuses to the nasal cavity. A clear understanding of this area promotes an insightful interpretation of sinonasal region images.
   b. Nasal septum.
      1) Like the palate, the nasal septum has both a hard and a soft mobile part.

Q#2

2) The hard portion of the nasal septum is primarily comprised of three components: the perpendicular plate of the ethmoid bone, the septal cartilage, and the vomer bone (Fig. 15-5).

3) The mobile septum comprises the medial limbs of the U-shaped alar cartilages as well as the skin and soft tissues between the tip of the nose and the anterior nasal spine.

4) The anterior aspect of the nasal septum normally may appear bulbous on coronal sinus CT scans. Avoid mistaking this for pathology.

c. Lateral nasal wall (Fig. 15-6).

1) The lateral wall of the nose is an undulating surface with three distinct projections: the superior, middle, and inferior turbinates. As the turbinates curl inferolaterally they define distinct air tunnels running from anterior to posterior: the superior, middle, and inferior meati.

2) Superior turbinate/meatus.

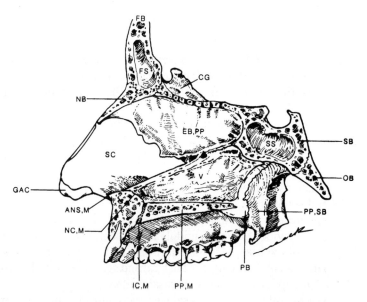

Fig. 15-5 Infrastructure of the nasal septum. From superior to inferior the abbreviations include: *FB*, frontal bone; *FS*, frontal sinus; *NB*, nasal bone; *CG*, crista galli; *EB,PP*, ethmoid bone, perpendicular plate; *SB*, sphenoid bone; *SS*, sphenoid sinus; *SC*, septal cartilage; *V*, vomer; *GAC*, greater alar cartilage; *ANS,M*, anterior nasal septum, membranous portion; *OB*, occipital bone; *NC,M*, nasal crest, maxilla; *IC,M*, incisive canal, maxilla; *PP,M*, palatine process, maxilla; *PB*, palatine bone; *PP,SB*, pterygoid process, sphenoid bone.

a) Only the posterior ethmoid air cells empty into the superior meatus. From there secretions drain via the sphenoethmoidal recess into the posterior nose.

b) The sphenoid sinus empties into the sphenoethmoidal recess but not into the superior meatus.

3) Middle turbinate/meatus.

a) The middle meatus is the most important anatomic area on the lateral wall of the nose. When diseased, a characteristic pattern of unilateral frontal, anterior, and middle ethmoid and maxillary sinus opacification is seen on coronal sinus CT scans (i.e., the ostiomeatal unit pattern).

b) Middle meatus contents (Figs. 15-1, 15-3, and 15-6).

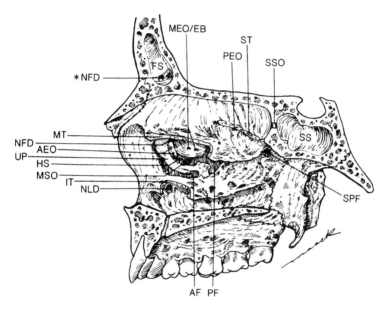

A

Fig. 15-6   **A**, Bones and ostia of the lateral wall of the nose. Compare this panel, which emphasizes bones and ostia only, with panel *B*, which illustrates these structures covered by mucosa. Abbreviations from superior to inferior include: *MEO/EB*, middle ethmoid sinus ostia; *ST*, superior turbinate cut end; *PEO*, posterior ethmoid ostia; *FS*, frontal sinus; *NFD**, nasofrontal duct proximal end; *SSO*, sphenoid sinus ostia; *SS*, sphenoid sinus; *MT*, middle turbinate cut edge; *NFD*, nasofrontal duct distal end; *AEO*, anterior ethmoid ostia; *UP*, uncinate process; *HS*, hiatus semilunaris; *MSO*, maxillary sinus ostia; *IT*, inferior turbinate; *NLD*, nasolacrimal duct; *SPF*, sphenopalatine foramen; *AF*, anterior fontanelle; *PF*, pos-

(continued)

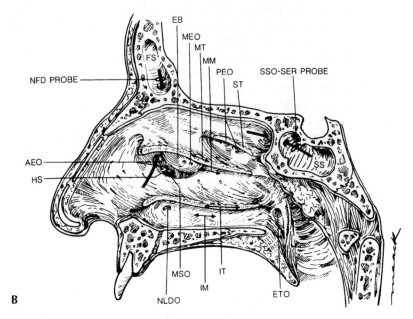

Fig. 15-6 (*continued*)   terior fontanelle. **B**, Lateral wall of the nose emphasizing mucosal surfaces. Compare this drawing with panel *A*, which depicts the underlying bones of the lateral wall of the nose. Abbreviations from superior to inferior include: *EB*, ethmoid bulla; *MEO*, middle ethmoid ostia; *MT*, middle turbinate cut edge; *MM*, middle meatus; *PEO*, posterior ethmoid ostia; *ST*, superior turbinate cut end; *NFD PROBE*, nasofrontal duct probe; *SSO-SER PROBE*, sphenoid sinus ostia–spenoethmoidal recess probe; *SS*, sphenoid sinus; *AEO*, anterior ethmoid ostia; *HS*, hiatus semilunaris; *MSO*, maxillary sinus ostia; *IT*, inferior turbinate cut edge; *IM*, inferior meatus; *ETO*, eustachian tube orifice; *NLDO*, nasolacrimal duct orifice.

    i)   The ethmoid bulla is nestled in the cephalad recess of the middle meatus. It receives drainage from the middle ethmoid air cells through multiple ostia.

   ii)   Located just inferior to the ethmoid bulla in the middle meatus, the hiatus semilunaris receives multiple ostia from the anterior ethmoid air cells in its anterior aspect. More posteriorly, the hiatus semilunaris receives the maxillary ostium–infundibulum, which is the single major drainage passage of the maxillary sinus.

  iii)   The frontal recess of the middle meatus receives the drainage from the frontal sinus via the nasofrontal duct.

  c) Concha bullosa. This is a pneumatized middle turbinate. It may be seen as a normal variant or may cause disease when too large or superinfected.

4) Inferior turbinate/meatus.
  a) Although the inferior meatus is the largest of the three nasal meati, its anatomy is the simplest.
  b) It receives the nasolacrimal duct in its anterior aspect (Figs. 15-1, 15-4, and 15-8).
    i) Because the nasoantral windows are placed in the inferior meatus, surgical injury of the nasolacrimal duct may occur if the window is located too anteriorly.

5) Ostiomeatal unit.
  a) Since the development of functional endoscopic sinus surgery (FESS), interest in the precise anatomy of the lateral nasal wall has intensified. The ostiomeatal unit is the center of this interest, because it is the crossroads of mucociliary drainage of the paranasal sinuses into the middle meatus of the nose.

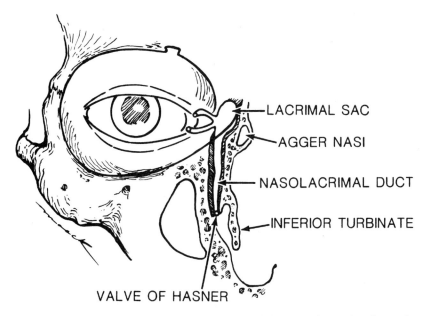

Fig. 15-7 Nasolacrimal apparatus. This coronal drawing shows the close relationship of the nasolacrimal sac to the agger nasi ethmoid air cell. Do not mistake the fluid-filled sac for an opacified agger nasi cell on coronal sinus CT scans. The nasolacrimal duct drains inferiorly into the anterior aspect of the inferior meatus (see Fig. 15-4).

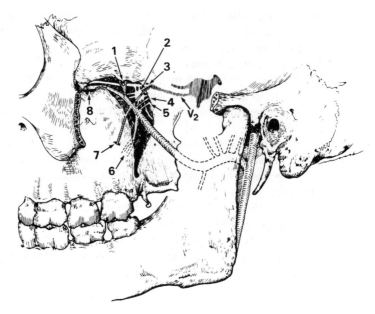

Fig. 15-8 Pterygopalatine fossa viewed through the pterygomaxillary fissure. Within the fossa the distal internal maxillary artery subdivides into the spheno-palatine artery (*1*), vidian artery (*4*), pharyngeal artery (*5*), descending palatine artery (*6*), posterior superior alveolar artery (*7*), and infraorbital artery (*8*). The maxillary division of the trigeminal nerve (*V₂*) exits the foramen rotundum (*3*), runs along the roof of the pterygopalatine fossa, and continues anteriorly as the infra-orbital nerve. The sphenopalatine ganglion (*2*) dangles from the maxillary nerve in the pterygopalatine fossa. (From Osborn AG: *Introduction to cerebral angiography.* Hagerstown, Md., 1980, Harper & Row. Used with permission.)

    b) The ostiomeatal unit is the area of superomedial maxillary sinus and middle meatus that conveys the mucociliary drainage of the frontal sinus, anterior and middle ethmoid sinuses, and maxillary sinus into the nose.

Q#3

    c) Important components of the ostiomeatal unit include the infundibulum, uncinate process, ethmoid bulla, hiatus semi-lunaris, and the middle meatus (Fig. 15-3).

    d) Maxillary infundibulum. Although the infundibulum appears on coronal sinus CT scans as a funnel-shaped tube connecting the maxillary sinus to the middle meatus, it actu-ally is a trough-shaped groove within the lateral nasal wall, running obliquely from anterosuperior to posteroinferior. The infundibulum is bounded superomedially by the hiatus semilunaris, posterosuperiorly by the ethmoid bulla, laterally by the inferomedial wall of the orbit, and inferomedially by the uncinate process (Fig. 15-3).

e) Uncinate process. This is a curvilinear bone in the lateral wall of the nose that runs along the inferior margin of the hiatus semilunaris. It represents the medial bony wall of the infundibulum (Fig. 15-3).

f) Hiatus semilunaris. This is the sigmoid-shaped groove in the lateral wall of the nose with the ethmoid bulla as its superior margin and the cephalad edge of the uncinate process as its inferior margin. The hiatus semilunaris is difficult to identify on coronal sinus CT.

g) The goal of FESS is to reestablish normal drainage through the ostiomeatal unit. This usually is accomplished by entering the hiatus semilunaris of the middle meatus with the endoscope and removing the uncinate process.

h) The normal mucociliary drainage pattern of the maxillary sinus (Fig. 15-3, *right*) creates a mucous flow from the maxillary sinus cavity superomedially through the maxillary ostium into the infundibulum. From there the mucus continues into the hiatus semilunaris of the middle meatus, then posteroinferiorly along the middle meatus into the posterior nares and nasopharynx (Fig. 15-4).

Q#3

i) The ostiomeatal unit is best visualized with coronal CT. Coronal sinus CT (see Section C2) has been devised to optimally display the intricate anatomy of the ostiomeatal units.

4. Sphenopalatine foramen and pterygopalatine fossa.

a. The sphenopalatine foramen connects the lateral nasal cavity with the pterygopalatine fossa. Because of the complex connections of the pterygopalatine fossa, nasal infection and tumors can access the orbit, nasopharyngeal masticator space, and intracranial space through this escape hatch.

b. Sphenopalatine foramen.

1) The sphenopalatine foramen is located in the high posterolateral wall of the nose (Fig. 15-1).

2) The foramen transmits the lateral nasal and nasopalatine nerves and vessels, and it is closed over in life by the mucous membrane of the lateral wall of the nose (Fig. 15-9).

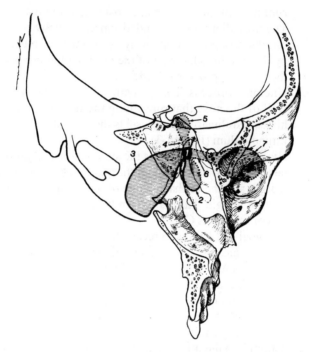

Fig. 15-9 Routes of tumor spread from the central position of the sphenopala-tine foramen (*1*). The classic example of tumor spreading out in the area of the sphenopalatine foramen is juvenile angiofibroma. Possible routes of spread include anteriorly into the nose (*2*), posteroinferiorly into the nasopharynx (*3*), posterosuperiorly through the foramen rotundum (*4*) into middle cranial fossa (*5*), and laterally through the pterygopalatine fossa (*6*) on into the nasopharyngeal masticator space (*7*) (i.e., infratemporal fossa).

3) Tumors involving the lateral wall of the nose tend to escape the nasal cavity by passing through the sphenopalatine foramen into the pterygopalatine fossa.
  a) The classic example of this phenomenon is juvenile angiofi-broma (Fig. 15-9). This tumor really is a primary nasal tumor. Because it usually demonstrates early spread to the pterygopalatine fossa, however, this lesion often is mistaken as originating in the fossa.
c. Pterygopalatine fossa.
  1) The pterygopalatine fossa is the major crossroads between the nasal cavity, nasopharyngeal masticator space (i.e., infratempo-ral fossa), orbit, and middle cranial fossa.

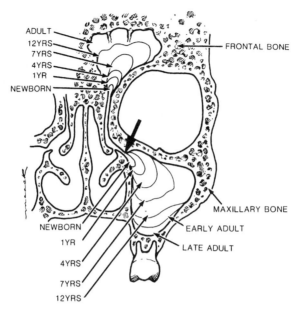

Fig. 15-10 **A,** Composite drawing showing the temporal and morphologic changes of maxillary and frontal sinus development in the coronal projection from birth to maturity. The maxillary sinus advances from the infundibulum (*large arrow*) in an inferolateral direction. It is the largest and most developed sinus group at birth. Maxillary pneumatization is complete when the permanent teeth erupt, allowing the sinus floor to extend below the level of the hard palate (early and late adult growth bands). The frontal sinus develops as an anterosuperior extension of the anterior ethmoid sinus into the frontal bone. It is not present radiologically in newborns. It is the last of the sinus groups to reach its full adult size, usually well after puberty.

B, Axial drawing showing the temporal and morphologic changes of ethmoid and sphenoid sinus development. The ethmoid and maxillary sinuses are present at birth, although the more anterior ethmoid air cells are larger than their posterior counterparts. The lateral walls of the ethmoid air cells go from concaved inward to straight to convex outward as the ethmoid air cells develop. The sphenoid sinus is undeveloped and nonaerated at birth. It develops embryologically from bilateral posterior invaginations of nasal mucosa into the sphenoid bone area of the skull base. At approximately 3 years of age aeration begins in the anterior portion of the sphenoid bone in the area known as the *presphenoid*, progressing posteriorly into the *basisphenoid* area until the aeration process reaches the anterior wall of the clivus. The sinus attains its mature size by approximately 12 to 14 years of age. The perpendicular plate of the ethmoid bone and vertical sphenoid septum have been *blackened* to illustrate fusion of the ethmoid labyrinth and sphenoid sinus. **C,** Composite drawing showing the temporal and morphologic changes of sphenoid sinus

(*continued*)

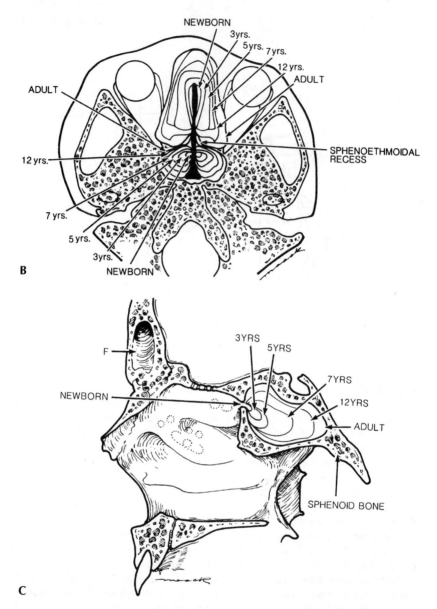

Fig. 15-10 *(continued)* development in the lateral projection from birth to maturity. At 3 years of age aeration of the presphenoid bone begins, progressing a variable distance into the basisphenoid area. The maximum degree of sphenoid pneumatization is seen when the process reaches as far as the anterior clival wall. It is normal to see the pneumatization arrest as far anterior as the anterior margin of the sella. Note that the sphenoid sinus ostium is nondependent. *F,* Frontal sinus. (From Scuderi AJ, Harnsberger HR, Boyer RS: Pneumatization of the paranasal sinuses: normal features of importance to the accurate interpretation of CT scans and MR images. *Am J Roentgenol* 160:1101–1104, 1993. Used by permission.)

2) Location. The pterygopalatine fossa is located between the posterior wall of the maxillary sinus, the pterygoid process of the sphenoid bone, and the vertical part of the palatine bone.
3) Contents.
    a) Distal internal maxillary artery.
    b) Pterygopalatine ganglion. This is the largest of the parasympathetic ganglia associated with the trigeminal nerve. It contains sensory roots from the palatine nerve (i.e., cranial nerve V_2 branch) and a motor root from the preganglionic parasympathetic nerve via the greater superficial petrosal nerve. From the sphenopalatine ganglion, peripheral branches are distributed to the lacrimal gland, nose, palate, and oropharynx.
    c) The main trunk of the second division of the trigeminal nerve (i.e., maxillary nerve) comes out of the foramen rotundum to cross the cephalad aspect of the pterygopalatine fossa.

Q#4

4) Communications between the pterygopalatine fossa and the surrounding adjacent spaces are:
    a) Directly lateral is the pterygomaxillary fissure, which leads to the nasopharyngeal masticator space (i.e., infratemporal fossa).
    b) Directly medial is the sphenopalatine foramen, which leads to the posterior aspect of the superior meatus of the nasal cavity.
    c) Anterosuperiorly, the pterygopalatine fossa communicates with the orbit through the inferior orbital fissure.
    d) Posterosuperiorly, it is connected to the middle cranial fossa via the foramen rotundum and the vidian canal.
    e) Inferiorly, the pterygopalatine fossa is in communication with the oral cavity through the pterygopalatine canal, which transmits the palatine vessels and nerves.

B. Paranasal sinus development.

1. Introduction.
    a. Developmentally, the paranasal sinuses represent nasal "diverticula." Hence, the mucosa of the sinuses and nose form one continuous sheet of tissue.
    b. Because the sinuses do not reach full size until the teenage years, radiologic interpretive errors (especially of plain films) result when understanding of the developmental sequence and rate of the paranasal sinuses is lacking.
    c. All of the paranasal sinuses normally may be opaque in an infant younger than 1 year of age.

1) No clear understanding of the histopathologic basis of this observation exists, but some authors suggest that "redundant mucosa" is responsible.
2) More recent, MRI-derived observations suggest that a bone will undergo pneumatization changes its marrow signal from "red marrow" (i.e., tissue intensity) to yellow marrow (i.e., fat intensity). After this change occurs the sinus begins to form, normally as an opacified structure (i.e., fluid intensity). The final phase of normal pneumatization is the change from opacified sinus to aerated sinus.

   d. No clinical significance can be attributed to sinus opacification alone in an infant younger than 1 year of age. Radiologic evaluation of the paranasal sinuses for inflammatory disease should be avoided during the first year of life.

   e. Children older than 3 years of age with paranasal-sinus opacification or air–fluid levels may be considered to have pathologically inflamed sinuses. Between the ages of 1 and 3 years, however, radiologic studies must be interpreted with considerable reservation.

2. Sinus development.

Q#5

   a. Maxillary sinuses.
1) The maxillary sinus is the first aerated sinus to be visualized on plain-film radiographs or CT scans (Fig. 15-10*A*).
   a) Small, aerated maxillary sinuses are present at birth.
   b) Lateral growth of the maxillary sinuses beneath the orbits continues until 15 years of age.
   c) After eruption of the adult upper teeth, the maxillary sinus completes its pneumatization process by extending inferiorly into the maxillary ridge.
2) Aplasia and hypoplasia of the maxillary sinuses in otherwise normal persons occurs with an incidence of 0.4% and 9.0%, respectively (Table 15-1).

   b. Ethmoid sinuses.
1) Small, aerated ethmoid sinuses may be present at birth. Because of their size, however, they may be difficult to identify on plain-film radiographs.
2) The ethmoid sinus air-cell formation extends from medial to lateral and from anterior to posterior (Fig. 15-10*B*).
3) Growth of ethmoid sinuses ceases in late puberty.

   c. Sphenoid sinuses.
1) Nonaerated sphenoid sinuses with a maximum diameter of 2 mm usually are present at birth. Aeration of the sphenoid sinuses generally is apparent by 3 years of age.

Table 15-1   Differential Diagnosis of Small or Absent Sinus

Congenital
  Congenital hypoplasia or aplasia
    Frontal sinus aplasia (4.0%)
    Maxillary sinus hypoplasia (9.0%)
    Maxillary sinus aplasia (0.4%)
  Cretinism
  Down syndrome
    Absent frontal sinuses (90.0%)
  Kartagener's syndrome
    Dextrocardia, bronchiectasis, absent frontal sinuses

Bony Sinus Wall Overgrowth
  Paget disease
  Fibrous dysplasia
  Hemolytic anemia

    2) Growth proceeds from anterior to posterior underneath the sella turcica and continues into early adulthood (Fig. 15-10*C*). The posterior border of the sphenoid sinus will never exceed the line of the sphenooccipital synchondrosis.

    3) As the sphenoid bone prepares to pneumatize, red marrow converts to yellow or fatty marrow. This focal, high-signal area on T1-weighted images often has been called *dermoid* by unwary radiologists.

  d. Frontal sinuses.

    1) The frontal sinuses are the last paranasal sinus group to be aerated. They usually are not visible on plain-film radiographs until 6 years of age (Fig. 15-10*A*). Pneumatization may progress well into adult life.

    2) Frontal sinus size ranges widely; 4% of the overall population has no frontal sinuses (Table 15-1).

  e. To summarize, the maxillary and ethmoid sinuses generally demonstrate some degree of aeration at birth. The sphenoid sinuses usually will be aerated on plain-film radiographs by 3 years of age. The frontal sinuses are the last group to appear, becoming visible by 6 years of age.

C. Imaging Techniques.

1. General remarks.

  a. The paranasal sinuses now can be imaged with a variety of methods, from the more inexpensive plain-film radiographs of the sinuses (i.e., single Water's view, sinus series) to the more expensive CT examinations (i.e., coronal sinus CT, multiplanar CT with contrast) to the most expensive technology, MRI.

  b. How does the radiologist decide among these methods? A few generalizations may help.

   1) If the clinical question is an initial evaluation or follow-up of inflammatory disease of the sinuses, plain-film radiography may suffice, but coronal sinus CT is necessary when any form of traditional or endoscopic surgery is anticipated. It is too easy to make a significant interpretive error with plain films alone to rely solely on their interpretation for surgical planning.

   2) Two clinical settings merit either multiplanar CT with contrast or MRI. These are radiologic evaluation of patients suspected of having serious regional complications of sinusitis (e.g., subdural empyema, brain abscess, and so on), and radiologic staging of malignant tumor of the sinuses where it is critical to evaluate fully the true deep-tissue extent (i.e., stage) of the tumor.

     a) In cases where coronal sinus CT reveals a mass with a destructive or infiltrative appearance, suggesting a primary malignancy of the sinonasal region, the CT scan should be extended immediately to multiplanar CT with contrast immediately. If the patient has already left the imaging area, MRI can be recommended to the referring physician.

  2. Coronal sinus CT.

  a. Indications.

   1) The principal indication for coronal sinus CT is preoperative planning before FESS in a patient suspected of having acute or chronic sinusitis.

   2) Coronal sinus CT also has proven to be useful in follow-up imaging of patients who have undergone sinus surgery for inflammatory disease but still have persistent symptoms.

  b. Patient preparation.

   1) In the weeks before CT examination, an attempt to treat reversible disease maximally should be made. A complete course of antibiotics is recommended. Nasal steroid spray or a short oral course of high-dose steroids may be indicated in some cases (e.g., sinonasal polyposis) as well.

   2) Fifteen minutes before coronal sinus CT, a vasoconstrictor spray should be applied in each nostril. Just before the patient is put on the CT scanner, a vigorous nose blow should be accomplished.

  c. Coronal sinus CT technique (Table 15-2).

   1) Scan plane. Coronal positioning ideally images structures of the ostiomeatal unit for the endoscopic sinus surgeon.

   2) Slice thickness/increment. Contiguous, 3-mm sections from the back of the sphenoid sinus to the front of the frontal sinus.

Table 15-2   Technique for Screening Sinus CT*

Patient Position

Prone coronal with head hyperextended, resting on chin, which keeps free fluid out of infundibulum). In patients unable to maintain a prone position or cases where questions arise from prone images, use a supine coronal position with the head hyperextended over edge of table.

Axial images may be obtained with spiral technique when a patient cannot tolerate neck flexion/extension, such as with infant or geriatric population. Coronal reconstructions in conjunction with initial axial images will provide sufficient diagnostic information in most cases.

Gantry Angle

Perpendicular to the hard palate to obtain direct coronal images. The actual coronal angle is not critical, with 15° perpendicular in either direction being adequate to visualize the ostiomeatal unit.

Scan Extent

Posterior margin of sphenoid sinus to anterior margin of frontal sinus.

Section Thickness

Contiguous, 3-mm sections represent the best balance of coverage and delineation of anatomic aspects of the ostiomeatal unit.

kVp

120.

mA (dose per slice)

200 (100 mA × 2-second scan time) or less. Low exposure can be used because of the bone algorithm technique with filming at intermediate window.

Imaging Algorithm

Bone (maximum edge-enhancement program)

Photography

Window width = 1500–2500 HU.
Window center = 100–300 HU.
Both bone and soft tissues are visualized on the single set of images.

Contrast

None

*These recommendations are for coronal sinus CT when evaluating inflammatory disease. In noninflammatory cases and extensive or complicated inflammatory cases, full sinus CT or MRI should be considered.

3) Intravenous contrast. None
4) Radiation dose. With use of the bone algorithm in this study, low-dose radiation can be used during the acquisition of these images. A total of 200 mA (i.e., 100 mA at 2 seconds) in combi-

nation with 120 kV is more than adequate for this examination. With this low tube load, dynamic CT techniques can be employed without the limitations from tube heating.

5) Image processing. Edge-enhancement program to maximize bone detail.

6) Photographing the image. Intermediate window settings in the 1200- to 1800-HU width and 100- to 250-HU center range emphasize bone changes without losing an appreciation of the different soft-tissue types (especially orbital fat versus muscle).

7) The coronal sinus CT should be extended into a standard multiplanar sinus CT with contrast whenever complicated inflammatory disease or a lesion suspicious for tumor are found.

   a) If the patient has already left the imaging area, they are called back with permission of the referring physician for either multiplanar enhanced CT or MRI.

8) Comment. The choice of section thickness is controversial. Slice thickness from 1.5 to 5.0 mm have been advocated by different authors. The choice is made based on the perceived needs of your referring physician.

   a) The goal of coronal sinus CT is to obtain precise information on the extent of inflammatory sinus disease, especially in the ostiomeatal unit, at approximately one half the cost of multiplanar sinus CT with contrast.

   b) I suggest 3-mm sections, because the balance of slice number (i.e., cost) and scan information is best achieved at this thickness.

3. Multiplanar sinus CT with contrast medium.

   a. Indications.

   1) Complex inflammatory disease.

      a) Extensive polyposis.

      b) Suspected osteomyelitis

      c) Persistent symptoms following multiple sinus surgeries.

   2) Benign or malignant tumor of the sinonasal region.

   3) Mass lesion identified on coronal sinus CT.

   b. Technique.

   1) Scan plan. Axial plane initially. Coronal plane is used freely to evaluate lesion interaction with the orbit, skull base, hard palate, and anterior and middle cranial fossae.

   2) Slice thickness/increment/extent. Axial images are obtained using contiguous, 3-mm scans from the hard palate to the top of the frontal sinus. Coronal images are obtained with contiguous, 3-mm images, at least through the area of lesion. If scans cannot

be checked, coronal images should be obtained from the anterior frontal sinus to the posterior sphenoid sinus.

3) Contrast strategy. Bolus-drip technique with a 50-mL bolus of 60% iodinated contrast medium and 100-ml rapid-drip infusion of 60% contrast.
4) Imaging processing. Both bone and soft-tissue image processing should be completed in both planes.
5) Photographing images. Bone windows are used for bone images; soft-tissue windows are used for soft-tissue images.
6) Comment. Either CT or MRI can answer the imaging questions raised by suspected disease that is more than routine sinusitis in the sinonasal region. Coronal images on CT often are more affected than MRI scans by dental amalgam artifact, but CT offers a better delineation of the bony structures of the region.

c. MRI of the sinonasal region.
1) Indications. Same as for multiplanar CT with contrast medium (discussed previously).
2) Technique.
a) Scan plane/coil. Axial and coronal/head coil.
b) Section thickness/increment. Series of 4-mm, no-skip images from the hard palate to the upper frontal sinus (axial) and from the anterior frontal sinus to the posterior sphenoid sinus (coronal).
c) Imaging parameters. T2-weighted images can be conventional, but fast spin echo should be used if it is available. TR of 2000 milliseconds or longer, with TE of 20 and 70 milliseconds. T1-weighted images can have variable TR of up to 800 milliseconds to achieve the desired number of slices. Postcontrast images should be fat saturated in one plane.
d) Contrast. MRI contrast is used to answer specific questions raised by the initial scans.

D. Sinonasal disease.

1. Congenital disease.
a. The anterior neuropore closes in the vicinity of the optic recess in the fourth-gestational-week fetus (Fig. 15-11). At this time the mesodermal tissue begins to form bone, cartilage, and connective tissue in the frontonasal region. The fetal ectoderm may become entrapped with the outgrowth of the frontonasal process, which probably explains the formation of ectopic (nasal) glioma, dermoid, and sinus tracts. Failure of this neuropore to close, however, is the best explanation for the formation of frontonasal, frontoethmoidal, and frontosphenoidal cephaloceles.

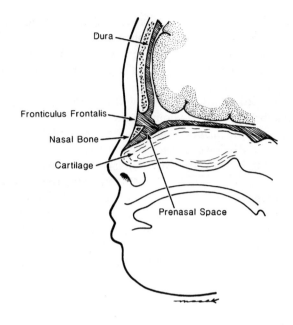

A

B

Fig. 15-11   Normal development of the midline area of the anterior skull base. **A,** Early in the development of this area a small fontanelle, the fonticulus frontalis, is briefly present between the developing frontal bones and the developing nasal bones. A second, prenasal space also is seen at the same time between the devel-

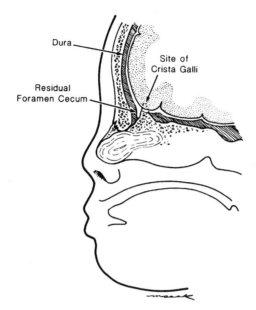

oping nasal bones and the cartilage of the developing nasal capsule. Both sites can become the location of a cephalocele (see Fig. 15-12*C,D*). **B,** Closure of the fonticulus frontalis slightly later in development. The prenasal space has narrowed because of the continued growth of the nasal processes of the frontal bones. The prenasal space is now referred to as the *foramen cecum,* as it is completely surrounded by bone. A dural stalk extends from the intracranial space through the foramen cecum. This dura projection comes into contact with the skin in the region of the bridge of the nose (*curved arrow*). Inadequate closure of this connection will lead to sinus tracts and/or dermoid formation in this region (see Fig. 15-12*B*). **C,** Normal midline anterior skull base development, again slightly later in the process. The dural stalk separates from the skin of the nose and retracts intracranially. After this, the foramen cecum partially fuses, and the prenasal space is obliterated. The foramen cecum does not finally become obliterated until a few years into postnatal life. (Adapted from Barkovich AJ, Vandermarck P, Edwards MSB, et al: Congenital nasal masses: CT and MR imaging features in 16 cases. *AJNR* 12:105–116, 1991. Used with permission.)

    b. Nasal glioma.
        1) An extracranial rest of glial tissue and not a neoplastic lesion.
        2) Only 15% of these lesions have a fibrous connection to the subarachnoid space. No cerebrospinal fluid connection exists.
        3) Radiologic features. Nonspecific, benign-appearing, soft-tissue mass in the nasal septum without associated bony destruction (Fig. 15-12*A*).

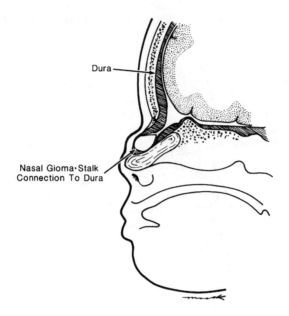

A

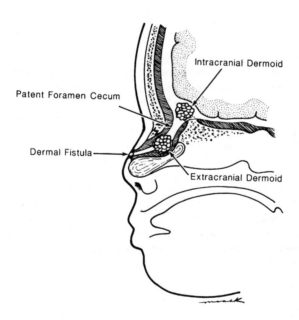

B

Fig. 15-12 Varied results of aberrant development of the anterior, midline skull base. **A**, If the dural projection passing through the foramen cecum does not retract and involute normally, leaving behind a glial rest, a nasal glioma with a fibrous band connecting it to the intracranial contents through the foramen cecum may occur. **B**, If the dural projection does not adequately involute, dermal sinuses may result. Any part of the dural projection may involute, producing complete and incomplete dermal sinuses. Desquamation of the lining of the dermal sinus any-

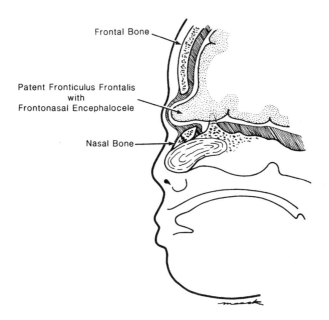

C

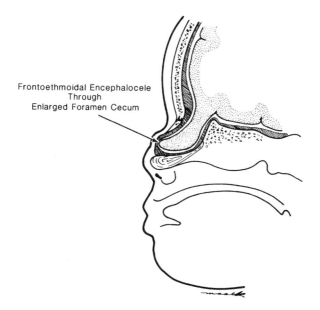

D

where along its course can result in a dermoid or epidermoid lesion. The dermoid or epidermoid may be intracranial or extracranial in location. **C,** If the fonticulus frontalis does not close, the result is a frontonasal cephalocele. **D,** A failure of closure of the prenasal space–foramen cecum results in a frontoethmoidal cephalocele. (Adapted from Barkovich AJ, Vandermarck P, Edwards MSB, et al: Congenital nasal masses: CT and MR imaging features in 16 cases. *AJNR* 12:105–116, 1991. Used with permission.)

   c. Nasal dermoid.
1) Clinical presentation. A dimple or fistula containing hair may be present over the dorsum of the nose (Fig. 15-12*B*).
2) Radiologic features. A fusiform mass of fat density is seen in the nasal septum. An enlarged foramen cecum, bifid crista galli, or broadened nasal septum may be seen when a dermal sinus tract exists between the intracranial space or the falx.

   d. Anterior cephaloceles.
1) Etiology. Cephaloceles are congenital or acquired lesions.
   a) Congenital cephalocele. These congenital lesions result from the failure of mesodermal ingrowth between the neural tube and the overlying ectoderm, with incomplete closure of the anterior neuropore. Abnormalities in the cranial and underlying meninges result.
   b) Acquired cephalocele. These are most commonly secondary to surgery or trauma. Posttraumatic cephalocele may be found involving any of the sinuses. A spontaneous form has been reported to occur in the sphenoid sinus area when the pterygoid wing is fully pneumatized, and in the petrous apex area when petrous apex aeration is present.
2) Cephalocele terminology.
   a) *Cephalocele* is a term used to denote herniation of meninges (i.e., *meningocele*) or meninges and brain substance (i.e., *encephalocele*) through the cranial defect.
   b) Visible cephaloceles are termed *sincipital*. Those that cannot be seen without the help of CT or MRI are called *basal*.
3) Congenital cephalocele location.
   a) Seventy percent of these lesions involve the occipital bone.
   b) Approximately 15% of all cephaloceles occur in the anterior cranial fossa.
   c) The anterior cephaloceles are named according to their craniofacial pathway.
     i) Frontonasal cephalocele (Fig. 15-12*C*).
     ii) Nasoethmoidal cephalocele (Fig. 15-12*D*).
     iii) Nasoorbital cephalocele.
     iv) Basal cephaloceles are grouped anatomically according to the location of the bony defect: transethmoidal, sphenoethmoidal, transphenoidal, sphenoorbital, and sphenomaxillary.
4) Clinical presentation.
   a) A high degree of suspicion is necessary if congenital basal (i.e., nonvisible) cephalocele is to be diagnosed before any surgical procedure is undertaken. A child with suspected

nasal polyp or nasopharyngeal mass or having recurrent bouts of bacterial meningitis (with or without cerebrospinal fluid rhinorrhea) should undergo CT or MRI before surgical intervention.

b) A child with a lump on the bridge of the nose also should undergo CT or MRI before surgical removal to look for possible frontonasal cephalocele.

c) The patient's status after temporal bone or sinonasal surgery with new appearance of a mass should be considered for possible diagnosis of postsurgical cephalocele.

d) Patients who have undergone significant skull base fractures also may develop posttraumatic cephalocele.

5) Imaging issues.

a) CT features. Axial and coronal CT bone images will clearly depict the bony defect through which the cephalocele passes. Soft-tissue components of the cephalocele, however, are not seen as well with CT as with MRI.

b) MRI features. Sagittal and coronal MRI scans best delineate the soft-tissue portion of the cephalocele, helping to determine what is herniated through the bony rent in the skull base. The location of the dura relative to the cephalocele also at times can be seen.

i) Because surgery will be extradural if possible, information from MRI scans is vital to effective surgical planning.

e. Choanal atresia.

1) The oronasal membrane normally perforates during the seventh fetal week. If it fails to complete this process, some degree of choanal atresia results.

2) Half of these lesions are isolated, and half are associated with other anomalies. The lesion may be unilateral or bilateral, membranous (15% of cases) or bony. In the least severe circumstance only stenosis is present.

2. Inflammatory disease and acute and chronic sinusitis.

a. Introduction.

1) Sinuses and backs are very similar. A tremendous number of people complain about both of these areas, but relatively few of them will benefit from surgical therapy.

2) Fortunately for the head and neck surgeon, there is not really a surgical equivalent to the "failed back syndrome" in sinus surgery. Litigation surrounding FESS, however, has grown at an alarming rate, because many patients do not seem to benefit significantly from the surgery.

3) Surgeons and insurance companies both are looking for CT images to provide additional clues beyond the clinical complaints as to who really will benefit from FESS. As the surgeon looks harder at these images, so must the radiologist so that patient care can be affected positively.

4) The initial contact of the radiologist with inspection and interpretation of coronal sinus CT can be frustrating and unsatisfying without a method to approach the CT images. The most common complaint is "I feel like I am just giving a long laundry list of areas where I see inflammatory change."

5) Once the anatomy of the mucociliary drainage routes of the lateral nasal wall is known and an appreciation for the major obstructive areas gained, patterns of inflammatory disease emerge.

6) Armed with this anatomic information along and an understanding of the major inflammatory patterns, radiologists find coronal sinus CT image interpretation significantly easier. When specific patterns of inflammatory sinonasal disease are identified, coronal sinus CT serves as a detailed guide for FESS, allowing an individually tailored surgical technique to be employed.

7) This segment constructs an anatomic framework for the understanding and interpretation of coronal sinus CT. The goal is to provide a method of interpreting such images that dovetails the FESS techniques of your surgical colleagues.

b. Coronal sinus CT and sinusitis.

1) Background information for coronal sinus CT image interpretation.

a) FESS has become widely used for the treatment of both acute and chronic sinusitis. This surgical technique restores normal mucociliary drainage to the paranasal sinuses.

b) The dramatic increase in use of FESS has produced an equally impressive increase in the volume of coronal sinus CT scans obtained during the presurgical assessment of paranasal sinuses and the nose.

c) The keystone of FESS is its ability to diagnose accurately and to treat even relatively minor changes in the areas of mucociliary drainage. Coronal sinus CT detects even more sinonasal inflammatory disease than diagnostic endoscopy, because it can "see through" the bony walls of the sinuses and assess the sinus contents. As a result coronal sinus CT has emerged as the diagnostic study of choice for patients under consideration for possible FESS.

     d) Any rational method of approach to interpretation of the coronal sinus CT examination must be founded on a clear understanding of the underlying anatomy of the sinuses and nose as it relates to the known patterns of mucociliary drainage in this area.

2) Previous sections have reviewed sinonasal anatomy by specific sinus and area of the nose.

3) The following discussion centers on the routes of mucociliary drainage from each sinus.

4) Once the major mucociliary drainage routes have been reviewed, they will be linked with our anatomic understanding to explain the patterns of inflammatory sinonasal disease often seen on coronal sinus CT scans.

5) The discussion concludes by reviewing the clinical and coronal sinus CT scan features of sinonasal polyposis and sporadic inflammatory sinus disease.

c. Interpreting coronal CT scans.

1) Coronal sinus CT is the standard method of examining a patient under evaluation for possible surgical treatment of inflammatory sinus disease. Let me begin by reviewing my standard method of analyzing images found on routine coronal sinus CT. Reporting follows the same general trend, with a short paragraph on the nose followed by a paragraph on the left and right ostiomeatal unit and paranasal sinuses.

2) First begin by looking at the nasal vault.

     a) Observe the nasal septum. Is it straight or deviated? Is a bony spur present?

     b) Identify three pairs of turbinates. Is there evidence for normal or diseased concha bullosa or agger nasi cells?

     c) Are there any bridging synechiae between the nasal septum and the turbinates?

     d) Is the nasal vault full of polypoid soft-tissue densities?

3) Next move to the area of the ostiomeatal unit.

     a) Is the maxillary infundibulum opacified?

     b) Are any Haller's cells present? Are they diseased?

     c) Are there secondary signs (e.g., mucosal thickening, sinus air cell opacification) of postobstructive ipsilateral maxillary, ethmoid, or frontal sinusitis?

     d) Can the sinus opacification be described as a postobstructive pattern such as an infundibular, nasofrontal, or ostiomeatal unit pattern (described later)?

4) Observe the area of the sphenoethmoidal recess.

     a) Is there obstruction of the sphenoethmoidal recess?

      b) Is postobstructive opacification of the sphenoid sinus present? Is the posterior ethmoid also opacified?

      c) Can a sphenoethmoidal recess, postobstructive inflammatory pattern be defined?

   5) Finally, look at each of the four sinuses.

      a) Are any of them partially or completely opacified? If so, do the associated bony wall changes suggest chronic sinusitis (i.e., thickened), osteomyelitis (i.e., thickened with patchy wall destruction), mucocele (i.e., thinned and expanded), or malignancy (i.e., destruction associated with mass)?

      b) Are any air–fluid levels seen that suggest acute sinusitis? Any fluid levels seen in the frontal, ethmoid, or sphenoid sinuses are immediately called to the referring physician's attention so that aggressive antibiotic therapy can be instituted.

d. Physiology and anatomy of mucociliary drainage.

   1) Physiology of mucociliary drainage.

      a) Normal mucociliary clearance moves all secretions toward the natural sinus ostia.

      b) Normal mucociliary drainage occurs only with patent sinus ostia.

      c) Wherever two opposing mucosal surfaces contact, normal mucociliary action is disrupted.

      d) This disruption allows mucous and debris to accumulate, creating increased potential for infection even when ostial closure is absent.

      e) Dysfunction of mucociliary drainage is cited as the most likely cause for recurring inflammatory sinonasal disease.

      f) The ability of the mucociliary action to clear secretions is pronounced, and successful FESS requires reestablishment of the normal physiologic route for mucous to be removed. This is the main goal of FESS.

   2) Anatomic considerations in mucociliary drainage.

      a) Specific drainage routes of the individual sinuses have been reviewed previously.

      b) These pieces of anatomic information now will be combined into groups based on intersecting mucociliary drainage patterns to explain the patterns of inflammatory disease seen on screening sinus CT scans.

      c) The simplest sinus drainage route is that of the maxillary sinus. The maxillary sinus mucous is swept superomedially by mucociliary action and funnels into the maxillary ostium. From there the mucous passes successively into the posteroinferior aspect of the maxillary infundibulum, through the hiatus semilunaris, and into the middle meatus (Fig. 15-4).

d) A lesion causing obstruction to mucociliary drainage in the maxillary ostium area or base of the infundibulum may result in isolated maxillary sinus inflammatory disease (i.e., infundibular pattern).

e) Similar to the maxillary sinus, the frontal sinus has a single channel for drainage of its secretion: the nasofrontal duct.

f) A lesion causing obstruction to the mucociliary drainage in the area of the nasofrontal duct may result in isolated frontal sinus inflammatory disease (i.e., nasofrontal duct pattern).

g) Mucociliary drainage through the ostiomeatal unit into the middle meatus region occurs with the anterior and middle ethmoid, maxillary and frontal sinuses (Fig. 15-4).

h) The middle meatus is the final common pathway for mucous arising from all five sinus groups. Obstruction to mucous movement within the middle meatus may result in opacification of all ipsilateral sinuses (i.e., ostiomeatal unit pattern).

i) Because variation exists in the precise patterns of ostial drainage for all sinus groups, it is unusual for all sinuses to be affected in each case.

j) Mucociliary drainage through the sphenoethmoidal recess is less well understood. The sphenoid sinus drains through its ostia directly into the sphenoethmoidal recess.

k) The posterior ethmoid complex first drains into the superior meatus and then secondarily into the sphenoethmoidal recess.

l) A smaller lesion of the sphenoethmoidal recess will create ipsilateral sphenoid sinus opacification (i.e., sphenoethmoidal recess pattern). A larger lesion will involve the posterior ethmoid complex along with the sphenoid sinus (Fig. 15-4).

m) It should be obvious that the constellation of afflicted sinuses identified on coronal sinus CT scans tells the interpreter where the obstructive lesion is on the lateral nasal wall.

e. Patterns of inflammatory disease as seen by coronal sinus CT.

1) The initial contact of the radiologist with inspection and interpretation of screening sinus CT scans can be frustrating and unsatisfying without a method of approach to these images.

a) The most common complaint voiced by the interpreting radiologist is "I feel like I am merely cataloging a list of inflammatory change without understanding of what I am seeing."

b) Once the anatomy of the drainage routes of the lateral nasal wall is known and an appreciation for the major obstructive areas gained, however, patterns of inflammatory disease can be identified by the radiologist.

c) Armed with this anatomic information and an understanding of major inflammatory patterns, the radiologist will find interpreting coronal sinus CT scans significantly easier.

d) When specific patterns of inflammatory sinonasal disease are identified, coronal sinus CT scans serve as a more detailed guide for FESS, allowing a tailored surgical technique.

2) The following discussion is based on my experience with over 4000 patients undergoing coronal sinus CT over the last 5 years as part of a pre-FESS evaluation.

a) Approximately 40% of coronal sinus CT scans were identified as normal in this group. This tells me that many patients complaining of symptoms suggesting sinusitis actually have some other problem unrelated to sinus disease.

b) Another 30% of this group had findings on coronal sinus CT that did not fit any of the more distinctive patterns and were therefore put into the sporadic, nonobstructive category.

c) The final 30% of this group had coronal sinus CT findings that could be assigned to an inflammatory pattern other than sporadic. It is this group that would be expected to benefit most from endoscopic sinus surgery.

3) Multiple patterns of inflammatory sinonasal disease can be identified during coronal sinus CT. These include:

I: Maxillary infundibular pattern.
II: Nasofrontal duct pattern.
III: Ostiomeatal unit pattern.
IV: Sphenoethmoidal recess pattern.
V: Sinonasal polyposis pattern.
VI: Sporadic (nonobstructive) pattern.

a) The first four of these patterns (I–IV) are obstructive, relating to blockage of the normal routes of mucociliary drainage.

4) Maxillary infundibular pattern (Fig. 15-13).

a) This is a limited form of inflammatory disease involving a focal area of the osteomeatal unit (i.e., maxillary infundibulum).

b) The term should be used only when the frontal and ethmoid sinuses on the side of the disease are normal. Only the maxillary infundibulum and the corresponding maxillary sinus are diseased in this pattern.

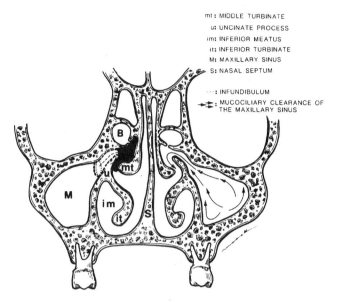

mt : MIDDLE TURBINATE
u: UNCINATE PROCESS
im: INFERIOR MEATUS
it: INFERIOR TURBINATE
M: MAXILLARY SINUS
S: NASAL SEPTUM

---: INFUNDIBULUM
: MUCOCILIARY CLEARANCE OF THE MAXILLARY SINUS

Fig. 15-13 Coronal drawing illustrating two of the major obstructive patterns seen on coronal sinus CT in patients with sinusitis. The ostiomeatal unit pattern of obstructive sinusitis is seen when the middle meatus is plugged (*black area*). In this case the frontal, anterior, and middle ethmoids as well as the maxillary sinus on the side of the obstruction are at risk to fill with mucous because of blockage of their normal mucociliary drainage pathways. When the blockage is more focal in the maxillary infundibulum (*dashed lines*), only the maxillary sinus is obstructed. In this case of infundibular pattern of obstructive sinusitis, only the ipsilateral maxillary sinus is diseased.

c) Coronal sinus CT findings. The maxillary infundibular pattern is seen when opacification of the maxillary infundibulum is found. Secondary inflammatory changes are seen within the maxillary sinus. Maxillary infundibular lesions include mucosal swelling, inflammatory debris, polyp, diseased Haller's cells, and hypoplastic maxillary sinus. When the maxillary sinus is hypoplastic, the maxillary infundibulum usually is longer and thinner than normal. Mucociliary drainage often fails to drain the hypoplastic maxillary sinus effectively, leading to partial or complete opacification early in life. The other sinuses usually are not affected.

d) Surgical implications. As the maxillary infundibular pattern represents limited sinus disease, the anticipated surgical result is excellent in this situation, where only an uncinectomy is necessary to relieve the problem. Surgical complications are rare.

5) Nasofrontal duct pattern.

a) This inflammatory pattern results from obstruction of a limited area of the osteomeatal unit (i.e., nasofrontal duct) (Fig. 15-1).

b) This pattern is only described when sinus disease is limited to the frontal sinus.

c) Coronal sinus CT findings. The nasofrontal duct pattern is seen as nasofrontal duct opacification in conjunction with ipsilateral, frontal sinus partial or complete opacification. Nasofrontal duct lesions include mucosal swelling, inflammatory debris, polyp, and diseased agger nasi cells.

d) Surgical implications. When an isolated nasofrontal duct pattern is recognized on coronal sinus CT scans, surgery can be focused to the anterior part of the ostiomeatal unit. If an associated, diseased agger nasi cell also is present, it must be dealt with at the time of surgery.

6) Ostiomeatal unit pattern.

a) This pattern is the best understood and most fully described pattern of inflammatory disease seen on coronal sinus CT scans. The offending lesion involves the middle meatus area.

b) The ostiomeatal unit pattern classically is thought to result from chronic inflammation of the anterior and middle ethmoid air cells, with infected material from the ethmoid secondarily infecting the maxillary and frontal sinuses.

c) If an obstructing lesion is present in the middle meatus, this pattern can result without the anterior/middle ethmoid sinuses being the cause.

d) Coronal sinus CT findings. The ostiomeatal unit pattern is seen as opacification of the middle meatal area of the lateral wall of the nose, with associated chronic or acute inflammatory change in the adjacent maxillary, anterior, and middle ethmoid and frontal sinuses (Fig. 15-13). The frontal sinus may be spared when disease in the middle meatus is limited or the nasal frontal duct passes anterior to the anterior ethmoid sinus. Middle meatal lesions that cause the ostiomeatal unit pattern include mucosal swelling, inflammatory debris, polyps, diseased concha bullosa, more severe forms of septal deviation with or without spur, intranasal adhesions, and nasal tumors.

e) Comment. Careful inspection of the middle meatus area by the radiologist to search for these potentially causal lesions is recommended when the ostiomeatal unit pattern is observed.

   f) Surgical implications. This pattern requires more surgery than the infundibular or nasofrontal patterns, because multiple sinuses are involved. Uncinectomy combined with ethmoid bullectomy, and perhaps more extensive intranasal ethmoidectomy, is required. Excision of the middle meatal lesion (if present) also is necessary (e.g., resection of a diseased concha bullosa).

7) Sphenoethmoidal recess pattern.

   a) In this inflammatory pattern the level of obstruction is within the sphenoethmoidal recess, with secondary sinus inflammatory changes seen primarily in the sphenoid sinus and, to a lesser extent, in the ipsilateral posterior ethmoid sinus.

   b) Coronal sinus CT findings. Opacification of the sphenoethmoidal recess is present (Fig. 15-4). Chronic and/or acute inflammatory changes are seen within the ipsilateral sphenoid sinus and infrequently within the posterior ethmoid sinus. The posterior ethmoid sinus is involved only when the offending lesion is large enough to fill both the sphenoethmoidal recess and superior meatus.

   c) Surgical implications. This is a more difficult area to reach via endoscope, so transnasal endoscopic surgery of this area is more difficult. An increased rate of surgical complications should be expected as well.

8) Sinonasal polyposis pattern.

   a) In this inflammatory pattern polyps fill the nasal vault and sinuses bilaterally, creating mixtures of all the obstructive inflammatory patterns mentioned previously.

   b) Coronal sinus CT findings. Features suggesting the diagnosis of sinonasal polyposis include polypoid masses filling the nasal vault, pansinus polypoid opacifications, enlarged maxillary infundibulae, convex (i.e., bulging) ethmoid sinus walls, attenuated nasal septum, and ethmoid trabeculae.

   c) Surgical implications. Because diffuse sinus involvement is the rule, surgical intervention quickly becomes extensive, with increased surgical complications resulting. Surgical landmarks are obscured by polyps, and vigorous bleeding is not unusual. As the process is naturally reactive, poorer surgical results can be anticipated, with revision surgery often being necessary.

9) Sporadic (nonobstructive) pattern.

a) This term is used when inflammatory changes do not appear to relate to known patterns of mucous drainage but instead seem to be spread randomly throughout the sinuses.

b) The most common form of sporadic pattern is seen when mild, chronic, inflammatory changes are seen throughout many sinuses without any dominant opacification or air–fluid levels.

c) Determining which of these patients might benefit from FESS is one of the most difficult tasks for the endoscopic sinus surgeon.

d) Individual lesions seen throughout the paranasal sinuses, such as retention cyst and mucoceles, also are included in the sporadic group. Retention cysts are thought to occur as a local complication of previous sinus infection that caused stenosis of a seromucinous gland duct in the sinus. Mucoceles occur when a major ostia to a sinus closes; the sinus continues to produce mucous, with resultant, gradual enlargement of the affected sinus cell.

e) Postsurgical changes are included in the sporadic group, because the normal anatomy and mucociliary drainage routes defining other inflammatory patterns have been disturbed by surgery.

f) Postsurgical coronal sinus CT images must be interpreted in light of the known type of previous surgery and bearing in mind possible revision surgery to finish the job.

g) Coronal sinus CT findings. These images most commonly show random, chronic inflammatory changes unrelated to known patterns of mucous drainage. Retention cysts are seen as randomly placed, well-circumscribed, soft-tissue masses, most commonly in the dependent portion of the maxillary sinus. Mucoceles are seen as complete sinus opacification with outwardly convexed, thinned, bony sinus walls.

h) Postoperative coronal sinus CT findings. Postsurgical changes most often are sporadic and without relationship to known patterns of mucociliary drainage. At times, however, meaningful postsurgical changes will be observed.

   i) Persistent sinus opacification despite known or visible surgical opening into the diseased sinus indicates either that material in the sinus is too viscous to be moved by mucociliary action or a membrane has formed at the surgical site.

   ii) Persistent maxillary sinus opacification despite partial uncinectomy often signals that the uncinectomy is too far posterior (i.e., not in the area where mucociliary action pumps the mucous).

    iii) "Trapped frontal sinus" after internal ethmoidectomy. The frontal sinus becomes opacified with or without an associated air–fluid level after internal (i.e., intranasal) ethmoidectomy has been completed. This finding means that internal ethmoidectomy has injured the nasofrontal duct. The injury results either from direct surgical involvement or the normal healing process sealing off the nasofrontal duct.

  i) Surgical implications. The approach is tailored to the individual affected site. Surgical results generally are good. The degree of difficulty and chances of complications vary greatly depending on the accessibility of the affected sinus and the type of lesion needing treatment.

f. Fungal sinusitis.

  1) Mucormycosis often is seen in the immunocompromised host or the patient with diabetes. Aspergillosis occurs in an otherwise healthy patient.

  2) *Mucor* sp. and *Aspergillus* sp. are the primary offending organisms.

  3) Plain-film and CT findings.

    a) Multiple sinuses are affected, with nodular mucoperiosteal thickening. Calcifications may be present.

    b) When the lesion is invasive, multiple areas of focal bony destruction give the appearance that an aggressive malignancy is present.

    c) *Aspergillus* sp. can cause a vasculitis that results in thrombosis and hemorrhagic infarction of the adjacent brain.

  4) MRI findings. Hypointensity on T1-weighted images and marked hypointensity on T2-weighted images are characteristic of fungal sinusitis. Preliminary reports suggest that mycelial iron or manganese is responsible for this finding.

g. Local–mucosal complications of sinusitis (Table 15-3).

  1) Inflammatory polyp.

    a) This is most common mucosal complication of chronic sinusitis.

    b) Pathophysiology. Mucous membrane hyperplasia from chronic inflammation is thought to cause inflammatory polyp. The nose and maxillary sinus are most frequently involved, but inflammatory polyposis may develop in any of the paranasal sinuses.

Table 15-3   Complications of Sinusitis

Local–mucosal
Polyps
Mucous retention cyst
Mucocele
Osteomyelitis

Regional–intracranial
Orbital cellulitis, abscess
Optic neuritis
Meningitis
Subdural empyema
Brain abscess
Cavernous sinus thrombosis
Cerebral vein thrombosis with or without cerebral infarction

i) Polyps usually are 3- to 10-mm in size. As a result they blend into the associated mucoperiosteal thickening in most cases and also are inseparable from it.
c) When polyps are extensive and cause obstruction of sinus drainage, the term *sinonasal polyposis* is used.
d) Isolated polyps do occur. They may be larger in their solitary form (i.e., 1–3 cm).
e) Coronal sinus CT features.
i) The coronal sinus CT appearance of pansinus polyps was described earlier in the section on sinonasal polyposis.
ii) When polyposis is severe, it may be mistaken by a less experienced radiologist as invasive malignancy because of the bone loss accompanying the polyp enlargement.
iii) When an isolated polyp is present, a polypoid, soft-tissue lesion is seen, with remodeling of affected bony surfaces apparent. When the polyp occurs at the site of a sinus ostium, postobstructive changes are seen in the parent sinus.
2) Mucous retention cyst.
a) Pathophysiology. Inflammatory obstruction of the seromucinous glands of the sinus lining causes the mucous retention cyst.
b) Radiologic appearance. Coronal sinus CT most commonly demonstrates a low-density, smooth-walled mass in the dependent portion of the affected sinus. The maxillary sinus

is the most commonly affected, but any sinus may be involved.

   c) Comment. It commonly is felt that antrochoanal polyp is in fact just a very large mucous retention cyst of the maxillary sinus that has come out through the maxillary infundibulum into the nose (Fig. 15-14).

3) Mucocele.

   a) Pathophysiology. Mucoceles most commonly result from inflammatory obstruction of the ostium in the affected sinus. Posttraumatic and neoplastic obstruction also can yield a secondary mucocele. The lesion represents a dilated, mucus-containing sac lined by mucous membrane that results from secretion into the obstructed sinus. The frontal sinus most commonly is affected. Mucopyocele is the diagnosis when the lesion is superinfected.

   b) Radiologic features.

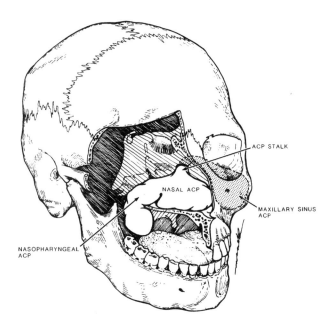

Fig. 15-14 Major imaging features of the antrochoanal polyp (*ACP*). The lesion begins by filling the maxillary sinus. It most commonly then herniates through the maxillary ostium–infundibulum into the middle meatus of the nose. From there it fills the nasal cavity, finally billowing into the ipsilateral nasopharyngeal airway. The patients sometimes come to clinical attention because of a "nasopharyngeal mass."

      i)   Plain-film radiographs show opacification of the involved sinus with loss of the normal mucoperiosteal line of the sinus wall.

      ii) CT findings are characteristic in most cases, with a nonenhancing, low-density, expansile mass seen in the affected paranasal sinus. When secretions become inspissated, contents of the mucocele become hyperdense on CT scans.

      iii) MRI scans show one of two patterns. In a mucocele that has not yet undergone inspissation, the expanded sinus is hyperintense on T1-weighted images (because of the high protein content in the secretions) and hyperintense on T2-weighted images (because of water in the secretions). When a mucocele has undergone inspissation, the signal changes dramatically to very hypointense on both T1- and T2-weighted images.

    c) Beware the inspissated mucocele on MRI scans. It may appear to be an aerated sinus to an unwary radiologist. Use CT to confirm the suspicion of a mucocele under these circumstances.

    d) Inflammatory polyps, benign tumors, and slow-growing malignant lesions can mimic mucocele in every way. The material in the sinus, however, generally is tissue density rather than fluid density.

  4) Osteomyelitis.

    a) Osteomyelitis of any sinus wall is possible if chronic bacterial sinusitis is not treated adequately. Realize before trying to assign this diagnosis to a patient that actual sinus wall osteomyelitis is far less common than the many bizarre-appearing sinus wall reactive changes associated with chronic sinusitis.

    b) Radiologic features. In chronic sinusitis the walls of the sinus often undergo reactive thickening. When thickening becomes focal with associated, destructive-appearing bony change but no tumor mass to explain this finding, osteomyelitis is the diagnosis.

    c) Comment. Patients with sinus wall osteomyelitis are at great risk for more serious regional–intracranial complications. Treatment must be aggressive.

h. Regional–intracranial complications of acute sinusitis (Table 15-3).

  1) These complications usually result from acute or chronic sinusitis of the frontal, ethmoid, or sphenoid sinuses. Spread of infection occurs through the emissary veins of the skull.

2) Regional–intracranial complications include:
    a) Orbital abscess (subperiosteal vs. retroglobar) or cellulitis.
    b) Optic neuritis from sphenoid sinusitis.
    c) Meningitis.
    d) Subdural empyema.
    e) Brain abscess.
    f) Cavernous sinus thrombosis.
3) Orbital cellulitis/abscess.
    a) Ethmoid sinusitis can lead to subperiosteal abscess along the medial wall of the orbit (Fig. 15-15).
    b) Orbital abscess of any kind as a complication of sinusitis is an indication for emergency surgical intervention. Pus collects behind the orbital septum and therefore can lead to ischemia of the optic nerve and blindness.
    c) Thin-section CT (3 mm, contiguous images) performed with contrast and filmed in soft tissue windows is necessary to diagnose the more subtle cases of subperiosteal abscess. If orbital involvement is suggested clinically but coronal sinus CT has been ordered, further imaging in the axial plane with contrast enhancement should be done.

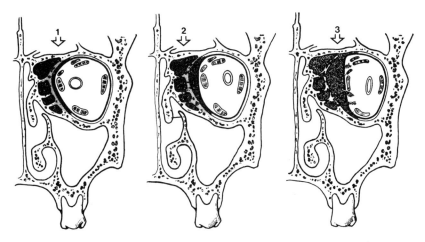

Fig. 15-15 Phases of subperiosteal abscess formation from ethmoid sinusitis. Initially the ethmoid sinus disease involves the lateral wall, including the periosteum, to create a process referred to as *orbital periostitis* (*1*). Left untreated the process evolves to orbital phlegmon, where the inflammatory process has begun to involve the subperiosteal area without the creation of walled-off pus (*2*). The term *subperiosteal abscess* (*3*) is used when frank pus is present in the subperiosteal area. Usually by this time loss of vision has occurred because of optic nerve ischemia.

4) Optic neuritis from sphenoid sinusitis. Sphenoid sinusitis may lead to optic neuritis. Swelling of the optic nerve in the optic canal can produce optic nerve ischemia and blindness.

5) Intracranial complications.

   a) As a group, the intracranial complications of sinusitis are much of the reason why a surgeon pursues the treatment of sinusitis so aggressively.

   b) Coronal sinus CT is not the way to diagnose these problems. Contrast-enhanced MRI is far superior to CT in identifying the presence of these diseases.

   c) Meningitis: As more MRI is done in patients with sinusitis, it has become clear that inflammation of the meninges by adjacent sinusitis is not as uncommon as was previously suspected. Contrast-enhancing meninges alone are not an indication for craniotomy. A meningeal phlegmon may progress to abscess but usually can be managed with intravenous antibiotics.

   d) Subdural empyema. If fluid is found in the extraaxial area of a patient with significant sinusitis, subdural empyema must be excluded. Surgical intervention is required immediately.

   e) Brain abscess. Brain abscess may be seen either in conjunction with subdural empyema or alone. MRI is much more sensitive than CT to this diagnosis. When discovered very early in the development of brain abscess (i.e., focal encephalitis without clear, walled-off fluid collection), clinical judgment is necessary to determine whether to operate or to wait and watch while treating with intravenous antibiotics.

   f) Cavernous sinus thrombosis. When the cavernous sinus is seeded by the organism or organisms causing the sinusitis, multiple cranial neuropathy (cranial nerves III, IV, VI, V_1, V_2) results. MRI scans show enlarged cavernous sinus with multiple, nonenhancing areas within the sinus itself (i.e., clots).

i. Surgical treatment of infectious inflammatory disease in the paranasal sinuses and nose.

1) FESS.

   a) Using an endoscope to recreate sinus drainage via a transnasal route is a relatively new and less invasive surgical technique.

   b) Coronal sinus CT is used to identify candidates for this procedure.

   c) The most common CT findings indicating the need for endoscopic surgery are an opacified ostiomeatal unit (especially the infundibulum) with associated chronic inflammatory changes in the ipsilateral maxillary, frontal, or anterior and middle ethmoid sinuses.

2) Nasoantral window and Caldwell-Luc procedure.
   a) This is the "gold standard" surgical technique for the treatment of maxillary sinusitis.
   b) The Caldwell-Luc portion of this procedure includes placement of a hole in the anterior maxillary sinus wall just above the roots of the teeth.
   c) The nasoantral window portion of the procedure is accomplished by creating a hole in the lateral wall of the nose in the anterior aspect of the inferior meatus. Nasolacrimal duct obstruction may result when the hole is placed too closely to this aperture.

3) Other surgical techniques include ethmoidectomy, sphenoid window, and frontal sinus obliteration.

4) Turbinectomy no longer is commonly performed. Loss of the humidifying function of the turbinate bones can create an arid nasal cavity prone to epistaxis.

3. Noninfectious sinusitis.
   a. As a group these lesions often are mistaken for malignancy of the paranasal sinus or nose, because the radiologic picture frequently is a mix of mass and destructive bony changes (Table 15-4).
   b. Wegener's granulomatosis.
      1) Clinical presentation. Necrotizing vasculitis involving the upper and lower respiratory tracts, necrotizing glomerulonephritis, and varying degrees of disseminated small-vessel vasculitis are associated with nose and paranasal sinus changes.
      2) Radiologic picture. Mucosal thickening and soft-tissue nodules are seen throughout the sinuses and nose. The maxillary sinus is the sinus most commonly affected. Extensive bony dissolution may occur without associated large, soft-tissue masses.
   c. Idiopathic midline granuloma.
      1) Pathologic features. Midline granuloma is more a lymphoreticular disorder that can lead to non-Hodgkin lymphoma than a "real" granulomatous disease.

Table 15-4   Lesions that Mimic Sinonasal Malignancy

Mucormycosis
Wegener's granulomatosis
Idiopathic midline granuloma
Cocaine nose

2) Radiologic features. Destructive mass in the nasal septum leading to perforation without significant sinus disease is typical in the initial stages. As the disease progresses, it may spread to the sinuses and orbit.

   d. Cocaine nose.
    1) Pathologic features. Cocaine-induced granuloma of the nasal septum is the primary component of this lesion.
    2) Radiologic features. Indistinguishable from idiopathic midline granuloma.
    3) Comment. It is important to seek out any history of cocaine abuse in this setting, because cocaine nose is treated with antibiotics and midline granuloma with radiation therapy.

4. Benign tumor.
  a. Many benign and malignant tumors of the sinonasal region can occur in either the nose or the sinus. This discussion, however, subdivides them into nasal and sinus groups where possible for construction of differential diagnoses.
  b. Evaluation of a sinonasal region mass.
    1) Consider whether the mass can be localized to the nose or the sinus. If the center is clearly within one or the other, the mass is said to originate from that structure. When the mass spans both, a useful clue to the origin of the mass is the direction of the convexity of the shared wall between the sinus and nose. If the bony wall is pushed toward the nose, the mass is almost certainly of sinus origin. If the bony wall is pushed away from the nose and nasal septum, the mass originates from the nasal cavity itself.
    2) Next attempt to designate the mass as either benign or malignant. A benign mass expands and remodels the adjacent bony walls. A malignant mass invades and destroys these walls.
    3) After completing this exercise review the differential diagnoses for nasal (Table 15-5) or sinus (Table 15-6) masses.
    4) It is imperative to remember that:
     a) Benign lesions may appear to "destroy bone" by causing focal compressive deossification. As a result reserve the term *destructive bony changes* for situations when bony changes have an aggressive, malignant appearance.
     b) Slow-growing, malignant lesions may only expand bone.

Q#6

     c) Certain nontumorous lesions may mimic nasal or sinus malignancy (Table 15-4).
  c. Benign sinus tumors.

Table 15-5   Differential Diagnosis of Nasal Masses

Pseudomass
Inferior turbinate engorgement

Congenital
Nasal glioma
Septal dermoid

Inflammatory
Rhinosinusitis
   Polyps with mucosal or turbinate hyperplasia
Cocaine nose

Benign Tumor
Juvenile angiofibroma
Angiomatous polyp
Inverting papilloma
Papilloma
Enchondroma

Malignant Tumor
Squamous cell carcinoma
Esthesioneuroblastoma
Exposure carcinoma
Chondrosarcoma
Non-Hodgkin lymphoma
Metastasis

Other
Idiopathic midline granuloma

1) Osteoma.
   a) Clinical presentation. Usually asymptomatic, but may be responsible for postobstructive sinusitis, pneumocephalus, or severe sinus pain associated with airplane flights.
   b) Pathologic features. Dense, compact bone or lamellar bone with intertrabecular fibrous tissue. Eighty percent are found in the floor of the frontal sinus.
   c) Radiologic features. Bone density, sharply circumscribed mass in the frontal or ethmoid sinus varying in size from a few millimeters to several centimeters.
   d) Osteoma complications. Osteomas are of limited clinical significance unless they block the nasofrontal duct, causing mucocele formation, or erode the posterior wall of the frontal sinus, resulting in pneumocephalus.

Table 15-6   Differential Diagnosis of Sinus Masses

Pseudomass
"Redundant mucosa" in infants

Inflammatory
Retention cyst
Mucocele
Wegener's granulomatosis

Benign Tumor
Osteoma
Papilloma
Antrochoanal polyp

Malignant Tumor
Squamous cell carcinoma
Non-Hodgkin lymphoma
Minor salivary gland malignancy
    Adenoid cystic carcinoma
    Mucoepidermoid carcinoma
Osteosarcoma or chondrosarcoma

---

    e) With the volume of presurgical coronal sinus CT now being ordered, incidental osteoma without associated postobstructive sinus opacification commonly is encountered. Finding a small, uncomplicated osteoma does not signal an absolute need for surgery.

2) Papilloma.

    a) Pathologic features. Papillomas are benign epithelial growths that may be polypoid or papillomatous in the sinus or nose. They frequently are mobile.

    b) Radiologic features. Nonspecific. Multiple areas of nodular mucosal thickening in the sinus and nose. May be indistinguishable from the more common chronic inflammatory sinonasal polyposis.

3) Antrochoanal polyp.

    a) Antrochoanal polyp is included as a benign tumor of the sinus, because in most cases it lacks any association with chronic or allergic sinusitis.

    b) Pathologic features. Focal, reactive mucosal process of the maxillary sinus similar to sinonasal polyps, except with a paucity of mucous glands and eosinophils. Some pathologists believe this lesion actually is just an overgrown maxillary sinus retention cyst that has grown into the nose through the maxillary infundibulum. (I share this opinion.)

c) Radiologic appearance. The appearance of antrochoanal polyp often is characteristic (Fig. 15-14). Unilateral opacification of the sinus and nose is seen on plain-film radiographs. A soft-tissue mass also may be seen on a lateral plain film of the nasopharynx. On CT scans a mucous density (i.e., near fluid density) mass is seen occupying the maxillary sinus, ipsilateral nasal cavity, and nasopharynx. The maxillary infundibulum and ostium are considerably enlarged by passage of the mass into the nose. MRI scans show the same features, with T1-weighted images revealing the lesion as hypointense and T2-weighted images as hyperintense.

d) Unusual radiologic features. Infrequently the antrochoanal polyp may herniate into the nose through a accessory maxillary ostium or the area of the posterior fontanelle. In this case the lesion will not enlarge the maxillary ostium.

4) Odontogenic cysts. See the mandible section in Chapter 8.
5) Fibrous dysplasia. See the fibrous dysplasia section in Chapter 16.

d. Benign nasal tumors.
  1) Juvenile angiofibroma.
      a) Clinical presentation. A male adolescent with a nasal mass and history of recurrent spontaneous epistaxis. Life-threatening epistaxis may result from office biopsy.
      b) Pathologic features. Benign tumor arising from a fibrovascular stroma on the posterolateral nasal wall adjacent to the sphenopalatine foramen.
      c) Radiologic features. CT scans reveal a hyperintense mass centered in the posterior nares. The lesion usually has a tongue of tissue extending through the sphenopalatine foramen into the pterygopalatine fossa. Other directions of tumor extension include (Fig. 15-9):
          i) Posteriorly into the nasopharynx.
          ii) Via the vidian canal and the foramen rotundum into the middle cranial fossa.
          iii) Laterally through the pterygomaxillary fissure into the nasopharyngeal masticator space (i.e., infratemporal fossa). MRI scans show the same features and routes of spread. Multiple flow voids within the tumor mark it as hypervascular.
      d) Radiologic classification.
          i) Type 1a. Tumor in the posterior nares and nasopharynx.

  ii) Type 1b. Tumor extends into a sinus.
  iii) Type 2a. Lateral extension of tumor through the sphenopalatine foramen into the pterygopalatine fossa.
  iv) Type 2b. Tumor continues laterally through the pterygo-maxillary fissure into the nasopharyngeal masticator space (i.e., infratemporal fossa).
  v) Type 3. Tumor extends intracranially.
  vi) Types 1 and 2 are treated with surgery alone. Type 3 usually is treated with radiation therapy.
2) Inverted papilloma.
  a) Clinical presentation. Nasal obstruction in an older patient (i.e., 50–70 years). Four times more common in males than in females.
  b) Pathologic features. This neoplastic epithelium inverts into the underlying stroma and is endophytic rather than exophytic from a microscopic viewpoint. This lesion is almost exclusively to a lateral wall of the nose and represents 4% of all nasal cavity tumors. Approximately 5% to 8% of such lesions either degenerate into or coexist with squamous cell carcinoma (SCCa).
  c) Radiologic features. CT identifies an enhancing mass on the lateral wall of the nose with its center in the hiatus semilunaris region. Spread of the tumor initially is into the maxillary and ethmoid sinuses.
  d) Comment. Because of the association of inverted papilloma with invasive recurrence and degeneration into carcinoma, use of CT for preoperative assessment of the disease extent is encouraged. Surgical removal of all radiologically suspect tissue is the goal of treatment.
5. Malignant tumor.
  a. Malignant sinus tumors (Table 15-6).
  1) SCCa.
    a) Clinical presentation.
      i) SCCa of the sinuses often is clinically silent until the disease course is advanced. Early symptoms usually result from secondary obstructive sinusitis.
      ii) SCCa of the maxillary sinus is the most common paranasal sinus cancer. Ethmoid sinus cancers are less common. SCCa of the sphenoid and frontal sinuses are so rare that no staging criteria are warranted.
    b) Pathologic features.
      i) SCCa is by far the most common (80% to 90% of cases) malignant tumor of the paranasal sinus and nose.

    ii) The maxillary sinus is most frequently involved (80%), with most remaining SCCa found in the ethmoid sinuses (10% to 20%). The frontal and sphenoid sinuses rarely are involved.

    iii) Approximately 18% of patients with maxillary sinus SCCa have malignant adenopathy at presentation. These patients usually have posterior maxillary sinus wall tumor or tumor invasive into the posterior ethmoids and/or sphenoid sinus. The most common lymph node group to be involved is the retropharyngeal chain.

c) Radiologic features.

    i) CT and MRI show a unilateral sinus mass, usually with associated aggressive, bony wall destruction. Expansion of the involved sinus is rare (as opposed to wall destruction). These are the features of any paranasal sinus malignancy. SCCa cannot be differentiated radiologically from lymphoma, glandular malignancy, or other malignancy in this area.

    ii) When tumor of the maxillary sinus is advanced, the primary roots for spread of SCCa must be looked for. These include posterior spread into the retroantral fat pad and pterygopalatine fossa. From the pterygopalatine fossa the tumor can spread into the orbit through the infraorbital fissure and to the middle cranial fossa through the foramen rotundum. Superior spread occurs through the orbital floor to the orbit proper. Inferiorly the tumor involves the maxillary alveolar ridge, buccal space, and hard palate. Medial spread occurs through the maxillary ostium into the nose.

d) Staging.

    i) The role of CT and MRI in paranasal sinus SCCa is initial radiologic staging and posttreatment follow-up for the diagnosis of early recurrence.

    ii) If the patient has a known SCCa of the sinonasal area and pretreatment radiologic staging is anticipated, MRI is the modality of choice because of its sensitivity to perineural tumor and intracranial spread as well as leptomeningeal invasion.

    iii) Radiologic staging criteria in maxillary sinus SCCa are presented in Table 15-7. They are based on a theoretic plane joining the medial canthus of the eye with the angle of the mandible, or the so-called *Ohngren's line* (Fig. 15-16). The area anteroinferior to this line is

Table 15-7   Staging Criteria for Maxillary Sinus Squamous Cell Carcinoma

T1:	Tumor limited to the antral mucosa with no erosion or destruction of bone
T2:	Tumor with destruction of the infrastructure,* including the hard palate or middle meatus of the nose; excludes posterior maxillary antral wall
T3:	Tumor invades any of the following: skin of cheek, posterior wall of the maxillary sinus, floor or medial wall of orbit, infratemporal fossa (i.e., nasopharyngeal masticator space), pterygoid plates, ethmoid sinuses
T4:	Tumor invades the orbital contents or any of the following: cribriform plate, posterior ethmoid or sphenoid sinuses, nasopharynx, soft palate, skull base.

*Ohngren's line is a theoretic plane joining the medial canthus of the eye with the angle of the mandible (Fig. 15-16). It divides the maxillary antrum into an anteroinferior portion (i.e., infrastructure) and a superoposterior portion (i.e., suprastructure).

referred to as the *infrastructure*, whereas that superoposterior is called the *suprastructure* of the maxillary antrum.

    e) Prognosis.
        i)   The overall survival rate is between 25% and 30%.
        ii) This statistic reflects the fact that most patients present with advanced (i.e., T3 or T4) primary tumors.

2) Non-Hodgkin lymphoma.
    a) Pathologic features. Sinonasal involvement with non-Hodgkin lymphoma represents an extranodal, extralymphatic manifestation of this disease.
    b) Radiologic features. Sinonasal non-Hodgkin lymphoma cannot be differentiated from SCCa unless multiple sites are seen on CT or MRI scans. An associated mass in Waldeyer's lymphatic ring or lymphadenopathy in the neck also provides a clue to the lymphomatous nature of a sinonasal mass.

3) Minor salivary gland malignant lesions.
    a) Pathologic features. Minor salivary glands are found in the mucosa throughout the upper aerodigestive tract. Adenoid cystic carcinoma, adenocarcinoma, or mucoepidermoid carcinoma may originate in these glands. The sinonasal region is no exception.
    b) Radiologic features. These malignant tumors cannot be differentiated on CT scans from the statistically more common SCCa. These "glandular tumors" do appear to have much more hyperintense signal than their SCCa counterparts on T2-weighted MRI scans.

4) Osteosarcoma and chondrosarcoma.

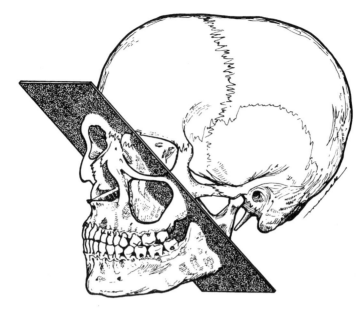

Fig. 15-16   Ohngren's line is a theoretic plane joining the medial canthus of the eye with the angle of the mandible. The area anteroinferior to this line is referred to as the *infrastructure,* whereas superoposterior to the line is called the *suprastructure* of the maxillary antrum. This term is used in staging squamous cell carcinoma (see Table 15-7).

    a) Osteosarcoma.
       i) Pathologic features. Within the head and neck region de novo osteosarcoma most frequently is found in the maxillary sinus, mandible, and calvarium. It is not seen as primary to the nose. Postradiation osteosarcoma is found at the edge of the previous radiation field. Osteosarcoma arises from undifferentiated connective tissue of bone, producing an osteoid matrix as it grows.
      ii) Radiologic features. Most maxillary de novo osteosarcomas arise from the alveolar ridge. The presence of tumor matrix mineralization, either osteoid or chondroid, with aggressive bone destruction and soft-tissue extension leads directly to the radiologic diagnosis of osteosarcoma. When the lesion has less aggressive margins and a chondroid matrix, it may be impossible to differentiate it radiologically from chondrosarcoma.
    b) Chondrosarcoma.

    i)   Pathologic features. Chondrosarcoma is a slow-growing, cartilaginous, malignant tumor representing approximately 1% of all malignant bone tumors. Sinonasal involvement, although it is the most common head–neck site of occurrence, is rare.

    ii) Radiologic features. These tumors occur in the wall of the maxillary sinus, at the junction of the nasal septum vomer with the sphenoid and ethmoid sinuses, and on the undersurface of the sphenoid bone. They are typically large, multilobulated, and sharply demarcated when first detected. Bone changes include erosion and destruction. Tumor matrix calcification (usually chondroid) virtually always is present and best visualized by CT.

b. Malignant tumors of the nose (Table 15-5).

  1) Any of the three sinus malignancies can originate from the nasal mucosa, which is identical to the mucosa of the sinus with the exception of the olfactory mucosa in the nasal vault. The cartilage of the nasal septum also provides the body with a second opportunity to create malignancy unique to the nose.

  2) Esthesioneuroblastoma (i.e., olfactory neuroblastoma).

    a) Clinical presentation. Most frequently seen in 10- to 20-year-old and 51- to 60-year-old patients. Nasal obstruction with repeated episodes of epistaxis is the rule, but symptoms of rhinorrhea, sinus pain, and headache often make these lesions clinically indistinguishable from inflammatory polyposis.

    b) Pathologic features. Esthesioneuroblastoma arises from neurosensory receptor cells in the olfactory epithelium of the high nasal vault. These tumors frequently are misdiagnosed as undifferentiated carcinoma on routine pathologic examination.

    c) Radiologic features. The tumor center is in the high nasal vault. Common routes of spread are into the ethmoid and sphenoid sinuses, up through the cribriform plate into the anterior cranial fossa, and through the ethmoid sinus into the orbit. Enhanced CT or MRI scans show a moderately enhancing mass centered in the cephalad nasal cavity with associated cribriform plate and sinus wall destruction. Punctate intratumoral calcification and hyperostosis of the turbinate bones and adjacent sinus walls also have been reported.

SUGGESTED READING

Aoki S, Dillon WP, Barkovich AJ, et al: Marrow conversion before pneumatization of the sphenoid sinus: assessment with MR imaging. *Radiology* 172:373–375, 1989.

Atar E, Mor C, Har-El Gadi, et al: Inverting papilloma of the nose and paranasal sinuses. *Laryngoscope* 96:394–398, 1986.

Babbel R, Harnsberger HR, Nelson B, et al: Optimization of techniques in screening CT of the sinuses. *AJNR* 12:849–854, 1991.

Babbel RW, Harnsberger HR, Sonkens J, et al: Recurring patterns of inflammatory sinonasal disease demonstrated by screening sinus CT. *AJNR* 113:903–912, 1992.

Barkovich AJ, Vandermarck P, Edwards MSB, et al: Congenital nasal masses: CT and MR imaging features in 16 cases. *AJNR* 12:105–116, 1991.

Batsakis JG: *Tumors of the head and neck: clinical and pathological considerations,* ed 2. Baltimore, 1979, Williams & Wilkins.

Becker GD, Hill S: Midline granuloma due to illicit cocaine use. *Arch Otolaryngol Head Neck Surg* 114:90–91, 1988.

Bilaniuk LT, Zimmerman RA: Computed tomography in the evaluation of the paranasal sinuses. *Radiol Clinic North Am* 20:51–66, 1982.

Bolger WE, Butzin CA, Parsons DS: Paranasal sinus bony anatomic variations and mucosal abnormalities: CT analysis for endoscopic sinus surgery. *Laryngoscope* 101:56–64, 1991.

Bryan RN, Sessions RB, Horowitz BL: Radiographic management of juvenile angiofibromas. *AJNR* 2:157–166, 1981.

Burke DP, Gabrielsen TO, Knake JE: Radiology of olfactory neuroblastoma. *Radiology* 137:367–372, 1980.

Carter BL, Bankoff MS, Fisk FD: Computed tomographic detection of sinusitis responsible for intracranial and extracranial infections. *Radiology* 147:739–742, 1983.

Chinwuba C, Wallman J, Strand R: Nasal airway obstruction. CT assessment. *Radiology* 159:503–506, 1986.

Diament MJ, Senac MO, Gilsanz V, et al: Prevalence of incidental paranasal sinuses opacification in pediatric patients: a CT study. *J Comput Assist Tomogr* 11:426–431, 1987.

Dillon WP, Som PM, Fullerton GD: Hypointense MR signal in chronically inspissated sinonasal secretions. *Radiology* 174:73–78, 1990.

Forbes WSC, Fawcitt RA, Isherwood I, et al: Computed tomography in the diagnosis of diseases of the paranasal sinuses. *Clin Radiol* 29:501–511, 1978.

Gamba JL, Woodruff WW, Djang WT, et al: Craniofacial mucormycosis: assessment with CT. *Radiology* 160:207–212, 1986.

Glasier CM, Ascher DP, Williams KD: Incidental paranasal sinus abnormalities on CT of children: clinical correlation. *AJNR* 7:861–864, 1986.

Harnsberger HR, Osborn AG, Smoker WRK: CT in the evaluation of the normal and diseased paranasal sinuses. *Semin Ultrasound CT MR* 7:68–89, 1986.

Hasso AN: CT of tumors and tumor-like conditions of the paranasal sinuses. *Radiol Clin North Am* 22:119–130, 1984.

Hasso AN, Vignaud J: *Normal anatomy of the paranasal sinuses, nasal cavity and facial bones.* In Newton TH, Hasso AN, Dillon WP, editors: *Computed tomography of the head and neck.* San Anselmo, Calif., 1988, Clavadel Press.

Hasso AN, Vignaud J: *Pathology of the paranasal sinuses, nasal cavity and facial bones.* In Newton TH, Hasso AN, Dillon WP, editors: *Computed tomography of the head and neck.* San Anselmo, Calif., 1988, Clavadel Press.

Hesselink JR, New PFJ, Davis KR, et al: Computed tomography of the paranasal sinuses and face. I: normal anatomy. *J Comput Assist Tomogr* 2:559–567, 1978.

Hesselink JR, New PFJ, Davis KR, et al: Computed tomography of the paranasal sinuses and face: II: pathological anatomy. *J Comput Assist Tomogr* 2:568–576, 1978.

Hesselink JR, Weber AL, New PFJ, et al: Evaluation of mucoceles of the paranasal sinuses with computed tomography. *Radiology* 133:397–400, 1979.

Kennedy DW, Zinreich SJ, Rosenbaum AE, et al: Functional endoscopic sinus surgery. *Arch Otolaryngol* 111:576–582, 1985.

Kennedy DW, Zinreich SJ, Shaalan H, et al: Endoscopic middle meatal antrostomy: theory, technique, and patency. *Laryngoscope* 97:1–9, 1987.

Laine FJ, Smoker WRK: The ostiomeatal unit and endoscopic surgery: anatomy, variations, and imaging findings in inflammatory diseases. *Am J Roentgenol* 159:849–857, 1992.

Lee YY, Tassel PV: Craniofacial chondrosarcoma: imaging findings in 15 untreated cases. *AJNR* 10:165–170, 1989.

Lee YY, Tassel PV, Nauert C, et al: Craniofacial osteosarcomas: plain film, CT and MR findings in 46 cases. *AJNR* 9:373–385, 1988.

Li C, Yousem DM, Hayden RE, et al: Olfactory neuroblastoma: MR evaluation. *AJNR* 14:1167–1171, 1993.

Lund VJ, Lloyd GAS: Radiological changes associated with inverted papilloma of the nose and paranasal sinuses. *Br J Radiol* 57:455–461, 1984.

Momose KJ, Weber AL, Goodman M, et al: Radiological aspects of inverted papilloma. *Radiology* 134:73–79, 1980.

Nino-Murcia M, Rao VM, Mikaelian DO, et al: Acute sinusitis mimicking antrochoanal polyp. *AJNR* 7:513–516, 1986.

Osborn AG: *The nose.* In Bergeron RT, Osborn AG, Som PM, editors: *Head and neck imaging excluding the brain.* St. Louis, 1984, Mosby–Year Book.

Osborn AG, McIff EB: Computed tomography of the nose. *Head Neck Surg* 4:182–199, 1982.

Paling MR, Roberts RL, Fauci AS: Paranasal sinus obliteration in Wegener's granulomatosis. *Radiology* 144:539–543, 1982.

Pollei S, Harnsberger HR: The radiologic evaluation of the sinonasal region. *Postgrad Radiol* 9:242–264, 1989.

Press AG, Weindling SM, Hesselink JR, et al: Rhinocerebral mucormycosis: MR manifestations. *J Comput Assist Tomogr* 12:744–749, 1988.

Scuderi AJ, Harnsberger HR, Boyer RS: Pneumatization of the paranasal sinuses: normal features of importance to the accurate interpretation of CT scans and MR images. *Am J Roentgenol* 160:1101–1104, 1993.

Shapiro MD, Som PM: MRI of the paranasal sinuses and nasal cavity. *Radiol Clin North Am* 27:447–475, 1989.

Slovis TL, Renfro B, Watts FB, et al: Choanal atresia: precise CT evaluation. *Radiology* 155:345–348, 1985.

Som P: *The paranasal sinus.* In Bergeron RT, Osborn AG, Som PM, editors: *Head and neck imaging excluding the brain.* St. Louis, 1984, Mosby–Year Book.

Som PM, Dillon WP, Fullerton GD, et al: Chronically obstructed sinonasal secretions: observations on T1 and T2 shortening. *Radiology* 172:515–520, 1989.

Som PM, Dillon WP, Sze G, et al: Benign and malignant sinonasal lesions with MR imaging. *Radiology* 172:763–766, 1989.

Som PM, Lawson W, Biller HF, et al: Ethmoid sinus disease: CT evaluation in 400 cases. I: nonsurgical patients. *Radiology* 159:591–597, 1986.

Som PM, Sacher M, Lawson W, et al: CT appearance distinguishing benign nasal polyps from malignancies. *J Comput Assist Tomogr* 11:129–133, 1987.

Som PM, Shapiro MD, Biller HF, et al: Sinonasal tumors and inflammatory tissues: differentiation with MR imaging. *Radiology* 167:803–808, 1988.

Som PM, Shugar JMA, Biller HF: The early detection of antral malignancy in the postmaxillectomy patient. *Radiology* 143:509–512, 1982.

Tadmor R, Ravid M, Millet D, et al: Computed tomographic demonstration of choanal atresia. *AJNR* 5:743–745, 1984.

Tassel PV, Lee YY, Jing BS, et al: Mucoceles of the paranasal sinuses: MR imaging with CT correlation. *AJNR* 10:607–612, 1989.

Terrier F, Weber W, Rufenacht D, et al: Anatomy of the ethmoid: CT, endoscopic, and macroscopic. *Am J Roentgenol* 144:493–500, 1985.

Towbin R, Dunbar JS: The paranasal sinuses in childhood. *RadioGraphics* 2:253–279, 1982.

Towbin R, Dunbar JS, Bove K: Antrochoanal polyps. *Am J Roentgenol* 132:27–31, 1979.

Weingarten K, Zimmerman RD, Becker RD, et al: Subdural and epidural empyema: MR imaging. *AJNR* 10:81–87, 1989.

Woodruff WW, Vrabec DP: Inverted papilloma of the nasal vault and paranasal sinuses: spectrum of CT findings. *Am J Roentgenol* 162:419–423, 1994.

Zinreich SJ, Kennedy DW, Malat J, et al: Fungal sinusitis: diagnosis with CT and MR imaging. *Radiology* 169:439–444, 1988.

Zinreich SJ, Kennedy DW, Rosenbaum AE, et al: Paranasal sinuses: CT imaging requirements for endoscopic surgery. *Radiology* 163:769–755, 1987.

Zinreich SJ, Mattox DE, Kennedy DW, et al: Concha bullosa: CT evaluation. *J Comput Assist Tomogr* 12:778–784, 1988.

IV

Imaging of the
Skull Base and Cranial Nerves

16

The Skull Base

CRITICAL IMAGING QUESTIONS: THE SKULL BASE

1. Can the skull base be evaluated adequately in the axial plane?
2. Name the five bones that compose the skull base. List the major components of each bone as well as the apertures and transmitted structures found in each.
3. Name the three perspectives for viewing diseases of the skull base.
4. What is a cephalocele? Name the two major types. Is CT or MRI preferred for evaluating these lesions?

Answers to these questions are found in the text beside the question (Q#) in the margin.

THE NORMAL SKULL BASE

A. Introduction.

1. The important aspect of normal anatomy of the skull base is found in the skull base apertures and their contents. The cranial nerves and brain vasculature traversing the skull base make knowledge of this anatomy essential.
2. Only after these passages and their contents are familiar can the radiologist begin to tackle diseases affecting the skull base.
3. Diseases of the skull base can be intrinsic to the area or affect the skull base from either above or below.
   a. Lesions affecting the skull base from the intracranial compartment are discussed elsewhere and only mentioned here.
   b. Lesions intrinsic to the skull base or affecting it from below are discussed thoroughly later in this chapter.
   c. This chapter focuses on normal anatomy of the skull base and its interaction with the deep facial spaces.

B. Technical considerations of skull base imaging.

1. The skull base is an undulating surface with minimal dimension in the craniocaudad direction. To image this area completely, section thickness must be kept to a minimum, especially in the axial plane.

Q#1

2. Because the plane of the skull base approximates the axial imaging plane, coronal images are mandatory to evaluate transgression of the skull base by a lesion.
3. When using CT to image the skull base, the following general guidelines are recommended:
   a. Section thickness: 3 mm.
   b. Slice increment: Contiguous.
   c. Scan planes: Axial and coronal.
   d. Imaging algorithm: Bone and soft tissue.
   e. Photography: Wide window settings (i.e., >2000 HU) for bone images; narrow settings (i.e., 200–400 HU) for soft-tissue images.
   f. Intravenous contrast: Designed to maximize intravascular contrast either by using an injector (30-mL load over 15 seconds followed by 2 mL/sec during scanning using 180 agent) or with a bolus-drip technique (bolus of 30–50 mL with rapid drip employed to end approximately 3 minutes before the scan ends).
      1) Total dose limits for contrast are defined relative to the weight and age of the patient. See the individual contrast agent's package insert.
4. When MRI is used to image the skull base region, the following guidelines are recommended:

a. Section thickness: 3 to 4 mm.

b. Increment: Contiguous or minimal interslice gap.

c. Scan planes: Axial and coronal.

d. MRI parameters: Short and long TR sequences.

    1) T2-weighted, fast spin echo is used preferentially over conventional T2-weighted, spin echo, because it is not as affected by susceptibility artifacts in the skull base area.

e. Contrast. MRI contrast frequently is helpful in imaging the skull base by providing contrast to the lesion. Intracranial and extracranial extension often is better appreciated on contrast-enhanced images.

    1) When contrast is used, fat suppression is added to the T1-weighted, spin echo sequence to remove the high signal contributed to the image by skull base fat.

f. MRA to emphasize venous anatomy (two-dimensional time of flight) and arterial anatomy (three-dimensional time of flight; multiple overlapping slab technique) is added to the examination when vascular imaging questions are posed.

C. Normal skull base.

Q#2

1. The adult skull base consists of five bones (Fig. 16-1*A*). The ethmoid, sphenoid, and occipital bones are unpaired. The remaining two actually are two pairs: the temporal and frontal bones.

2. The adult skull base extends from the root of the nose anteriorly to the superior nuchal line posteriorly. The most complex and clinically important part of this region is between the anterior aspect of the sella and the posterior lip of the foramen magnum, or the basisphenoid and basiocciput. The cranial nerves and cerebral vasculature traverse the skull base here.

3. Although intracranial anatomy is discussed from the viewpoint of anterior, middle, and posterior fossa, the concept of fossa does not work well for the skull base. This is because the bony anatomy spills over from one fossa to the next. It is easier to approach the skull base from the perspective of the individual bones that combine to form this complex structure (Fig. 16-1, Table 16-1). Each bone can be described in terms of its important components, apertures (Fig. 16-1*B*), and their transmitted structures (Fig. 16-2).

D. Bones of the skull base.

1. Occipital bone.

Q#2

    a. The occipital bone forms the floor of the posterior fossa.

    b. Three distinct areas of the occipital bone can be identified.

        1) Basiocciput (i.e., clivus and jugular tubercles).

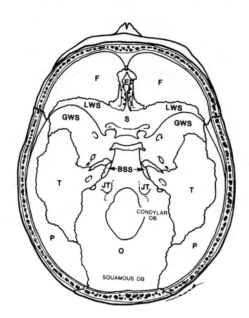

A

FORAMEN CAECUM
CRISTA GALLI

POSTERIOR BORDER OF LESSER WING
TUBERCULUM SELLAE
HYPOPHYSEAL FOSSA
DORSUM SELLAE

FORAMEN LACERUM

GROOVE FOR SUP. PETROSAL SINUS
HYPOGLOSSAL CANAL

B

INTERNAL OCCIPITAL
PROTUBERANCE

CRIBRIFORM PLATE
OPTIC CANAL

ANTERIOR CLINOID
PROCESS
FORAMEN ROTUNDUM
FORAMEN OVALE
FORAMEN SPINOSUM

CAROTID GROOVE
POSTERIOR CLINOID PROCESS
GROOVE FOR INF. PETROSAL SINUS

JUGULAR TUBERCLE

GROOVE FOR
TRANSVERSE SINUS

Fig. 16-1 **A**, The five bones that compose the normal skull base: paired frontal (*F*) and temporal (*T*) bones, and unpaired ethmoid (*E*), sphenoid (*S*), and occipital (*O*) bones. The sphenoid bone has two distinct areas: the greater wing (*GWS*), and the lesser wing (*LWS*). The occipital bone also has two areas of interest: the condylar and the squamous occipital bone (*OB*). *BSS*, Basisphenoid synchondrosis; *JT*, jugular tubercle; *P*, parietal bone. **B**, Skull base from an endocranial viewpoint emphasizing its topographic bony landmarks and apertures. Compare with panel **A** to identify apertures by the specific bone of the skull base.

Table 16-1   Bones of the Skull Base

Occipital Bone
  Basiocciput
    Clivus, jugular tubercle
  Condylar part
  Squamous part

Temporal Bone
  Petrous pyramid
  Mastoid process

Sphenoid Bone
  Basisphenoid
  Greater wing of sphenoid
  Lesser wing of sphenoid

Frontal Bone
  Orbital plate

Ethmoid Bone
  Cribriform plate
  Crista galli

    2) Condylar (i.e., lateral) portion.
    3) Squamous (i.e., posterior) portion.
  c. Important occipital bone apertures (Table 16-2).
    1) Foramen magnum.
    2) Posterior condylar canal.
    3) Hypoglossal canal.
2. Temporal bone.

Q#2
  a. The petrous pyramid and mastoid process form most of the skull base between the posterior and middle cranial fossae.
  b. The apex of the petrous pyramid joins the anterolateral margin of the clivus (i.e., basiocciput) and the posteromedial margin of the greater wing of the sphenoid along the basisphenoid synchondrosis (Fig. 16-1).

Q#2
  c. Important temporal bone apertures (see Table 16-2).
    1) Jugular foramen.
    2) Facial nerve canal.
    3) Internal auditory canal.
    4) Eustachian tube.
    5) Petrous carotid canal.

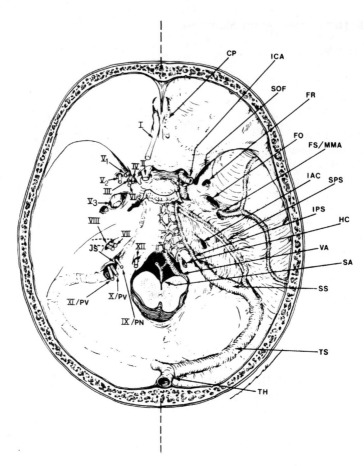

Fig. 16-2 Anatomic drawing of the endocranial aspects of the skull base. *Left,* Cranial nerves I through XII exit the skull base. *Right,* Critical openings and vascular anatomy. See page 423 for the key to numbered and lettered structures. (From Osborn AG, Harnsberger HR, Smoker WRK: Base of skull imaging. *Semin Ultrasound CT MR* 7:91–106, 1986. Used with permission.)

    d. The jugular foramen is an anatomically complex area of the skull base that requires further delineation.
        1) Although the discussion of the temporal bone includes the jugular foramen, it actually is located in the floor of the posterior fossa, between the petrous temporal bone anterolaterally and the occipital bone posteromedially.
        2) The jugular foramen is divided into a smaller anteromedial compartment (i.e., pars nervosa) and a larger posterolateral compartment (i.e., pars vascularis) (Fig. 16-3).

Table 16-2   Major Apertures of the Skull Base and Their Contents

Skull-Base Aperture	Location in Skull Base	Fissure/Transmitted Structure(s)
Cribriform plate	Medial floor of the anterior cranial fossa	Olfactory nerve (I) Ethmoid arteries
Optic canal	Lesser wing of sphenoid bone	Optic nerve (II) Ophthalmic artery Subarachnoid space, cerebro-spinal fluid, dura by optic nerve
Superior orbital fissure	Between lesser and greater sphenoid wings	Cranial nerves III, IV, V_1 and VI Superior ophthalmic vein
Foramen rotundum	Medial cranial fossa floor inferior to roof of pterygopalative fossa	Maxillary division of V (V_2) Emissary veins Artery of foramen rotundum
Foramen ovale	Floor of middle cranial fossa lateral to sella	Mandibular division of V (V_3) Emissary veins from carvernous sinus to pterygoid plexus Accessory meningeal branch of maxillary artery
Foramen spinosum	Posterolateral to foramen ovale	Middle meningeal artery Recurrent (meningeal) branch, mandibular nerve
Foramen lacerum	Base of medial pterygoid plate at petrous apex	Meningeal branches of ascending pharyngeal artery; not internal carotid artery
Vidian canal	In sphenoid bone inferomedial to foramen rotundum	Vidian artery Vidian nerve
Carotid canal	Within petrous temporal bone	Internal carotid artery Sympathetic plexus
Jugular foramen	Posterolateral to carotid canal, between petrous temporal bone and the occipital bone	Pars nervosa Inferior petrosal sinuses Glossopharyngeal nerve Jacobsen's nerve Pars vascularis Internal jugular vein Vagus and spinal accessory nerves Arnold's nerve

(continued)

Table 16-2 *(continued)*

Skull-Base Aperture	Location in Skull Base	Fissure/Transmitted Structure(s)
		Small meningeal branches of ascending pharyngeal and occipital arteries
Stylomastoid foramen	Behind styloid process	Facial nerve
Hypoglossal canal	Base of occipital condyles	Hypoglossal nerve
Foramen magnum	Floor of posterior fossa	Medulla and its meninges Spinal segment of cranial nerve XI Vertebral arteries and veins Anterior and posterior spinal arteries

a) Cranial nerves X, and XI travel through the pars vascularis along with the jugular vein. The pars nervosa only contains cranial nerve IX, contrary to its name implication.

b) Note that the hypoglossal nerve travels through the skull base in its own canal (i.e., the hypoglossal canal). This canal can be found just anterior and inferior to the jugular foramen.

3. Sphenoid bone.

   a. The sphenoid bone forms the midsection of the skull base and the anterior wall of the middle cranial fossa.

Q#2

   b. The sphenoid bone is divided into three components.

   1) Basisphenoid (i.e., dorsum sella, posterior clinoids, sella turcica, tuberculum sella, sphenoid sinus).

      a) In an adult the basisphenoid is fused to the clivus. In children it is separated from the clivus by the easily identified sphenooccipital synchondrosis.

   2) Greater wing of sphenoid.

      a) Forms the medial two thirds and the anterior wall of the middle cranial fossa floor.

   3) Lesser wing of sphenoid.

      a) Forms the medial and superior aspects of the anterior wall of the middle cranial fossa and the anterior clinoids.

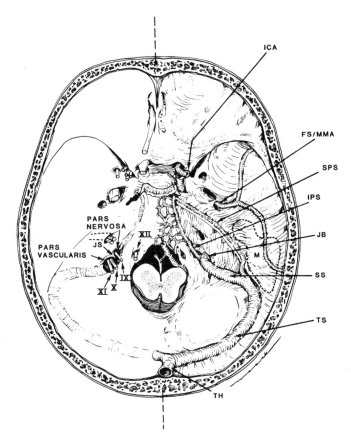

Fig. 16-3   Skull base viewed from above with the normal jugular foramen and contents on the left and normal arteries and veins on the right. The pars nervosa contains the glossopharyngeal nerve (*IX*) and the inferior petrosal sinus (*IPS*), whereas the pars vascularis has the vagus (*X*) and the spinal accessory (*XI*) nerves within it, as well as the jugular bulb (*JB*). Note the relationship of the mastoid air cells (*M*) to the sigmoid sinus (*SS*). More serious mastoid infections can cause thrombosis of the sigmoid sinus. *FS/MMA*, Foramen spinosum/middle meningeal artery; *ICA*, internal carotid artery; *JS*, jugular spine; *SPS*, superior petrosal sinus; *TH*, torcular Herophili; *TS*, transverse sinus; *XII*, hypoglossal nerve. (From Swartz J, Harnsberger HR: The Temporal Bone. Used with permission.)

      b) The lesser wing also creates the superior and medial edges of the superior orbital fissure.

Q#2

    c. Important apertures of the sphenoid bone (Fig. 16-2, Table 16-2):

      1) Foramen ovale.

2) Foramen spinosum.
3) Foramen rotundum.
4) Optic canal.
5) Superior orbital fissure.
6) Precavernous carotid canal.
7) Foramen lacerum.
   a) The foramen lacerum is not a true foramen. It is a thinning of the skull base, filled with fibrocartilage in life and seen only as a hole in the dried skull.
4. Frontal bone.

Q#2
   a. The anterior cranial fossa is bounded laterally and anteriorly by the frontal bone. Although not strictly subdivided into pieces, the majority of the anterior cranial fossa floor is comprised of the orbital plate of the frontal bone (Fig. 16-1*A*).
   b. An indentation in the medial anterior frontal bone, called the *foramen cecum*, is normal and should not be confused with cephalocele, which is sometimes present in this location.
      1) The foramen cecum has a complete bony floor, whereas a cephalocele will protrude through a gap in the frontal bone.
      2) The foramen cecum is prominent at birth and gradually shrinks over the first 10 years of life to become almost invisible on axial CT scans.
5. Ethmoid bone.
   a. The roof of the ethmoid bone forms the medial floor of the anterior cranial fossa.

Q#2
   b. Two distinct pieces of the ethmoid bone are discernible: the cribriform plate, and the crista galli.
      1) The cribriform plate is perforated by approximately 20 holes on each side of the crista galli.
      2) The nerve fibers of the olfactory nerve (i.e., cranial nerve I) pass from the nasal mucosa to the olfactory bulb.
      3) The crista galli serves as the anchor for the anterior margin of the falx cerebri.

E. Apertures and transmitted structures.
1. The normal skull base apertures and their contents are summarized in Table 16-2 and Figure 16-2.
2. The normal cranial nerves, their passages through the skull base, and their functions are presented in Table 16-3 and Figures 16-2 through

Table 16-3   Cranial Nerve Skull-Base Passages

Cranial Nerve Number	Cranial Nerve Name	Skull Base Passage
I	Olfactory	Cribriform plate
II	Optic	Optic canal
III	Oculomotor	Superior orbital fissure
IV	Trochlear	Superior orbital fissure
V	Trigeminal	
V_1	Ophthalmic division	Superior orbital fissure
V_2	Maxillary division	Foramen rotundum
V_3	Mandibular division	Foramen ovale
VI	Abducens	Superior orbital fissure
VII	Facial	Stylomastoid foramen
VIII	Vestibulocochlear	Internal auditory canal
	Cochlear	Modiolus
	Vestibular	Superior and inferior vestibular apertures
IX	Glossopharyngeal	Jugular foramen Pars nervosa
X	Vagus	Jugular foramen Pars vascularis
XI	Spinal accessory	Jugular foramen Pars vascularis
XII	Hypoglossal	Hypoglossal canal

16-4. Each cranial nerve is discussed comprehensively in Chapters 18 and 19.

F. Skull base interaction with deep facial spaces.

1. The spaces of the deep face, which abut the skull base, are important to recognize, because both infections and tumors of these spaces frequently are responsible for the radiographic changes seen in the skull base. In addition, lesions distant from the skull base in the lower face can reach the skull base and intracranial region by tracking cephalad along these spaces.

2. The deep facial spaces that abut the skull base include (Fig. 16-4):

   a. Parapharyngeal space.

   b. Masticator space.

   c. Carotid space.

   d. Retropharyngeal space.

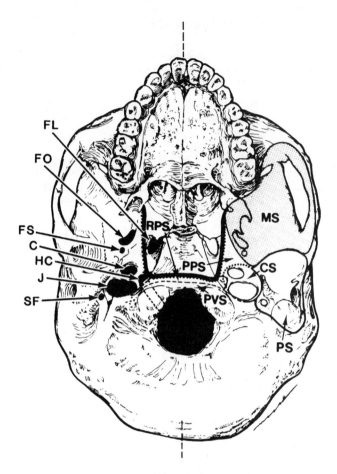

Fig. 16-4 Extracranial aspects of the skull base. *Left,* Critical openings. *Right,* Nasopharyngeal spaces as they abut the skull base. *Heavy line,* pharyngobasilar fascia; *light line,* superficial layer of deep cervical fascia; *dotted line,* middle layer, deep cervical fascia (buccopharyngeal fascia); *dashed line,* deep layer, deep cervical fascia (prevertebral fascia); *dotted–dashed line,* carotid sheath. See page 423 for the key to lettered structures. (From Osborn AG, Harnsberger HR, Smoker WRK: Base of skull imaging. *Semin Ultrasound CT MR* 7:91–106, 1986. Used with permission.)

    e. Perivertebral space.
3. These spaces are discussed briefly in this section. Detailed accounts of the deep facial spaces are provided by Chapters 2 through 7.
4. Parapharyngeal space.
    a. Although only a small wedge of parapharyngeal space abuts the skull base, it nonetheless is important. This space provides a natural

"elevator shaft" through which tumor or infection can reach the skull base from any site in the suprahyoid neck.

b. The parapharyngeal space spans the distance from the submandibular space below to the skull base above. It contains only fat, which is a natural medium for infection and an easy substance for tumor to traverse.

5. Masticator space.

    a. The masticator space connects the mandible to the skull base, creating a tube through which odontogenic infection and oropharyngeal squamous cell carcinoma (SCCa) can reach the skull base.

    b. Perineural tumor running along the mandibular division of the trigeminal nerve (i.e., cranial nerve V_3) accesses the skull base in the region of the foramen ovale. The intracranial compartment also is reached via perineural tumor spread when the tumor continues along the nerve into Meckel's cavity.

        1) Comment. An important imaging guideline is always to image the entire trigeminal nerve when a lesion is found within the masticator space to avoid missing intracranial perineural tumor.

6. Carotid space.

    a. The carotid space is important in skull base imaging because of the types of lesions primary to it. Vascular lesions (i.e., jugular vein thrombosis) and neural tumors (i.e., schwannoma, neurofibroma, paraganglioma), which are common to this space, are longitudinal lesions that often involve the carotid space simultaneously with the jugular foramen of the skull base.

7. Retropharyngeal and perivertebral spaces.

    a. These midline spaces become extremely attenuated as they approach the skull base.

    b. In their normal state, the area of skull base they abut is limited (Fig. 16-4). Only when involved by infection or tumor do these spaces swell with disease.

    c. Clival destruction in conjunction with a deep facial lesion indicates that disease has reached the skull base via one of these two spaces.

THE DISEASED SKULL BASE

A. General concepts.

1. The skull base represents the dividing line between surgical territories of the ear, nose, and throat (ENT) surgeon and the neurosurgeon.

2. Most ENT surgeons operate comfortably below the skull base and the neurosurgeon above it.

3. The skull base can be operated on by surgeons of either specialty. It is common to see a team of surgeons including a more aggressive ENT surgeon and a neurosurgeon operating on lesions of the skull base.

Q#3

4. Diseases of the skull base can be divided into three categories based on this surgical division of labor.

   a. Diseases involving the skull base from above (i.e., "top-down lesions").

   b. Diseases intrinsic to the skull base.

   c. Diseases involving the skull base from below (i.e., "bottom up lesions").

5. This discussion focuses on intrinsic lesions of the skull base.

   a. "Top-down lesions" are fully discussed in Osborn's *Neuroradiology Handbook*.

   b. "Bottom-up lesions" are discussed in the chapters on the suprahyoid neck that begin this book.

B. Lesions intrinsic to the skull base.

1. General remarks.

   a. A lesion is judged to be intrinsic to the skull base if the volume of the primary mass is centered in the plane of the skull base.

   b. Intrinsic lesions of the skull base are rare.

   c. These lesions may spread either cranially to involve the brain or caudally to involve the deep facial spaces of the suprahyoid neck.

   d. The differential diagnosis of lesions intrinsic to the skull base is best thought of as a single, large list (Table 16-4), with a smaller list of those pertinent to the jugular foramen (Table 16-5).

2. Intrinsic lesions.

   a. Pseudomasses of the skull base.

      1) Complex flow in the jugular bulb.

         a) The most commonly misdiagnosed pseudomass in the skull base is seen in the many varied signals that may be seen associated with the jugular bulb on MRI scans.

         b) The complex flow (slow, turbulent, jetting) may create high signal in the normal jugular bulb on T1-weighted images. The high signal catches the eye of the radiologist, who then observes the other sequences and may find the area "enhancing" on T1-weighted, contrast-enhanced images that usually results from slow venous flow. At this point the misdiagnosis of a jugular foramen mass ("probable glomus jugulare paraganglioma") is offered.

         c) MRI findings. The key MRI sequence is the T2-weighted sequence. No signal will come from the jugular foramen; in other words the jugular foramen will appear black. Infrequently there also will be signal from the bulb on T2-weighted images. At this point two-dimensional time of

Table 16-4   Intrinsic Lesions of the Skull Base

Pseudomasses
Jugular bulb complex flow
Petrous apex air cell fluid

Congenital
Primary cholesteatoma

Inflammatory
Apical petrositis
Mucocele of petrous apex air cell or sphenoid/ethmoid sinus
Cholesterol granuloma

Trauma
Skull base fracture with or without dural tear

Tumor, Benign
Paraganglioma (i.e., glomus jugulare)
Neural sheath tumor (i.e., schwannoma, neurofibroma)
Meningioma
Chordoma
Benign primary bony tumors

Tumor, Malignant
Metastasis
Non-Hodgkin lymphoma and leukemia
Myeloma
Malignant primary bone tumors

Metabolic and Dysplastic Lesions
Fibrous dysplasia
Paget disease
Anemias
Histiocytosis X

Table 16-5   Masses of the Jugular Foramen

Vascular
Pseudomass from venous flow phenomenon
Pseudomass from venous vascular normal variant (i.e., high jugular bulb)
Jugular vein thrombosis

Tumor
Paraganglioma (i.e., glomus jugulare)
Neural sheath tumor (i.e., schwannoma, neurofibroma)
Meningioma
Metastasis

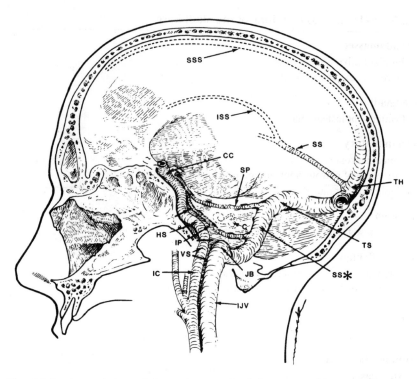

Fig. 16-5 Lateral view of the major vessels of the temporal bone and jugular foramen. *SSS*, superior sagittal sinus; *ISS*, inferior sagittal sinus; *SS*, straight sinus; *SS**, sigmoid sinus; *JB*, jugular bulb; *IJV*, internal jugular vein; *SP*, superior petrosal sinus; *IP*, inferior petrosal sinus; *IC*, internal carotid artery; *VS*, vertical segment, ICA; *HS*, horizontal segment, ICA; *CC*, cavernous internal carotid artery; *C*, cochlea. (From Swartz J, Harnsberger HR: *Imaging of the temporal bone*, ed 2. New York, 1992, Thieme Medical Publishers, p. 155. Used with permission.)

flight and/or phase-contrast MRA can be used to prove there is no tumor in the jugular foramen.

    d) If after all MRI sequences and MRA doubt still lingers about the true nature of the jugular bulb, thin-section (i.e., 3-mm contiguous), bone-algorithm CT scans through the skull base can clear up any problems by demonstrating normal bony anatomy including preservation of the jugular spine.

  2) Petrous apex air cell fluid.

    a) In approximately 33% of cases the petrous apex is pneumatized.

   b) Recurrent ear infections may result in ostial occlusion, which isolates these air cells and leaves them filled with old, sterile fluid that may be discovered incidentally later in life during head MRI scans for other clinical indications.
   c) MRI findings. Fluid in the petrous apex air cells most commonly follows the expected signal of water (cerebrospinal fluid [CSF]): low on T1-weighted and high on T2-weighted sequences. When the protein content is high, the higher signal on a T1-weighted sequences may be disturbing.
   d) If a question lingers regarding this finding, thin-section (i.e., 3-mm contiguous), axial, bone-algorithm CT scans will show normal but opacified petrous apex air cells. All internal trabeculae should be present to label such an area as incidental and of no clinical importance.
   e) Comment. The relationship of the postinflammatory fluid collections of the petrous apex air cell to the entity known as *cholesterol granuloma* is not known. I have speculated for years that these fluid collections rarely have associated hemorrhage, which leads into a cycle that eventually results in a cholesterol granuloma. If you subscribe to this theory as well, long-term follow-up either with CT or MRI on this patient group may be justified.
b. Congenital.
   1) Primary or congenital cholesteatoma.
      a) Squamous epithelial rest of embryonal origin.
      b) Occurs in the temporal bone (i.e., petrous apex, middle ear/mastoid), other skull bones, within the meninges, brain, or any other part of the body.
      c) In the skull base it most commonly is found in the petrous apex and the middle ear/mastoid areas.
      d) Terminology. Within the skull base this lesion is referred to as a *congenital cholesteatoma*. When found in the cisterns, the term *epidermoid cyst* or *epidermoidoma* is applied. Pathologically these lesions are indistiguishable.
c. Trauma.
   1) Skull base fractures are best seen on high-resolution CT scans.
   2) Fracture sequelae include cerebrospinal fluid leakage from a dural tear, cranial neuropathy, internal carotid artery pseudo-aneurysm or thrombosis, and intracranial infection.
   3) A suspected dural tear is best evaluated with thin-section, high-resolution, coronal CT scans (i.e., 3-mm contiguous slices). Contrast is not used initially, because in most cases the fracture location signals the site of the CSF leak.

        a) The most common sites for CSF leakage include the tegmen of the temporal bone (i.e., CSF otorrhea) and the cribriform plate/fovea ethmoidalis (i.e., CSF rhinorrhea).

        b) Intrathecal contrast medium is only used when there is extensive damage to the skull base and the focal site of the CSF leak is in question.

  d. Benign tumor.

    1) Paraganglioma (i.e., glomus jugulare).

        a) This tumor is located in the adventitia of the jugular bulb along the tympanic branch of the glossopharyngeal nerve (i.e., Jacobson's nerve).

        b) Clinical presentation. Complex cranial neuropathy including cranial nerves IX, X, and XI is the most common presentation of tumors in the jugular foramen. In addition paraganglioma of the middle ear (i.e., tympanicum type) and the jugular foramen (i.e., jugulare type) may be associated with pulsatile tinnitus.

        c) CT appearance. Enhancing mass in the jugular foramen with erosion of the jugular spine and adjacent permeative bony changes.

        d) MRI appearance. T1-weighted scans show a mixed-intensity mass in the jugular foramen with serpiginous flow voids within the mass that appear as black lines and/or dots (i.e., "pepper"). This appearance is best seen on the nonenhanced, T1-weighted MRI scans. If enhancement is used, fat suppression should accompany the T1 pulse sequence.

        e) Comment. Tumor that extends into the temporal bone is termed a *glomus jugulotympanicum*. This type of paraganglioma usually presents with pulsatile tinnitus and a vascular retrotympanic mass.

        f) Treatment considerations. Total resection is the goal. In older, infirm patients, however, radiation may be used as the primary treatment. In this case stabilization or reduction of the tumor size, decreased enhancement, diminished flow voids, and reduced T2-weighted signal all should be construed as MRI evidence for local control.

    2) Neural sheath tumor.

        a) This term refers to the group of benign neural sheath tumors.

        b) Primary lesions in this group include schwannoma and neurofibroma.

        c) Schwannoma. A solitary, encapsulated tumor sometimes associated with neurofibromatosis type II.

    d) Neurofibroma. This can be either multiple or single. It is unencapsulated and associated with neurofibromatosis type I in approximately 50% of cases.

    e) Any of the cranial nerves exiting the skull base may be involved with either of these lesions, but the most common site of occurrence is the jugular foramen (i.e., cranial nerves IX, X, and XI).

    f) CT appearance. Bone detail scan shows smooth, scalloped enlargement of the affected passage. A fusiform soft-tissue mass is seen within this passage.

    g) MRI appearance. Fusiform mass with uniform intensity, usually matching that of brain, filling the enlarged neural foramen. Contrast usually will cause uniform enhancement of these lesions.

3) Meningioma.

    a) May arise anywhere from the leptomeninges.

    b) When arising from the entrance or within a neural foramen, meningioma may appear intrinsic to the skull base.

    c) CT appearance. Uniformly enhancing, dural-based mass that may be partially calcified and associated with skull base hyperostosis.

    d) MRI appearance. Brain intensity, dural-based mass, often with calcification and hyperostosis. May be difficult to see on standard imaging sequences. Marked enhancement with gadolinium is the rule.

4) Chordoma.

    a) This is a rare bone tumor that arises from remnants of the cranial end of the primitive notochord.

    b) Thirty-five percent are intracranial, usually located in the clivus; 50% are sacrococcygeal; and 15% arise from a vertebral body.

    c) The principal intracranial location is the sphenooccipital synchondrosis. Other skull base locations that may be involved include the basisphenoid and basiocciput.

    d) CT features. Destructive midline mass in or adjacent to the clivus, with associated bone destruction (95% of cases) and tumor calcification (50%).

    e) MRI appearance. T1-weighted images show tumor to be isointense to hypointense to brain. T2-weighted image shows hyperintensity. The soft-tissue component usually is disproportionately larger than the area of bony involvement.

    f) Although MRI may not show tumor calcification, its ability to delineate the full extent of the chordoma, coupled with its display of normal adjacent vasculature, makes it the ideal imaging tool for chordoma.

    g. Comment. A midline lesion involving the clivus with very high signal on T2-weighted images showing heterogeneous enhancement with contrast, and associated with erosive bony changes strongly favors the diagnosis of chordoma.

  5) Benign bony tumors.
    a) Rarely of clinical significance unless strategically located.
    b) This group includes chondroma, osteoma, giant cell tumors.
  6) Primary cholesteatoma and cholesterol granuloma.
    a) See Chapter 17.

e. Malignant tumor.
  1) Metastatic tumor.
    a) Metastasis is the most common cause of malignant tumor of the skull base.
    b) Disease spreads to the skull base either directly (i.e., orbit, sinonasal, nasopharyngeal carcinoma) or hematogenously.
    c) The most common primary sites are the lung, breast, and prostate gland.
    d) CT appearance. Destructive mass infiltrating the skull base.
    e) MRI appearance. T1-weighted scans show a "muscle" intensity mass within the skull base with loss of normal, low intensity cortical bone signal.
  2) Non-Hodgkin lymphoma and leukemia.
    a) Focal lesions seen throughout the extracranial head and neck region.
    b) CT and/or MRI scans are characterized by multifocal masses that may be discrete or infiltrative in the skull base. Only lymphoma in a single site cannot be differentiated from other malignant skull base tumors.
  3) Myeloma.
    a) Multiple myeloma or solitary plasmacytoma is possible.
    b) Multiple myeloma is indistinguishable from osteolytic metastatic disease on CT or MRI scans.
      i) In the diffuse form, all bones of the skull base are involved, with permeative changes.
    c) Solitary myeloma (i.e., plasmacytoma) is indistinguishable from a single metastatic focus in the skull base.
  4) Malignant primary bone tumors.
    a) Extremely rare in the skull base region.
    b) Primarily chondrosarcoma and osteosarcoma.
    c) Chondrosarcoma. Rare, slow-growing, skull base malignancy that most commonly occurs in the area of the parame-

dian basisphenoid synchondrosis (Fig. 16-1*A*). CT scans show chondroid matrix mineralization in less than 50% of cases while MRI scans show signal heterogeneity in approximately 60%. Signal heterogeneity on MRI scans is thought to result from matrix mineralization, fibrocartilaginous elements, or both.

   f. Diffuse intrinsic lesions (Tables 16-6 and 16-7).

      1) Fibrous dysplasia.

         a) Clinical features. Relatively common, benign, developmental skeletal disorder typically seen in adolescents and young adults (i.e., 75% present before 30 years of age). May be asymptomatic or present with painful swelling, stress, or overt fracture. Cafe-au-lait spots situated predominantly on the trunk are present in 50% of patients with the polyostotic form of fibrous dysplasia.

         b) Pathophysiology. The medullary cavity of the affected bone fills and expands with fibrous tissue. The fibrous tissue then variably ossifies.

         c) CT appearance. Thickened, sclerotic bone. Usually uniform in density but may have cystic regions, especially in the early, active phase of the disease.

         c) MRI appearance. Expanded, low-intensity areas of bone. A lesion usually is seen as hypointense on both T1- and T2-weighted images. Active lesions may have complex signal with high- and low-signal areas seen on both T1- and T2-weighted sequences.

         d) Albright's syndrome. Polyostotic, unilateral form of fibrous dysplasia with ipsilateral cafe-au-lait spots and endocrine dysfunction that produces precocious puberty in girls.

      2) Paget disease.

         a) Clinical features. Bone disease of uncertain etiology but most commonly thought to be of viral origin that may be uni-

---

Table 16-6   Generalized Skull Base Involvement

Paget disease

Fibrous dysplasia

Metastatic tumor

Histiocytosis X

Multiple myeloma

Anemias

Table 16-7   Diseases Causing Skull Base Sclerosis

Osteoblastic metastases
Paget disease
Fibrous dysplasia
Meningioma en plaque
Osteopetrosis

---

focal or multifocal. Affects 10% of the population over 85 years of age.

b) Pathophysiology. Imbalance between bone resorption and formation, leading to osseous deformity. The course of bone disease usually includes an early destructive phase, an intermediate combined destructive and healing phase, and a late sclerotic (i.e., quiescent) phase.

c) Radiologic findings. May involve any bone. At times it is discovered incidentally on radiologic study done for other clinical indications. Both CT or MRI scans show expanded bone of the skull base associated with calvarial involvement. MRI better demonstrates the basilar invagination often seen with Paget disease because of bone softening.

d) Specific MRI findings. High-signal foci representing fat collections are seen on T1-weighted sequences. High-signal foci secondary to fibrovascular marrow in active Paget disease are seen on T2-weighted sequences.

3) Histiocytosis X.

a) Histiocytosis X is a group of granulomatous reticuloendothelioses, including eosinophilic granuloma, Hand-Schüller-Christian disease, and Letterer-Siwe disease. Children and young adults primarily are affected.

b) The common pathologic denominator is the histiocyte. Eosinophilic granuloma involves only bone; involvement of soft tissues indicates Hand-Schüller-Christian or Letterer-Siwe disease.

c) Radiologic features. Single or multiple areas of pure osteolysis are seen in the skull base and calvarium of children (i.e., eosinophilic granuloma). A soft-tissue mass may be associated (i.e., Hand-Schüller-Christian or Letterer-Siwe disease).

C. Lesions involving the skull base from above (Table 16-8).

1. Most of these lesions are discussed elsewhere. The chapters on cranial nerves describe lesions of the leptomeninges and cisterns most fully.

Table 16-8   Lesions Involving the Skull Base from Above

Congenital
Cephalocele (meningocele, encephalocele)
Arachnoid cyst

Vascular Lesions
Carotid–cavernous aneurysm
Dural arteriovenous malformation

Tumor, Benign
Meningioma
Nerve sheath tumors
Dermoid cyst
Pituitary adenoma
Rathke's pouch cyst

Tumor, Malignant
Primary brain tumor
Hypothalamic–opticochiasmatic glioma

2. The cephaloceles merit discussion here, because although they originate intracranially, these lesions traverse the skull base and cause both clinical and imaging problems in the extracranial head and neck.
3. Cephaloceles.
   a. Etiology. Cephaloceles are congenital or acquired lesions.
      1) Congenital cephalocele. These lesions result from failure of mesodermal ingrowth between the neural tube and the overlying ectoderm. Abnormalities in the cranium and underlying meninges result.
      2) Acquired cephalocele. These most commonly are secondary to surgery or trauma. A spontaneous form has been reported to occur in the sphenoid sinus area, when the pterygoid wing is fully pneumatized, and in the petrous apex area, when petrous apex aeration is present.
   b. Terminology.

Q#4
      1) *Cephalocele* is used to denote herniation of meninges (i.e., *meningocele*) or meninges and brain substance (i.e., *encephalocele*) through the cranial defect.
      2) Visible cephaloceles are termed *sincipital*. Those that cannot be seen without the help of CT or MRI are called *basal*.
   c. Congenital cephalocele location.

1) Seventy percent involve the occipital bone. Most are in the squamous portion, with cephaloceles in the basiocciput occurring rarely.

2) Approximately 15% of all cephaloceles occur in the anterior cranial fossa. These are named according to their craniofacial pathway.

   a) Nasofrontal cephalocele (see Fig. 15-12C).

   b) Nasoethmoidal cephalocele (see Fig. 15-12D).

   c) Nasoorbital cephalocele.

   d) Basal cephaloceles are grouped anatomically according to the location of the bony defect: transethmoidal, sphenoethmoidal, transphenoidal, sphenoorbital, and sphenomaxillary.

d. Clinical presentation.

1) A high degree of suspicion is necessary if congenital cephalocele is to be diagnosed before any surgical procedure is undertaken.

2) Any child with suspected nasal polyp or nasopharyngeal mass, recurrent bouts of bacterial meningitis (with or without CSF rhinorrhea), or lump on the bridge of the nose must undergo CT or MRI before surgical intervention.

Table 16-9   Lesions Involving the Skull Base from Below

Inflammatory

Skull base osteomyelitis from:
   Sinus infection
   Malignant otitis externa
   Deep facial space abscess
Aggressive sinonasal polyposis

Tumor, Benign

Nasal tumors
   Juvenile angiofibroma
   Inverting papilloma
   Nasal dermoid
Sinus osteoma

Tumor, Malignant

Nasopharyngeal carcinoma
Non-Hodgkin lymphoma
Esthesioneuroblastoma
Rhabdomyosarcoma
Parotid gland malignancies
Perineural squamous cell carcinoma (cranial nerves V_3 and VII)

3) Appearance of a new mass after temporal bone or sinonasal surgery should be considered a possible postsurgical cephalocele.
4) Patients who have undergone significant skull base fractures also may develop posttraumatic cephalocele.
   e. Imaging issues.
1) CT features. Axial and coronal CT bone images will depict clearly the bony defect through which the cephalocele passes. Soft-tissue components of the cephalocele are not so well seen with CT as with MRI.
2) MRI features. Sagittal and coronal MRI best delineate the soft-tissue portion of the cephalocele, helping to determine what is herniated through the bony rent in the skull base. The location of the dura relative to the cephalocele also at times can be seen.
   a) Because surgery will be extradural if possible, MRI information is vital to effective surgical planning.

D. Lesions involving the skull base from below (Table 16-9).

1. Lesions involving the skull base from the deep facial spaces are best grouped according to the space of origin. Each of these spaces has a unique differential diagnosis.
   a. Figure 16-3 summarizes the areas where each of the deep facial spaces abuts the skull base. For a complete discussion of the diseases emanating from these spaces, see Chapters 2 through 7.
2. In addition to the deep facial spaces, the sinonasal region and temporal bone are sites of specific lesions that affect the skull base secondarily.

KEY TO CHAPTER 16 FIGURES

Arteries

MMA = middle meningeal artery
SA = spinal artery
VA = vertebral artery
ICA = internal carotid artery

Canals

C = carotid canal
H = hypoglossal canal
IAC = internal auditory canal

Cranial Nerves

I = olfactory
II = optic
III = oculomotor
IV = trochlear

V_1 = trigeminal, ophthalmic division
V_2 = trigeminal, maxillary division
V_3 = trigeminal, mandibular division
VI = abducens
VII = facial
VIII = vestibulocochlear
IX = glossopharyngeal
X = vagus
XI = spinal accessory
XII = hypoglossal

Foramina

FL = foramen lacerum
FO = foramen ovale
FR = foramen rotundum
FS = foramen spinosum

J = jugular foramen	*PPS* = parapharyngeal space
SF = stylomastoid foramen	*PS* = parotid space
	PVS = perivertebral space
Sinuses	*RPS* = retropharyngeal space
IPS = inferior petrosal sinus	
SPS = superior petrosal sinus	**Miscellaneous**
SS = sigmoid sinus	*CP* = cribriform plate
TS = transverse sinus	*JS* = jugular spine
	PN = pars nervosa
Spaces	*PV* = pars vascularis
CS = carotid space	*SOF* = superior orbital fissure
MS = masticator space	*TH* = torcular Herophili

SUGGESTED READING

Normal Skull Base

Chusid JG: *Correlative neuroanatomy and functional neurology,* ed 19. Los Altos, Calif., 1985, Lange Medical Publications.

Daniels DL, Schenck JF, Foster T, et al: Magnetic resonance imaging of the jugular foramen. *AJNR* 6:699–703, 1985.

Daniels DL, Williams AL, Haughton KVM: Jugular foramen: anatomic and computed tomographic study. *Am J Roentgenol* 142:153–158, 1984.

Gilman S, Newman SW: *Manter and Gatz's essentials of clinical neuroanatomy and neurophysiology*, ed 7. Philadelphia, 1987, FA Davis.

Hans JS, Huss RG, Benson JE, et al: MR imaging of the skull base. *J Comput Assist Tomogr* 8:944–952, 1984.

Harnsberger HR: CT and MRI of masses of the deep face. *Curr Probl Diagn Radiol* 16:147–173, 1987.

Lo WWM, Solti-Bohman LG: High-resolution CT of the jugular foramen. Anatomy and vascular anomalies. *Radiology* 150:743–747, 1984.

Mancuso AA, Hanafee WN: *Computed tomography and magnetic resonance imaging of the head and neck*, ed 2. Baltimore, 1985, Williams & Wilkins.

Osborn AG, Harnsberger HR, Smoker WRK: Base of skull imaging. *Semin Ultrasound CT MR* 7:91–106, 1986.

Smoker WRK, Gentry LR: Computed tomography of nasopharynx and related spaces. *Semin Ultrasound CT MR* 7:107–130, 1986.

Whelan MA, Reede VL, Meisler W, et al: CT of the base of the skull. *Radiol Clin North Am* 22:177–217, 1984.

Diseased Skull Base

Brown RV, Sage MR, Brophy BP: CT and MR findings in patients with chordoma of the petrous apex. *AJNR* 11:121–124, 1990.

Daffner RH, Kirks DR, Gehweiler JA, et al: CT of fibrous dysplasia. *Am J Roentgenol* 139:943–948, 1982.

Diebler C, Dulac O: Cephaloceles: clinical and neuroradiological appearance. *Neuroradiology* 25:199–216, 1983.

Elster AD, Branch CL: Transalar sphenoidal encephaloceles: clinical and radiologic findings. *Radiology* 170:245–247, 1989.

Geoffray A, Lee YY, Jing BS, et al: Extracranial meningioma of the head and neck. *AJNR* 5:599–604, 1984.

Holtas S, Monajati A, Utz R: CT of malignant lymphoma involving the skull. *J Comput Assist Tomogr* 9:725–727, 1985.

Kransdorf MJ, Moser RP, Gilkey FW: Fibrous dysplasia. *RadioGraphics* 10:519–537, 1990.

Lo WWM, Solti-Bohman LG, Lambert PR: High-resolution CT in the evaluation of glomus tumors of the temporal bone. *Radiology* 150:737–742, 1984.

Mafee MF: MRI and CT in the evaluation of acquired and congenital cholesteatomas of the temporal bone. *J Otolaryngol* 22:239–248, 1993.

Manelfe C, Cellerier P, Sobel D, et al: Cerebrospinal fluid rhinorrhea: evaluation with metrizamide cisternography. *Am J Roentgenol* 138:471–476, 1982.

Meyer JE, Oot RF, Lindfors KK: CT appearance of clival chordomas. *J Comput Assist Tomogr* 10:34–38, 1986.

Meyers SP, Hirsch WL, Curtin HD, et al: Chondrosarcomas of the skull base: MR imaging features. *Radiology* 184:103–108, 1992.

Meyers SP, Hirsch WL, Curtin HD, et al: Chordomas of the skull base: MR features. *AJNR* 13:1627–1636, 1992.

Moore T, Ganti SR, Mawad ME, et al: CT and angiography of primary extradural juxtasellar tumors. *Am J Roentgenol* 145:491–496, 1985.

Mukherji SK, Kasper ME, Tart RP, et al: Irradiated paragangliomas of the head and neck: CT and MR appearance. *AJNR* 13:357–363, 1994.

Olsen WL, Dillon WP, Kelly WM, et al: MR imaging of paraganglioma. *AJR Am J Roentgenol* 148:201–204, 1987.

Osborn AG, Harnsberger HR, Smoker WRK: Base of skull imaging. *Semin Ultrasound CT MR* 7:91–106, 1986.

Oot RF, Melville GE, New PFJ, et al: The role of MR and CT in evaluating clival chordomas and chondrosarcomas. *AJNR* 9:715–723, 1988.

Pollock JA, Newton TH, Hoyt WF: Transsphenoidal and transethmoidal encephaloceles. *Radiology* 90:442–453, 1968.

Roberts MC, Kressel HY, Fallon MD, et al: Paget disease: MR imaging findings. *Radiology* 173:341–345, 1989.

Schreiman JS, McLeod RA, Kyle RA, et al: Multiple myeloma: evaluation by CT. *Radiology* 154:483–486, 1985.

Silver AJ, Mawad ME, Hilal SK, et al: CT of the carotid space and related cervical spaces. II: neurogenic tumors. *Radiology* 150:729–735, 1984.

Sze G, Uichano LS, Brant-Zawadzki MN, et al: Chordoma: MR imaging. *Radiology* 166:187–191, 1988.

Tjon-A-Tham RTO, Bloem JL, Falke THM, et al: MRI in Paget disease of the skull. *AJNR* 6:879–881, 1985.

Van Gils APG, Van den Berg R, Falke THM, et al: MR diagnosis of paraganglioma of the head and neck: value of contrast enhancement. *AJR* 162:147–153, 1994.

West SW, Russell EJ, Breit R, et al: Calvarial and skull base metastases: comparison of nonenhanced and Gd-DTPA-enhanced MR images. *Radiology* 174:85–91, 1990.

17

The Temporal Bone: External, Middle, and Inner Ear Segments

CRITICAL IMAGING QUESTIONS: THE TEMPORAL BONE

Normal temporal bone:

1. What are the five bony components of the normal adult temporal bone?
2. What are the three adjacent structures found along the posterior mesotympanum of the middle ear cavity? In which of these structures does cholesteatoma sometimes hide?
3. Where is Prussak's space? Why is it important to be able to identify it on CT evaluation of the temporal bone?
4. Name the three segments of the facial nerve (i.e., cranial nerve VII) within the temporal bone. What are the three branches of the facial nerve in the temporal bone? What functions do these branches subserve?

Diseased temporal bone:

5. Name the two most important CT observations in the setting of external and middle ear atresia that will help the ear, nose, and throat surgeon to predict the response to reconstructive therapy.
6. What five important radiologic questions must be answered when cholesteatoma is found in the middle ear?
7. When a "vascular retrotympanic mass" is found on otoscopic examination, what two abnormalities that do not require surgery may be seen on CT scans?

Answers to these questions are found in the text beside the question number (Q#) in the margin.

NORMAL TEMPORAL BONE

A. General comments.

1. With its ability to image the fine bony structures of the temporal bone, CT is the primary imaging tool for the diagnosis of temporal bone disease in the external and middle ear. MRI has begun to replace CT in the evaluation of inner ear pathology.
2. In replacing plain mastoid films and standard tomograms, CT has changed the rules for diagnosis of temporal bone disease from the use of late (i.e., bone) changes to early (i.e., soft tissue) changes.
3. The goal of the radiologist is to provide the surgeon with a precise preoperative picture of the pathology that is present. There should no longer be any intraoperative surprises during temporal bone surgery.
4. As the reader reviews this section on the normal anatomy of the temporal bone, a temporal bone monogram should be perused simultaneously to fix in mind the CT appearance of the structures. Two widely used monograms are contained in *CT of the temporal bone, vol 60, no 3* (Eastman Kodak, 1984) and *Direct multiplanar CT of the petrous temporal bone* (Philips, 1983). Alternatively, Swartz and Harnsberger's *Imaging of the temporal bone* (1992) can be used for this purpose.

B. Anatomy.

Q#1

1. The adult temporal bone is made up of five bony parts: the squamous, mastoid, petrous, tympanic, and styloid portions.
2. Squamous portion. This functions as the bony floor of the adult suprazygomatic masticator space (i.e., temporal fossa) and the lateral wall of the middle cranial fossa.
3. Mastoid portion.
   a. The mastoid portion has three important anatomic landmarks: the mastoid antrum, the aditus ad antrum (Latin for "entrance to cavity"), and Körner's septum.
      1) The *aditus ad antrum* connects the epitympanum (i.e., attic) of the middle ear cavity to the mastoid antrum.
      2) *Körner's septum* is part of the petrosquamosal suture that runs posterolaterally through the mastoid air cells.
         a) It serves as a barrier to the extension of infection from the lateral mastoid air cells to the medial mastoid air cells.
         b) It also functions as an important surgical landmark within the mastoid air cells.
   b. The mastoid portion of the temporal bone develops after birth. Because the mastoid eminence protects the facial nerve from harm,

this nerve is relatively unprotected until it has formed. This is why
the facial nerve is so vulnerable to birth trauma, especially during
delivery using forceps.

4. Petrous portion.

   a. The inner ear (i.e., otic capsule) is contained within the petrous portion of the temporal bone. It often is referred to as the *petrous pyramid*, because it is shaped like a pyramid with anterior, posterior, and
inferior surfaces.

   b. The two important structures on the anterior surface of the petrous
pyramid are:

      1) The tegmen (Latin for "cover") tympani is the roof or cover of
the tympanic cavity.

      2) The arcuate eminence is the bone prominence over the superior
semicircular canal.

         a) The arcuate eminence is a surgical landmark as the surgeon
cuts along the floor of the middle cranial fossa.

   c. The posterior surface of the petrous portion of the temporal bone contains the porus acusticus and the vestibular and cochlear aqueducts.

      1) The porus acusticus is the opening (or "mouth") of the internal
auditory canal.

      2) Relevant anatomy in the internal auditory canal includes the
modiolus (Latin for "hub"), which is the entrance to the cochlea
through which the cochlear nerve passes, and the crista falciformis, which is the horizontal bony septum in the lateral 3 mm
of the internal auditory canal fundus (see Figs. 20-1 and 20-2).

      3) The vestibular aqueduct transmits the endolymphatic duct and
runs parallel to the line of the petrous ridge.

      4) The cochlear aqueduct transmits the perilymphatic duct and is
located vertically below the internal auditory canal running parallel to it.

   d. The inferior surface of the petrous temporal bone helps to form the
carotid canal and jugular foramen.

   e. The petrous apex is separated from the clivus by the petrooccipital
fissure and the foramen lacerum.

5. Tympanic portion. This portion of the temporal bone is a U-shaped bone
forming the majority of the adult bony external auditory canal.

6. Styloid portion.

   a. The styloid portion of the temporal bone forms the styloid process.

   b. Like the mastoid process, the styloid process develops after birth.

C. Normal external auditory canal.

1. The external auditory canal is comprised of fibrocartilage laterally and
of bone medially.

  a. First branchial cleft anomalies with associated sinus tracts drain into
      the external auditory canal at this bony cartilaginous junction.
2. The medial border of the external auditory canal is formed by the tympanic membrane. The scutum is the bony projection to which the tympanic membrane attaches superiorly; it attaches to the tympanic annulus
   inferiorly (Figs. 17-1 and 17-2).
  a. The tympanic annulus serves as an important coronal CT landmark
      to determine if a lesion is in the external or middle ear.
3. Nodal drainage of the external auditory canal and adjacent scalp is to the
   parotid lymph nodes.
  a. This drainage pattern is important when evaluating a parotid mass,
      because the mass may represent nodal metastasis from an external
      auditory canal squamous cell carcinoma or melanoma.

D. Normal middle ear.

1. The three distinct regions of the middle ear are the epitympanum, or
   attic; the mesotympanum, or tympanic cavity proper; and the hypotympanum.

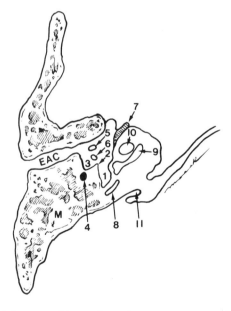

Fig. 17-1 Normal axial temporal bone through mesotympanum. *EAC,* External
auditory canal; *M,* mastoid air cells; *1,* sinus tympani; *2,* pyramidal eminence; *3,*
facial nerve recess; *4,* mastoid portion of facial nerve; *5,* manubrium of malleus; *6,*
long process of incus; *7,* tensor tympani; *8,* posterior semicircular canal; *9,* first turn
of cochlea; *10,* second turn of cochlea; *11,* vestibular aqueduct.

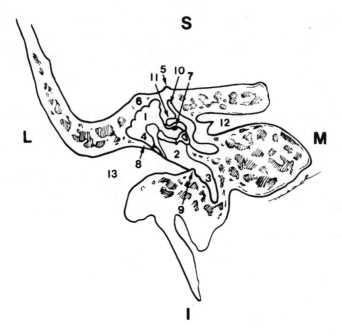

Fig. 17-2 Normal coronal temporal bone relationships. *I,* inferior; *L,* lateral; *M,* medial; *S,* superior; *1,* epitympanum; *2,* mesotympanum; *3,* hypotympanum; *4,* Prussak's space; *5,* arcuate eminence; *6,* tegmen tympani; *7,* horizontal (tympanic) portion of cranial nerve VII; *8,* scutum; *9,* tympanic annulus; *10,* superior semicircular canal; *11,* lateral semicircular canal; *12,* internal auditory canal; *13,* external auditory canal.

2. The normal middle ear cavity has six important walls:
   a. Anterior wall, or "carotid wall."
   b. Posterior wall, or "mastoid wall."
      1) The upper part of the posterior wall is absent. The aditus ad antrum connects the epitympanum to the mastoid antrum here.

Q#2
      2) The lower part of the mesotympanic portion of the posterior wall is comprised of three important structures: the pyramidal eminence, the sinus tympani, and the facial nerve recess (Fig. 17-1).
         a) The *pyramidal eminence* contains the belly and tendon of the stapedius muscle.
         b) The *sinus tympani* is a clinical blind spot during a standard mastoid surgical approach to the temporal bone. Cholesteatoma can hide here as a result.
         c) The *facial nerve recess* contains the descending facial nerve, either dehiscent or with a bony cover.

   c. Superior wall, or tegmen tympani.
     1) The bony roof separates lesions of the middle ear from the middle cranial fossa.
     2) Loss of this bony separation can lead to leptomeningeal or brain parenchymal involvement with infection or tumor.
   d. Inferior wall, or "jugular wall."
     1) The bony plate that separates the middle ear cavity from the jugular bulb may be normally dehiscent (i.e., dehiscent jugular bulb).
     2) This normal variant must be noted so that the surgeon can avoid the protuberant vein.
   e. Lateral wall, or "membranous wall."
     1) The tympanic membrane forms the lateral wall of the middle ear cavity.
     2) It slopes inferomedially from its scutum attachment above to the tympanic annulus below (Fig. 17-2).
3. Epitympanum (Fig. 17-2).
   a. Definition. The epitympanum is the tympanic cavity above the line drawn between the inferior tip of the scutum and the tympanic portion of the facial nerve.
   b. Contents. Within the epitympanum are the malleus head and the body and short process of the incus.
   c. Prussak's space.

Q#3

     1) Prussak's space is the area between the incus and the lateral, side wall of the epitympanum.
     2) This is the most common site for pars flaccida cholesteatoma.
4. Mesotympanum.
   a. Definition. The mesotympanum is the tympanic cavity or cleft proper. It extends from the inferior tip of the scutum above to the line drawn parallel to the inferior aspect of the bony external auditory canal.
   b. Contents. Within the mesotympanum are the remainder of the ossicles and the two muscles of the middle ear: the tensor tympani, and stapedius muscle.
     1) The ossicle portions within the mesotympanum are the manubrium of malleus, the long process of the incus, and the entire stapes.
     2) Middle ear muscles function to dampen sound.
       a) The tensor tympani is innervated by the third division of the trigeminal nerve (i.e., cranial nerve V_3). It is located in an anterior bony canal above the osseous eustachian tube (Fig.

17-1). It courses posteriorly to take a 90° bend at the cochleariform process, inserting on the manubrium of the malleus.

b) The stapedius muscle is innervated by the facial nerve. This muscle is contained within the pyramidal eminence, with its tendon reaching from the tip of the pyramidal eminence to the posterior surface of the head of the stapes.

5. Hypotympanum.
   a. Definition. The hypotympanum is a shallow trough in the floor of the middle ear.
   b. Contents. The hypotympanum contains no vital structures.

E. Normal inner ear.

1. The inner ear contains the membranous labyrinth, which is set within the bony labyrinth (i.e., otic capsule).
2. The membranous labyrinth consists of the vestibule (i.e., utricle and saccule), semicircular channels, endolymphatic duct, cochlear duct, and multiple communicating channels.
3. The bony labyrinth forms the cochlea, vestibule, semicircular canals, and both the vestibular and cochlear aqueducts.
4. CT visualizes the bony labyrinth. MRI displays the fluid spaces of the membranous labyrinth.
5. The cochlea has approximately two and one-half turns.
   a. The basal first turn and the apical second turn are readily visible on routine CT scans of the temporal bone.
   b. The basal first turn opens posteriorly into the round window niche.
   c. The entire cochlea encircles a central bony axis, also called the *modiolus*. The cochlear nerve enters the cochlea through the modiolus on its way to the multiple spiral ganglia.
6. The vestibule is the largest part of the membranous labyrinth.
   a. Subunits of the vestibule are the utricle and saccule.
   b. The utricle is the more cephalad portion of the vestibule and the saccule the inferior part.
   c. High-resolution MRI is beginning to distinguish the parts of the vestibule as well as the inner chambers of the cochlea.
   d. The vestibule is separated laterally from the middle ear by the oval window niche.
   e. Superiorly, the vestibule leads to the superior semicircular canal.
   f. Medially, the lamina cribrosa separates the vestibule from the fundus of the internal auditory canal.
7. The semicircular canals project off the superior, posterior, and lateral aspects of the vestibule.
   a. The upper bony margin of the superior semicircular canal forms a convexity on the petrous pyramid roof, called the *arcuate eminence*.

    b. The posterior semicircular canal points posteriorly along the line of the petrous ridge.

    c. The lateral (i.e., horizontal) semicircular canal juts into the epitympanum. As a result the typical epitympanic cholesteatoma has a propensity to fistulize the membranous labyrinth by eroding the lateral cortex of the lateral semicircular canal.

       1) The midtympanic portion of the facial nerve passes along the undersurface of the lateral semicircular canal.

8. The cochlear aqueduct contains the perilymphatic duct.

    a. The cochlear aqueduct is approximately 8-mm long, extending from the basal turn of the cochlea to the lateral border of the jugular foramen.

    b. As it runs medially to laterally, the cochlear aqueduct flares gradually.

    c. Because it parallels the internal auditory canal, it is sometimes mistaken for this structure by novice temporal bone imagers.

    d. The function of the cochlear aqueduct is obscure. Some believe it regulates cerebrospinal and perilymphatic fluid pressures.

    e. The cochlear aqueduct serves as an entryway for microorganisms to access the labyrinth when suppurative labyrinthitis develops from meningitis.

    f. Some authors believe that when the cochlear aqueduct is abnormally patent, a "stapes footplate gusher" may result.

9. The vestibular aqueduct encompasses the endolymphatic duct.

    a. The vestibular aqueduct extends from the vestibule, coursing posteroinferiorly approximately 1 cm to the posterior wall of the petrous pyramid where it joins the endolymphatic sac.

    b. The endolymphatic duct and sac is thought to equilibrate endolymphatic fluid pressures.

F. Normal peripheral facial nerve (see Fig. 19-2).

1. Whenever the temporal bone is imaged, the entire facial nerve canal must be visualized and inspected.

2. A lesion affecting the facial nerve should be localized precisely to one of the following facial nerve segments:

    a. Cisternal segment. Facial nerve from brain stem to porus acusticus.

    b. Internal auditory canal segment. Facial nerve in the anterosuperior portion of the canal.

Q#4

    c. Labyrinthine segment. Short segment of facial nerve curling anteriorly over the top of the cochlea.

       1) The labyrinthine segment terminates in the anterior genu (i.e., geniculate ganglion).

    2) This segment characteristically is banana shaped on axial CT or MRI scans. On coronal imaging it is the medial of the two circular "eyes" directly above the cochlea.

  d. Tympanic segment. Facial nerve from anterior genu to posterior genu.

    1) The tympanic segment of the facial nerve travels just under the lateral (i.e., horizontal) semicircular canal in the medial wall of the middle ear cavity.

  e. Mastoid segment. Facial nerve from posterior genu to stylomastoid foramen.

  f. Parotid segment. Extracranial segment of the facial nerve, dividing the parotid gland into superficial and deep lobes.

3. The facial nerve is comprised of a larger motor root and a smaller sensory-parasympathetic root (i.e., nervus intermedius).

  a. The motor root of the facial nerve supplies innervation to the muscles of facial expression, the stapedius, platysma, and the posterior belly of the digastric muscles.

  b. The nervus intermedius contains both general visceral efferent secretomotor fibers to the lacrimal, submandibular, and sublingual glands as well as the special visceral afferent fibers conveying taste from the anterior two thirds of the tongue.

4. The facial nerve has four major functions that may be used to localize topographically a lesion along its course (see Fig. 19-2).

  a. From central to peripheral these four functions are:

    1) Lacrimation (via greater superficial petrosal nerve).

    2) Stapedius reflex. Sound dampening.

    3) Taste, anterior two thirds of the tongue (via chorda tympani nerve to lingual nerve to oral tongue).

    4) Facial expression.

5. Some generalizations allow focused imaging along the facial nerve.

  a. If cranial nerve VI also is involved with peripheral nerve VII, the brain stem is the site of the lesion (i.e., VII circles the VI nerve nucleus on its way out of the brain stem; scc Fig. 19-2).

  b. If cranial nerve VIII also is involved, the cerebellopontine angle–internal auditory canal area needs careful inspection.

  c. If the first three special functions are variably involved with an isolated peripheral nerve VII, temporal bone disease is suspected.

  d. Finally, if cranial nerve VII is involved by itself with preservation of the three special functions, extracranial nerve VII (i.e., intraparotid) is implicated.

6. When imaging peripheral facial nerve paralysis with either CT or MRI, the most common error is to complete an unfocused scan of the brain without attempting to localize the lesion topographically.

a. In this case the brain scan is judged normal, and the occult offending lesion remains undiagnosed in the temporal bone or parotid gland.
7. Table 17-1 provides a differential diagnosis of the lesions that cause peripheral facial nerve paralysis organized by anatomic segments of the nerve.

Table 17-1   Differential Diagnosis of Peripheral Facial Nerve Paralysis

Intracranial
Intraaxial
  Cavernoma
  Brain stem glioma
  Metastasis
  Multiple sclerosis
  Cerebrovascular accident
  Hemorrhage
Extraaxial (cisternal)
  Cerebellopontine angle tumor: acoustic neuroma, meningioma, epidermoid
  Cerebellopontine angle inflammation: sarcoidosis, meningitis
  Vascular: vertebrobasilar dolichoectasia, arteriovenous malformation, aneurysm

Intratemporal
Trauma: fracture through the facial nerve canal
Bell's palsy (facial neuritis)
Otitis media
Cholesteatoma
Paraganglioma
Hemangioma
Facial nerve schwannoma
Metastasis

Extracranial (parotid)
Forceps delivery
Penetrating facial trauma
Malignant otitis externa
Parotid surgery
Parotid malignancy

Miscellaneous
Möbius syndrome
Diabetes mellitus
Myasthenia gravis
Hyperparathyroidism

DISEASED TEMPORAL BONE

A. General comments.

1. This section focuses on the few statistically common types of temporal bone lesions for which imaging plays an important part in evaluation.
2. This section is organized by temporal bone area (i.e., external auditory canal, middle ear, and inner ear) to facilitate its use as a ready reference.
3. The more global subjects of trauma to the temporal bone and otodystrophies are discussed at the end of this section.
4. Differential diagnoses are presented for:
    a. Mass lesions of the external auditory canal.
    b. Mass lesions of the middle ear.
    c. Lesions causing conductive hearing loss.
    d. Lesions causing pulsatile tinnitus.
    e. Lesions causing "vascular retrotympanic mass."
    f. Mass lesions of the inner ear.

B. Diseases of the external auditory canal.

1. The principal lesions of the external auditory canal (EAC) are listed in Table 17-2.
2. Congenital deformities (i.e., dysplasias).
    a. To deal with imaging questions that arise when assessing a congenital ear deformity, it is necessary to understand the major components of normal ear embryology.

Table 17-2   Masses of the External Auditory Canal

Congenital
  Atresia

Inflammatory
  Chronic external otitis
  Malignant otitis externa
  Keratosis obturans
  Cholesteatoma

Benign Tumor
  Exotoses (surfer's ear)
  Osteoma

Malignant Tumor
  Basal cell carcinoma
  Squamous cell carcinoma
  Melanoma
  Parotid malignancy (local invasion)

b. Normal ear development.
   1) Three developmentally separate parts compose the ear.
      a) The external and middle ear derive from the first and second branchial arch apparatus.
      b) The inner ear derives from the ectodermal plate (i.e., otocyst).
      c) The internal auditory canal derives from the third embryonic nidus.
   2) The external and middle ear develop separately from the inner ear. As a result, deformities of these two areas generally are separate from one another as well.
   3) Combined external, middle, and inner ear deformities are rare and seen only in such conditions as craniofacial dysplasias and trisomies 13, 18, and 21.
c. External and middle ear deformities (i.e., EAC atresia).
   1) Relevant statistics. Male gender in 61% of cases, bilateral in 29%, and a family history in 14%. Incidence of one in 10,000 births. Often associated with other anomalies.
   2) The patient has pinna deformity and a stenotic or absent EAC.
   3) CT scans define the severity of the deformity and thereby help the surgeon to decide whether the ear is salvageable.
d. Critical CT questions in congenital ear deformity.
   1) Is the EAC plug bony or membranous? If bony, how thick is it?
      a) Comment. EAC abnormalities range in severity from canal stenosis to membranous plug to thick, bony atresia. The thicker the bony atresia plate, the more difficult the surgery.

Q#5

   2) How small is the middle ear cavity?
      a) Comment. The more coarcted (i.e., smaller) the residual tympanic cavity, the poorer the surgical result.
   3) What is the status of the ossicles?
      a) Comment. Ossicular changes include rotation, fusion, or absence. The more severe the ossicular changes, the poorer the surgical end result.
   4) Is the facial nerve in the normal position?
      a) Comment. Ectopic nerve VII often is associated with EAC atresia. The portion usually out of place includes the posterior tympanic and mastoid segments. If this observation is not made before surgery, the surgical creation of a new EAC will result in facial nerve paralysis.
   5) What is the status of the oval and round windows?
      a) Comment. Because the medial wall of the middle ear represents the margin between the embryologic subunits of the

external middle ear and the inner ear, the oval and round windows at times do not form normally in cases of EAC atresia. Hypoplasia or aplasia of the oval or round window may be identified on coronal CT scans of the temporal bone.

6) Can a congenital cholesteatoma be identified?
   a) Comment. Congenital cholesteatoma is associated with EAC atresia only in a minority of cases, but it should be searched for in all patients with atresia.

7) What is the appearance of the inner ear structures?
   a) The inner labyrinth most commonly is not affected in EAC atresia.
   b) If the surgeon can recreate a functioning conduction system to connect to the inner ear, the patient may hear quite well from the repaired ear.

3. Inflammatory diseases of the EAC.
   a. Three inflammatory EAC processes must be recognized and understood: malignant otitis externa, keratosis obturans, and EAC cholesteatoma.
   b. Malignant otitis externa.
      1) Clinical considerations.
         a) Malignant otitis externa occurs in older patients with insulin-dependent diabetes and immunocompromised patients.
         b) The principal organism responsible for the infection is *Pseudomonas aeruginosa.*
         c) In its fulminant form, this condition may cause facial nerve or cranial nerve IX, X, and XI malfunction.
      2) Pathophysiology.
         a) Malignant otitis externa begins at the bony–cartilaginous junction of the EAC.
         b) The primary route for spread of infection is downward into the parotid space and inferomedially into the nasopharyngeal masticator space and skull base.
      3) Imaging features.
         a) CT is the method of choice for radiographic evaluation and follow-up of malignant otitis externa.
         b) A bolus-drip or injector-designed contrast technique to maintain maximum intravascular contrast during CT examination is desired.
         c) Both soft-tissue evaluation of the deep facial spaces and careful bone detail analyses of the skull base and temporal bone must be accomplished.
         d) The role of CT is to evaluate the bone detail images of the temporal bone and skull base for areas of destruction indicating osteomyelitis.

e) Soft-tissue CT images are searched for foci of frank pus in the adjacent deep facial spaces (i.e., parotid, masticator, parapharyngeal) that may need surgical drainage.

c. Keratosis obturans.

1) Keratosis obturans occurs in younger patients (i.e., <40 years), usually as a bilateral process associated with chronic sinusitis and bronchiectasis.

2) CT scans show a keratin plug occluding the EAC with widening of the bony EAC without bone erosion.

d. Cholesteatoma of the EAC.

1) EAC cholesteatoma occurs in older patients (i.e., >40 years), usually as a unilateral process without other associated disease.

2) In contrast to those of keratosis obturans, these CT scans show an EAC canal mass with bony erosion, usually seen as focal scalloping underneath the cholesteatoma mass.

4. Benign tumors.

a. Exostosis.

1) Bony exostosis is not a true tumor.

2) It occurs as a response to irritation by cold water and therefore is referred to as *Surfer's ear*.

3) CT scans demonstrate bony stenosis of the EAC with increased bone density in the thickened wall.

b. Osteoma. Typically solitary, unilateral, pedunculated bony growths that appear as a submucosal blockage of the external auditory canal.

5. Malignant tumors.

a. The three tumors of importance, which are basal cell carcinoma, squamous cell carcinoma, and melanoma, can be considered together.

b. Nodal drainage from the EAC is to the parotid and periparotid nodal group. In invasive cases, the parotid space should be imaged simultaneously with the EAC.

c. When invasive parotid malignancy occurs in the cephalad aspect of the parotid gland, it may invade the EAC and present as a mass in this area.

C. Diseases of the middle ear and mastoid.

1. Lesions of the middle ear are listed in Table 17-3.

2. Congenital lesions.

a. Congenital middle ear deformities are associated with EAC dysplasias (see section B2).

b. Congenital cholesteatoma (i.e., primary).

1) Clinical presentation. Conductive hearing loss in a child with no history of inflammatory ear disease suggests a congenital cholesteatoma. Cholesteatoma seen through an intact tympanic membrane also may be reported by the clinician.

Table 17-3   Masses of the Middle Ear

Congenital Vascular Pseudomass
Aberrant internal carotid artery
Dehiscent jugular bulb

Congenital Mass
Congenital cholesteatoma

Inflammatory
Acquired cholesteatoma
Cholesterol granuloma
Inflammatory debris
Granulation tissue
Histiocytosis X (pediatric population)

Benign Tumor
Paraganglioma (glomus tympanicum, glomus jugulotympanicum)
Facial nerve schwannoma
Hemangioma
Choristoma
Meningioma

Malignant Tumor
Squamous cell carcinoma
Adenocarcinoma
Adenoid cystic carcinoma
Rhabdomyosarcoma (pediatric population)
Metastasis

---

    2) Pathogenesis. Arises from aberrant epithelial rests.
    3) CT features.
       a) Originally thought to occur mostly in the petrous apex, this lesion is now known to be seen most commonly in the epitympanum of the middle ear cavity.
       b) Primary and secondary cholesteatoma are indistinguishable on CT scans.
       c) A globular mass with bony scalloping and ossicular destruction is characteristic.
    4) MRI features. T1-weighted signal is isointense to brain; T2-weighted signal is variable but usually slightly hyperintense to brain. Contrast enhancement does not occur except as a fine line on the periphery of the lesion.
   c. Aberrant internal carotid artery.
    1) Clinical features. "Vascular retrotympanic mass" sometimes associated with pulsatile tinnitus.

2) Imaging issues.
   a) The surgeon wants to know whether a lesion seen on otoscopic examination is a paraganglioma.
   b) As congenital vascular pseudomasses both aberrant internal carotid artery and dehiscent jugular bulb are lesions that are "leave-me-alone lesions."
   c) Clinical differentiation of these two groups often is impossible, leaving the decision to biopsy or to leave alone entirely up to the radiologist.
   d) Beware! The clinician often may be certain that a lesion seen at otoscopy is a paraganglioma, whereas the radiologist's diagnosis is an aberrant internal carotid artery. Hold your ground! Biopsy of an aberrant internal carotid artery can be disastrous.

3) CT features (Fig. 17-3).
   a) CT findings are diagnostic.
   b) CT features are a rounded, tubular, soft-tissue density that enters the middle ear cavity posterolateral to the cochlea, crosses the mesotympanum along the cochlear promontory, and exists anteromedially to become the horizontal portion of the carotid canal.
   c) On a few coronal CT images the lesion may appear to be focal, sitting on the cochlear promontory. Only by looking at all of the images will it be clear that the lesion is indeed tubular.

4) MRI features.
   a) Conventional MRI sequences will not allow the diagnosis of aberrant internal carotid artery. The signal loss from flowing blood and nonmobile protons in the temporal bone combine to create no tissue contrast.
   b) Both source images and projection images from MRA (three-dimensional time of flight or overlapping slab techniques) make the diagnosis of aberrant internal carotid artery.
   c) MRA projection images show the abnormal posterolateral segment of the aberrant internal carotid artery.

d. Dehiscent jugular bulb.
   1) Clinical features.
      a) The patient often has no symptoms but may complain of a pulsatile vascular sound in the ear.
      b) "Vascular retrotympanic mass" may be noted on otoscopic examination.
   2) Imaging issues. See section C2.

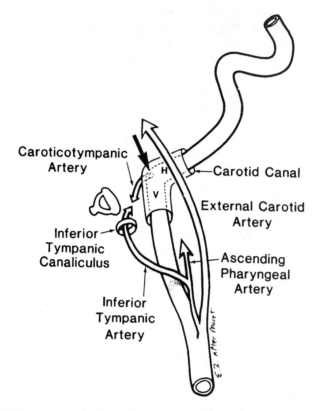

A

Fig. 17-3 **A,** Course of the normal adult cervical and intrapetrous internal carotid artery. Observe the normal vertical (*V*) and horizontal (*H*) segments of the petrous internal carotid artery. In the normal anatomic arrangement the inferior tympanic artery passes cephalad through the inferior tympanic canaliculus, while the caroticotympanic artery traverses posterolaterally through the caroticotympanic canaliculus (*arrow*). These two arteries normally anastomose on the cochlear promontory. **B,** Connections that constitute the aberrant internal carotid artery. This artery arises when the cervical portion of the internal carotid artery fails to develop. Instead, the inferior tympanic artery enlarges to feed into the caroticotympanic artery, which connects this alternative vascular channel to the posterior margin of the horizontal petrous internal carotid artery. The obvious results of such an arrangement include enlargement of the inferior tympanic canaliculus, reversal of flow in the caroticotympanic artery (hyoid artery), and enlargement of the caroticotympanic canaliculus. The aberrant artery ends up entering the middle ear cavity immediately adjacent to the stylomastoid foramen, crossing the middle ear at the level of the cochlear promontory, and reentering the

(*continued*)

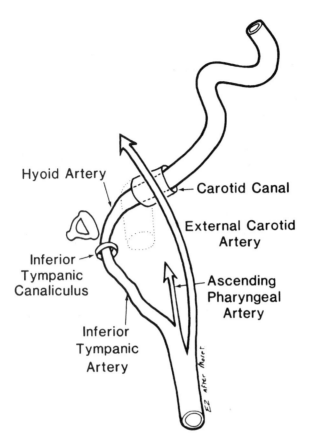

B

Fig. 17-3 (*continued*)   petrous internal carotid artery at its posterior horizon-tal margin. At times this point of reentry is stenotic and may cause jetting with resultant pulsatile tinnitus. (From Lo WM, Solti-Bohman LG, McElveen JT: Aberrant carotid artery: radiologic diagnosis with emphasis on high-resolution CT. *RadioGraphics* 5:985–994, 1987. Used by permission.)

3) CT features.
   a) Nondehiscent, high jugular bulb (i.e., jugular megabulb deformity). The jugular bulb ascends to or above the level of the floor of the external auditory canal with preservation of the bony plate separating the bulb from the middle ear cavity.
   b) Dehiscent, high jugular bulb. The bony plate separating the bulb from the posteroinferior middle ear is absent, with the contents of the jugular foramen being contiguous with the middle ear soft-tissue mass. The adjacent jugular fora-

men demonstrates no bony abnormality to suggest paraganglioma.

 4) MRI features.

  a) Two-dimensional time of flight MRA allows the identification of a high jugular bulb.

  b) Defining the relationship of the jugular bulb to the middle ear cavity (i.e., is there dehiscence or not) can be difficult or impossible on MRI sequences.

  c) If questions remain about the relationship of the bulb to the middle ear cavity, CT scans of the temporal bone may be needed.

3. Inflammatory lesions.

 a. Acquired cholesteatoma.

  1) Clinical presentation.

   a) Patient of any age, but usually under 30 years, with a history of recurrent otitis media associated with tympanic membrane rupture or tympanostomy tube placement.

  2) Pathogenesis.

   a) Acquired cholesteatoma occurring in the middle ear cavity results from ingrowth of squamous epithelium through the eardrum, either through a marginal perforation or invagination of a retraction pocket.

   b) The accumulation of squamous and keratin debris within the middle ear produces a mass effect that erodes the bony walls and ossicles.

  3) Two types of acquired cholesteatoma have been described.

   a) Pars flaccida cholesteatoma. The most common form of acquired cholesteatoma. Also referred to as *attic* or *primary acquired cholesteatoma*. The cholesteatoma herniates into Prussak's space in the lateral attic, and it may extend from there into the posterolateral attic, then through the aditus ad antrum into the mastoid antrum.

   b) Pars tensa cholestcatoma. The far less common type of acquired cholesteatoma. Also referred to as *secondary acquired cholesteatoma*. It usually results from posterosuperior retraction pockets. Because it begins in the posterior mesotympanum, the sinus tympani and ossicles often are involved.

  4) CT features.

   a) If the patient has conductive hearing loss and a retraction pocket (i.e., no diagnosis of cholesteatoma is made before imaging), the question is can the diagnosis of cholesteatoma be made based on CT findings?

b) Comment. When CT scans show a nondependent, homogeneous mass associated with bone erosion or ossicular destruction, 90% of cases are cholesteatoma. This constellation is present, however, in only 50% of cholesteatomas.
c) If the cholesteatoma can be seen by the clinician or CT findings permit the diagnosis of cholesteatoma to be made, the radiologist must identify the location and extent of the cholesteatoma mass.
d) In the presence of known cholesteatoma, CT is used for preoperative evaluation and planning. In each case a series of questions must be asked.

Q#6

  i) Is the tegmen tympani intact or dehiscent? Temporal lobe complications occur through a dehiscent tegmen tympani.
  ii) Is there potential for fistula? That is, is the lateral semicircular canal eroded, or does other evidence exist for fistula formation into the membranous labyrinth?
  iii) Is the facial nerve canal adjacent to or eroded by the cholesteatoma? If the facial nerve canal is dehisced by cholesteatoma, risk of a surgical complication involving the facial nerve is high.
  iv) Is there tissue in the sinus tympani? The sinus tympani is a clinical blind spot and cannot be seen through a standard mastoid surgical approach.
  v) What is the relationship of the mass to the ossicles? Pars flaccida cholesteatoma usually is lateral to the ossicles; pars tensa cholesteatoma ordinarily is medial to the ossicles.
5) Complications.
   a) All complications of cholesteatoma are secondary to bony erosion.
   b) Complications within the temporal bone include ossicular destruction, facial nerve paralysis (1% of cases), labyrinthine fistula, automastoidectomy, and complete hearing loss.
   c) Intracranial complications include meningitis, sigmoid sinus thrombosis, temporal lobe abscess, and cerebrospinal fluid rhinorrhea.
6) MRI features.
   a) MRI is not used routinely in patients with suspected cholesteatoma.

      b) If any intracranial complication of cholesteatoma is clinically suspected, MRI is the principal adjunctive study.

      c) MRI scans show the cholesteatoma as a nonenhancing mass with rim enhancement.

   7) In a patient with a "retraction pocket" and conductive hearing loss, the concern is that a cholesteatoma is present beyond otoscopic vision. Search the CT scan for any cause of conductive hearing loss (Table 17-4).

  b. Inflammatory debris.

   1) In the inflamed or infected middle ear, it is not possible to differentiate debris and granulation tissue from early acquired cholesteatoma on CT scans.

   2) CT usually demonstrates inflammatory debris as linear strands partially opacifying the middle ear cavity without bony erosion. When the debris is globular, however, it cannot be differentiated from early cholesteatoma, where scalloping has not yet taken place.

  c. Cholesterol granuloma.

   1) Clinical features. Otoscopic examination reveals a "blue (vascular) tympanic membrane" in the absence of pulsatile tinnitus when the lesion is in the middle ear. When in the inner ear, symptoms involving cranial nerves VII and VIII may result from involvement of the internal auditory canal.

Table 17-4   Lesions Causing Conductive Hearing Loss

Congenital
  Stapes fixation
  Ossicular deformity
  Cholesteatoma

Otodystrophies
  Fenestral otosclerosis

Inflammatory
  Cholesteatoma
  Ossicular fixation
  Tympanosclerosis

Trauma
  Ossicular disruption behind intact tympanic membrane

Tumor
  Facial nerve schwannoma
  Paraganglioma
  Hemangioma
  Malignant tumor (primary or metastatic)

2) Pathologic findings. Specialized form of postinflammatory granulation tissue. Brownish fluid contains cholesterol crystals and blood.

3) CT features. Middle ear mass does not enhance with contrast administration. Although the mass fills the middle ear cavity, the ossicles are intact. An inner ear lesion looks like an expansile mass in the petrous apex.

4) MRI features. Because of hemoglobin breakdown products and cholesterol content, both T1- and T2-weighted images will show the lesion to be hyperintense.

5) Compare the MRI features of cholesterol granuloma with those of primary cholesteatoma. These lesions often are confused both clinically and radiographically. Both may occur in the middle or inner ear, but the MRI signals are distinctly different. The T1-weighted signal of cholesterol granuloma is hyperintense, and that of cholesteatoma isointense to brain.

4. Benign tumors.
   a. Paraganglioma: glomus tympanicum versus glomus jugulotympanicum.
      1) Definition. Glomus tympanicum paraganglioma is a benign, neural crest tumor localized to the cochlear promontory of the middle ear cavity.
      2) Definition. Glomus jugulotympanicum paraganglioma originates in the jugular foramen, then invades the middle ear cavity.
      3) Clinical presentation. Pulsatile tinnitus (Table 17-5) and vascular retrotympanic mass (Table 17-6) characteristically are seen in both glomus tympanicum and jugulotympanicum paraganglioma.

Table 17-5   Lesions Causing Pulsatile Tinnitus*

Congenital Vascular Pseudomass
   Aberrant internal carotid artery
   Dehiscent or high jugular bulb

Vascular
   Arteriovenous malformation or fistula in temporal bone region
   Aneurysm in temporal bone region
   High grade stenosis of internal or external carotid artery

Tumor
   Paraganglioma
   Hemangioma
   Meningioma

*This differential diagnosis is similar to that of Table 17-6, with the addition of the vascular causes and absence of the inflammatory causes.

Table 17-6   Causes of Vascular Mass Behind the Tympanic Membrane*

Congenital Vascular Pseudomass
Aberrant internal carotid artery
Dehiscent jugular bulb

Inflammatory
Inflammatory debris with hemorrhage
Cholesterol granuloma

Tumor
Paraganglioma
  Glomus tympanicum
  Glomus jugulotympanicum
Hemangioma
Meningioma

---

*The term *vascular tympanic membrane* or *vascular retrotympanic mass* is used to describe the otoscopic impression of a vascular mass behind the eardrum. The membrane may in fact be pink, red, or blue.

4) CT appearance.
 a) Glomus tympanicum. Globular, soft-tissue mass abutting the cochlear promontory in the middle ear cavity. Intense enhancement with bolus-contrast infusion is seen. Inferior walls of the middle ear cavity are intact.
 b) Glomus jugulotympanicum. Intensely enhancing mass extending superolaterally from the jugular foramen below into the middle ear cavity. Bony floor of the middle ear cavity is invaded, and the jugular spine of the jugular foramen is eroded.
5) MRI appearance.
 a) Glomus tympanicum. Focal soft-tissue mass is seen in the low middle ear cavity adjacent to the cochlear promontory, signaled by the fluid space of the cochlear membranous labyrinth. T1-weighted, enhanced images show uniform, intense enhancement.
 b) Glomus jugulotympanicum. Larger jugulotympanicum paraganglioma will show multiple punctate and serpiginous signal voids within the tumor because of larger, feeding arterial branches. Following enhancement on T1-weighted images, the tumor uniformly enhances (like a meningioma). Use of fat saturation techniques along with T1-weighted enhancement allows the imager to track the tumor into the skull base with a high degree of confidence. T2-weighted, fast spin echo techniques combined with fat-saturation techniques

may allow adequate delineation of the tumor without use of contrast in the near future.

Q#7

6) In most cases the head and neck surgeon cannot clinically differentiate this tumor from the congenital mimics of aberrant internal carotid artery and dehiscent jugular vein. Only the tumor needs surgical intervention, and the radiologist must determine when this intervention is required.

7) Radiologic work-up of vascular tympanic membrane or pulsatile tinnitus.

   a) The main diagnostic considerations are paraganglioma (either glomus tympanicum or glomus jugulotympanicum), aberrant internal carotid artery, dehiscent jugular bulb, and (in the case of pulsatile tinnitus) dural arteriovenous fistula.

   b) The initial study in patients with a vascular retrotympanic mass or pulsatile tinnitus is MRI with MRA.

   c) If objective pulsatile tinnitus (i.e., both the physician and patient hear the sound) is present but MRI is negative, catheter angiography of the ipsilateral carotid and vertebral arteries is done to look for the small, strategically located, dural arteriovenous fistula.

   d) If subjective tinnitus (i.e., only the patient can hear the sound) is present and MRI is negative, catheter angiography is undertaken to complete the work-up only if the referring physician has a high degree of clinical suspicion that a dural arteriovenous fistula may be present.

   e) If the presenting sign is vascular retrotympanic mass, MRI with MRA is the initial study of choice, because it readily differentiates paraganglioma from the nonsurgical, vascular variants. Conventional MRI sequences all show the anatomic detail needed, while MRA (and magnetic resonance venous) sequences provide any needed vascular information.

   f) CT has little role in the initial work-up of patients with either pulsatile tinnitus or vascular tympanic membrane. Only after MRI has diagnosed a larger vascular tumor such as glomus jugulotympanicum or hemangioma is CT sometimes completed to help identify surgical bony landmarks.

b. Facial nerve schwannoma.

   1) Clinical features. Depending on the location and size of the mass, the most common presenting symptoms relate to mass effect such as conductive hearing loss (i.e., ossicular interaction)

and otitis media/mastoiditis (i.e., attic or aditus ad antrum block). Surprisingly, peripheral facial nerve paralysis usually is not an important symptom in the initial presentations.

2) CT appearance. Tubular mass scalloping and enlarging the facial nerve canal anywhere along its length. The schwannoma may occur in the cerebellopontine angle—internal auditory canal (CPA-IAC) area and mimic an acoustic neuroma.

3) MRI appearance. Contrast-enhancing, T1-weighted MRI scans show a uniformly enhancing, tubular mass enlarging the facial nerve canal.

4) Pitfalls in image interpretation.

   a) In younger patients this lesion may be confused with congenital cholesteatoma, which also sometimes grows along the facial nerve canal.

   b) When the schwannoma is found in the IAC-CPA area, look for the tail enlarging the labyrinthine segment of the facial nerve canal. If this "tell-tail" sign can be found, the imager can differentiate facial schwannoma from acoustic neuroma. Without this tail, there is no radiologic difference between facial and acoustic schwannoma in the IAC-CPA area.

c. Hemangioma (i.e., ossifying hemangioma).

   1) Clinical features. Often occurs with chronic, progressive, peripheral facial nerve paralysis. Pulsatile tinnitus sometimes is present.

   2) CT appearance. Intensely enhancing mass with a honeycomb and/or spiculated appearance with intratumoral bone flecks. Extends along the facial nerve canal. Most common sites of involvement are the labyrinthine segment of the facial nerve and the geniculate fossa area.

   4) MRI appearance. T1-weighted, contrast-enhanced MRI scans show an intensely enhancing, invasive appearing mass that tracks along the facial nerve canal. Focal mass is present in the geniculate fossa and/or the area of the labyrinthine segment of the facial nerve canal.

   5) Major considerations in differential diagnosis include facial nerve schwannoma (i.e., tubular, smooth bony margins) and Bell's palsy (i.e., enhancing facial nerve that may be prominent but shows no focal mass effect).

d. Choristoma.

   1) Pathologic findings. Ectopic, mature, salivary tissue.

   2) Clinical features. Patient treated for chronic otitis media because of glandular secretions.

   3) No differential CT or MRI features.

5. Malignant tumors.
    a. Multiple rare lesions.
    b. In each case CT scans show a destructive mass in the middle ear cavity.
    c. Check to see if the lesion is coming up the facial nerve from the parotid gland (i.e., perineural parotid malignancy).

D. Inner ear diseases.

1. Congenital deformities.
    a. With this group of lesions the structures of the inner ear are variably involved. It is prudent to describe the lesion individually in each patient.
    b. Mondini malformation (cochlear dysplasia).
        1) The term *Mondini malformation* has been used to describe any dysplasia of the inner ear. This book uses the term only when the primary lesion seen on CT or MRI scans is loss of the normal two and one-half turns to the cochlea.
        2) CT or high-resolution MRI scans reveal the cochlea to be "cystic." In the less severe form, closer inspection reveals that the basal first turn has developed, but the apical and middle turns occupy a common, nondeveloped space. In the more severely affected cochlea, no turns are discernible.
    c. Michel's aplasia. Poorly documented, extremely rare disorder characterized by complete lack of development of the inner ear.
    d. Vestibular aqueduct syndrome.
        1) Clinical presentation. The child usually hears during the first few years of life but then begins to have progressive sensorineural hearing loss. Hearing loss may begin as late as the teenage years.
        2) CT appearance. Enlargement of the vestibular aqueduct, sometimes in association with enlargement of the upper vestibule (i.e., utricle area). May be unilateral or bilateral.
        3) MRI appearance. Enlarged endolymphatic duct and sac. Upper vestibular enlargement also can be seen.
        4) Most commonly missed cause of congenital deafness.
2. Inflammatory lesions.
    a. Labyrinthine ossificans.
        1) Clinical presentation. Patients are profoundly deaf and are evaluated for possible cochlear implantation.
        2) Pathogenesis. Postinflammatory ossification of the membranous labyrinth.
        3) Labyrinthine ossificans can occur secondary to middle ear infection (i.e., tympanogenic), meningitis (i.e., meningogenic), or

mumps and measles (i.e., hematogenic). Also can occur after temporal bone trauma or labyrinthectomy.
4) CT diagnosis is made when the normal membranous labyrinth space is compromised by bony deposition.
5) Other CT observations.
   a) Labyrinthine ossificans may be bilateral (i.e., meningogenic) or unilateral (i.e., tympanogenic).
   b) May be cochlear or noncochlear.
   c) Only bilateral cochlear labyrinthine ossificans will prevent multichannel cochlear implantation.
   b. Petrous apicitis (i.e., Gradenigo's syndrome).
   1) Clinical presentation. The patient has retroorbital pain, sixth nerve palsy, and otorrhea.
   2) CT features. Destructive (osteomyelitic) lesion of the petrous apex, often with fluid in the ipsilateral middle ear and mastoid.
3. Tumors.
   a. Masses of the inner ear are summarized in Table 17-7. Most of these occur more frequently in the middle ear cavity (see sections C2 and C3).
   b. Endolymphatic sac tumors.
   1) Clinical presentation. Sensorineural hearing loss, disequilibrium, tinnitus, facial twitching, and facial weakness. May be associated with von Hippel-Lindau disease.
   2) Pathologic considerations. Previously referred to as *papillary adenomatous tumors of the temporal bone.* The contemporary term for this tumor group is *endolymphatic sac tumor.*

Table 17-7   Masses of the Inner Ear

Congenital
Congenital cholesteatoma

Inflammation
Cholesterol granuloma
Petrous apicitis (Gradenigo's syndrome)

Tumor
Paraganglioma (glomus jugulotympanicum)
Facial nerve schwannoma
Hemangioma
Endolymphatic sac tumors
Metastases
Larger cerebellopontine angle tumors

3) CT appearance. Tumor seen on the posterior wall of the petrous pyramid in the expected, normal location of the endolymphatic sac. Erosion of the temporal bone in this location with intratumoral bone that may appear stippled, reticular, or spiculated.

4) MRI appearance. Tumor seen in the endolymphatic sac with multiple foci of high signal throughout secondary to either methemoglobin and/or proteinaceous cystic components.

5) Angiographic appearance. Hypervascular tumor with arterial blood supply from the external carotid branches and the anterior inferior cerebellar artery.

E. Otodystrophies of the temporal bone.

1. Otosclerosis (i.e., otospongiosis).
   a. Clinical features.
      1) Fenestral type. Progressive conductive hearing loss with normal findings on otoscopic examination. Two thirds of patients have tinnitus early in the course of disease. Bilateral in 85% of patients.
      2) Cochlear type. Progressive sensorineural hearing loss.
      3) If both types exist simultaneously, a mixed pattern of hearing loss is observed.
   b. Pathogenesis.
      1) Early. Enchondral bone is replaced by foci of spongy new bone.
      2) Late. Decalcified foci recalcifies into a dense, ossific plaque.
   c. Fenestral otosclerosis.
      1) Most common type (80% to 90% of cases).
      2) Thought to begin in the fissula antefenestrum (i.e., anterior oval window margin).
      3) CT findings.
         a) New bone formation (i.e., plaque) seen on the anterior oval window margin is the most common CT finding.
         b) Plaque also may be found on the posterior oval window margin and the round window.
         c) In the early lytic phase the oval window may appear too wide, resulting from osteoclastic resorption of its margins.
         d) In 2% of cases complete plugging of the oval window (i.e., obliterative otosclerosis) may occur.
   d. Cochlear otosclerosis (i.e., retrofenestral type).
      1) Much less common than fenestral otosclerosis.
      2) Invariably associated with fenestral otosclerosis when present.
      3) Thought to cause cytotoxic enzyme diffusion into the fluid of the membranous labyrinth. The net effect is to cause sensory hearing loss.

    4) CT findings.
      a) Focal lucencies in the otic capsules.
      b) May appear as a "third turn" to the cochlea on axial CT scans.
      c) Late stages of the disease may not be visible on CT scans.
      d) CT may not pick up the more subtle cases of this disease.
    5) MRI findings.
      a) Preliminary reports describe focal areas of punctate enhancement in the otic capsule on contrast-enhanced, T1-weighted MRI scans.
      b) Little is known about the sensitivity of either MRI or CT to the presence of this disease. Pathologic literature suggests that this disease is present far more than it is diagnosed by either CT or MRI.

2. Paget disease.
    a. Paget disease (i.e., osteitis deformans) is an inherited, progressive, bony disease that primarily affects the axial skeleton. It may be monoosteitic or polyostotic (the more common form). Patients usually are older than 40 years of age and male (80% of cases).
    b. Pathogenesis. Active, pagetic bone undergoes waves of osteoclastic resorption and regeneration. The skull commonly is involved (i.e., osteoporosis circumscripta) and the temporal bone less commonly.
    c. Clinical presentation. Membranous labyrinth poisoning by the adjacent pagetoid bone results in sensorineural or mixed hearing loss. This process is poorly understood.
    d. CT findings. Diffuse demineralization of the bony labyrinth with associated fluffy, cotton–wool appearance is the rule.

3. Fibrous dysplasia.
    a. Fibrous dysplasia is a slowly progressing, inherited bony disease that is monoostotic when it involves the temporal bone.
    b. Pathogenesis. The cause of fibrous dysplasia is obscure. The normal reparative process seen in bone after injury is not present in bone involved with fibrous dysplasia. Fibroosseous tissue is found in the interior of the affected bone.
    c. Clinical presentation. Usually conductive hearing loss with EAC bony stenosis.
    d. CT features. Enlargement of the temporal bone identifies the lesion as fibrous dysplasia. The affected bone is dense in most cases, although cystic changes have been reported. Overgrowth of the bony EAC may be seen. Sparing of the membranous labyrinth, facial nerve canal, and internal auditory canal is the rule. A EAC cholesteatoma can develop medial to the stenotic EAC.

4. Osteogenesis imperfecta.

    a. The tarde (i.e., delayed) form of osteogenesis imperfecta manifests by painless fracture following minor trauma.

    b. Pathogenesis. Osteogenesis imperfecta tarde and otosclerosis are thought by many to result from a common genetic abnormality. Based on this assumption, otosclerosis may be a form of osteogenesis imperfecta involving only the temporal bone.

    c. Clinical manifestations. Symptoms of osteogenesis imperfecta are the same as for otosclerosis.

    d. CT findings. When osteogenesis imperfecta involves the temporal bone, CT features are identical to those seen in fenestral and cochlear otosclerosis.

    e. Comment. The combination of osteogenesis imperfecta, otosclerosis, and blue sclera is known as *van der Hoeve's syndrome.*

F. Temporal bone trauma.

1. Specific areas of concern when inspecting CT scans of the temporal bone in patients with trauma to that area include, from medial to lateral:

    a. Carotid canal. Fracture here may cause traumatic occlusion of the internal carotid artery.

    b. Bony labyrinth. Fracture through the labyrinth may cause acute labyrinthine dysfunction, including vertigo and immediate, irreversible deafness.

    c. Facial nerve canal. Peripheral facial nerve paralysis may result either immediately in the case of laceration or later if edema sets in.

    d. Ossicles. Any ossicle may be dislocated, but the incudostapedial joint is the weakest and therefore most susceptible to injury.

    e. Tegmen tympani. If associated with dural laceration, fracture here results in cerebrospinal fluid leak, either from the EAC canal with a tympanic membrane tear or via the eustachian tube into the nasopharynx.

    f. Mastoid air cells, medial wall. Fracture in this region may result in cerebrospinal fluid leak, recurring meningitis or abscess, or sigmoid sinus thrombosis.

2. Classification of temporal bone fractures.

    a. Longitudinal. Fracture along the long axis of the temporal bone accounts for 70% to 80% of cases.

    b. Transverse (i.e., vertical). Fracture at right angles to the long axis of the temporal bone accounts for 20% of cases.

        1) Transverse fractures usually present with anakusis, vertigo, and facial nerve injury.

    c. Complex or mixed. Fracture in orthogonal planes.

3. CT technique in trauma.

    a. It is essential to try to obtain both axial and coronal planes in the setting of trauma to identify any hidden fracture lying in one of the scan planes.

    b. In a patient with skull base fracture involving the temporal bone, CT is the method of choice in fracture evaluation. Even when facial nerve paralysis is associated, MRI does not have a role in the initial assessment. Blood in the middle ear cavity will prevent MRI identification of the facial nerve. Fracture lines in the region of the facial nerve seen on CT scans are much more useful as a clue to where the surgeon should look for facial nerve injury.

SUGGESTED READING

Normal Temporal Bone

Bergeron RT: *The temporal bone.* In Bergeron RT, Osborn AG, Som PM, editors: *Head and neck imaging, excluding the brain.* St. Louis, 1984, Mosby–Year Book.

Disbro MA, Harnsberger HR, Osborn AG: Peripheral facial nerve dysfunction: CT evaluation. *Radiology* 155:659–663, 1985.

Swartz JD: Current imaging approach to the temporal bone. *Radiology* 171:309–317, 1989.

Swartz JD: High-resolution CT of the middle ear and mastoid. Parts I, II, III. *Radiology* 148:449–464, 1983.

Swartz JD, editor: State of the art temporal bone imaging. *Semin Ultrasound CT MR* 10:177–301, 1989.

Swartz JD, Harnsberger HR: *Imaging of the temporal bone.* New York, 1992, Thieme Medical Publishers.

Teresi LM, Kolin E, Lufkin RB, et al: MR imaging of the intraparotid facial nerve: *normal anatomy and pathology. Am J Roentgenol* 148:995–1000, 1987.

Teresi L, Lufkin R, Wortham D, et al: MR imaging of the intratemporal facial nerve using surface coils. *AJNR* 8:49–54, 1987.

Virapongse C, Rothman SLG, Kier EL, et al: CT of the temporal bone. *Am J Roentgenol* 139:739–749, 1982.

Diseased Temporal Bone

Chen JC, Tsuruda JS, Halbach VV: Suspected dural arteriovenous fistula: results with screening MR angiography in seven patients. *Radiology* 183:265–271, 1992.

Curtin HD, Jensen JE, Barnes L, et al: "Ossifying" hemangioma of the temporal bone: evaluation with CT. *Radiology* 164:831–835, 1987.

De Marco JK, Dillon WP, Halbach VV, et al: Dural arteriovenous fistula: evaluation with MR imaging. *Radiology* 175:193–199, 1990.

Dietz RR, Davis WL, Harnsberger HR, et al: MR imaging and MR angiography in the evaluation of pulsatile tinnitus. *AJNR* In press, 1994.

Greenberg JJ, Oot RF, Wismer GL, et al: Cholesterol granuloma of the petrous apex: MR and CT evaluation. *AJNR* 9:1205–1214, 1988.

Griffin C, DeLaPaz R, Enzmann D: MR and CT correlation of cholesterol cyst of the petrous bone. *AJNR* 8:825–829, 1987.

Harnsberger HR, Dart DJ, Parkin JL: Cochlear implant candidates: assessment with CT and MR imaging. *Radiology* 164:53–57, 1987.

Holland BA, Brant-Zawadski M: High resolution CT of temporal bone trauma. *AJNR* 5:291–295, 1984.

Inoue Y, Tabuchi T, Hakuba A, et al: Facial nerve neuromas: CT findings. *J Comput Assist Tomogr* 11:942–947, 1987.

Jackler RK, Dillon WP: CT and MRI of the inner ear. *Otolaryngol Head Neck Surg* 99:300–310, 1988.

Jackler RK, Dillon WP, Schindler RA: Computed tomography in suppurative ear disease: a correlation of surgical and radiographic findings. *Laryngoscope* 94:334–340, 1984.

Johnson DW, Hasso AN, Stewart CE, et al: Temporal bone trauma: high resolution CT evaluation. *Radiology* 151:411–415, 1984.

Johnson DW, Voorhees RL, Lufkin RB, et al: Cholesteatomas of the temporal bone: role of CT and MR imaging. *Radiology* 171:443–448, 1983.

Lo WM, Shelton C, Waluch V, et al: Intratemporal vascular tumors: detection with CT and MR imaging. *Radiology* 171:443–448, 1983.

Lo WM, Solti-Bohman LG, McElveen JT: Aberrant carotid artery: radiologic diagnosis with emphasis on high-resolution CT. *RadioGraphics* 5:985–994, 1987.

Lo WWM, Applegate LJ, Carberry JN, et al: Endolymphatic sac tumors: radiologic appearance. *Radiology* 189:199–204, 1993.

Mafee MF, Henrickson GC, Deitch RL, et al: Use of CT in stapedial otosclerosis. *Radiology* 156:709–714, 1985.

Mafee MF, Valvassori GE, Deitch RL, et al: Use of CT in the evaluation of cochlear otosclerosis. *Radiology* 156:703–708, 1985.

Mancuso AA, Hanafee WN: *Temporal bone*. In Mancuso AA, Hanafee WN, editors: *Computed tomography and magnetic resonance imaging of the head and neck*, ed 2. Baltimore, 1985, Williams & Wilkins.

Martin N, Sterkers O, Mompoint D, et al: Facial nerve neuromas: MR imaging. *Neuroradiology* 34:62–67, 1992.

Martin N, Sterkers O, Nahum H: Haemantioma of the petrous bone: MRI. *Neuroradiology* 34:420–422, 1992.

Mehra YN, Dubey SP, Mann SBS, et al: Correlation between high-resolution CT and surgical findings in congenital aural atresia. *Arch Otolaryngol Head Neck Surg* 114:137–141, 1988.

Mendelson DS, Som PM, Mendelson MH, et al: Malignant external otitis: the role of CT and radionuclides in evaluation. *Radiology* 149:745–749, 1983.

Nardis PF, Teramo M, Giunta S, et al: Unusual cholesteatoma shell: CT findings. *J Comput Assist Tomogr* 12:1084–1087, 1988.

Parnes LS, Lee DH, Peerless SJ: MR imaging of facial nerve neuromas. *Laryngoscope* 101:31–35, 1991.

Phelps PD, Lloyd GA: Vascular masses in the middle ear. *Clin Radiol* 37:359–364, 1986.

Remley KB, Coit WE, Harnsberger HR, et al: Pulsatile tinnitus and the vascular tympanic membrane: CT, MR and angiographic findings. *Radiology* 1974: 388–389, 1990.

Remley KB, Harnsberger HR, Jacobs JM, et al: The radiologic evaluation of pulsatile tinnitus and the vascular tympanic membrane. *Semin Ultrasound CT MR* 10:236–250, 1989.

Rubin J, Curtin HD, Yu VL, et al: Malignant external otitis: utility of CT in diagnosis and follow-up. *Radiology* 174:391–394, 1990.

Sekhar LN, Pomeranz S, Janecka IP, et al: Temporal bone neoplasms: a report on 20 surgically treated cases. *J Neurosurg* 76:578–587, 1992.

Silver AJ, Janecka I, Wazen J, et al: Complicated cholesteatomas: CT findings in inner ear complications of middle ear cholesteatomas. *Radiology* 164:47–51, 1987.

Stewart KL: Paragangliomas of the temporal bone. *Am J Otolaryngol* 14:219–226, 1993.

Swartz JD, Faerber EN: Congenital malformations of the external and middle ear: high-resolution CT findings of surgical import. *Am J Roentgenol* 144:501–506, 1985.

Swartz JD, Faerber EN, Wolfson RJ, et al: Fenestral otosclerosis: significance of preoperative CT evaluation. *Radiology* 151:703–707, 1984.

Swartz JD, Glazer AU, Faerber EN, et al: Congenital middle-ear deafness: CT study. *Radiology* 159:187–190, 1986.

Swartz JD, Mandell DW, Berman SE, et al: Cochlear otosclerosis (otospongiosis): CT analysis with audiometric correlation. *Radiology* 155:147–150, 1985.

Swartz JD, Mandrell DW, Faerber EN, et al: Labyrinthine ossification: etiologies and CT findings. *Radiology* 157:395–398, 1985.

Swartz JD, Zwillenberg S, Berger AS: Acquired disruptions of the incustostapedial articulation: diagnosis with CT. *Radiology* 171:779–781, 1989.

Vogl T, Brüning R, Schedel H, et al: Paraganglioma of the jugular bulb and carotid body: MR imaging with short sequences and GD-DTPA enhancement. *AJNR* 10:823–827, 1989.

18

The Upper Cranial Nerves

CRITICAL IMAGING QUESTIONS: UPPER CRANIAL NERVES

1. What is the most common cause of isolated oculomotor neuropathy with loss of pupillary reflex? Should CT, MRI, or angiography be used to image this lesion?
2. Name the four trigeminal nerve nuclei. What is the upper brainstem extent and lower cervical cord extent of the trigeminal nuclei?
3. Name the three major branches of the trigeminal nerve and the openings they pass through on their way across the skull base.
4. Which of the three major trigeminal nerve branches carries both sensory and motor fibers? Name the four muscles of mastication that receive motor innervation from the masticator nerve.
5. When a malignant tumor is found in the masticator space of the deep face, what nerve must be imaged from the mandibular foramen to Meckel's cavity?

Answers to these questions are found in the text beside the question number (Q#) in the margin.

UPPER CRANIAL NERVES (I–VI)

A. Introduction.

1. Because they are responsible for the complex functions found in the extacranial head and neck, cranial nerves are included in this book. Without a thorough understanding of cranial nerve anatomy, function, malfunction, and diseases, many imaging problems will be misimaged and misinterpreted.

   a. The cranial nerves are subdivided into upper (i.e., cranial nerves I through VI) and lower (i.e., cranial nerves VII through XII) groups to simplify the task of relearning this material.

2. The ability of MRI to define the detailed anatomy of the brain stem, basal cisterns, and skull base has revolutionized the evaluation of both simple and complex cranial neuropathy. As MRI technology continues to advance, so does our understanding of the lesions that affect the cranial nerves.

   a. MRI has completely replaced CT as the diagnostic modality of choice for investigating cranial neuropathy.

3. Cranial nerves now can be seen in the cisterns and skull base passages, and the location of their brain stem nuclei can be identified through association with visible brain stem contours and internal landmarks. The diagnostic radiologist must be familiar with cranial nerve anatomy and the unique imaging problems of this area.

4. In this chapter cranial nerves I through VI are viewed from their nuclear origins to their end plates (i.e., from inside out). The reader may find it helpful to think of the cranial nerves based on their area of brain stem origin (Fig. 18-1):

Brain Stem Segment	Cranial Nerve
Diencephalon	II
Mesencephalon (i.e., midbrain)	III and IV
Pons	V, VI, VII, and VIII
Medulla	IX, X, XI, and XII

5. Cranial nerves I through VI are discussed individually regarding anatomy, function, malfunction, imaging issues, and lesions along the course of each nerve.

B. Olfactory nerve (i.e., cranial nerve I)

1. Anatomy.

   a. The structures of the central nervous system involved in the process of smelling as a group are referred to as the *rhinencephalon* (Greek, *rhinnose* and *enkephalos*, for "brain").

   b. The olfactory system is comprised of the olfactory epithelium, bulbs, and tracts, together with the olfactory areas of the brain (Fig. 18-2).

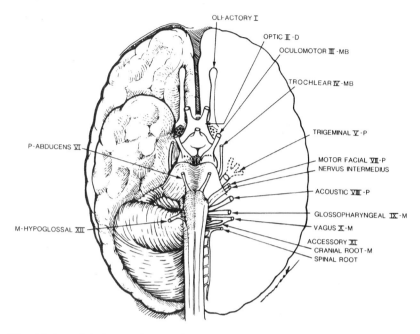

Fig. 18-1 Global cranial nerve drawing. Cranial nerve II is associated with the diencephalon (*D*). Cranial nerves III and IV arise from the midbrain (*MB*). Cranial nerves V, VI, VII, and VIII have their nuclear origins in the pons (*P*), and nerves IX, X, XI, and XII arise from the medulla (*M*).

1) The olfactory epithelium is found in the roof of the nasal cavity, extending inferolaterally on the superior turbinate and inferomedially on the nasal septum.
   a) Esthesioneuroblastoma is a high nasal tumor, because it arises from the olfactory epithelium.
2) The olfactory bulb is the rostral enlargement of the olfactory tract. It is a bulbous structure that lies on the intracranial surface of the cribriform plate.
   a) Both the olfactory bulb and tract can be visualized with high-resolution, coronal T1-weighted MRI.
3) The olfactory tract is comprised of the centrally projecting axons, which convey olfactory information to the medial and lateral olfactory areas.
4) The two main central projections of the rhinencephalon are the medial olfactory area and the lateral olfactory area.
   a) The medial olfactory area is found in the subcallosal region of the medial surface of the frontal lobe. The medial olfac-

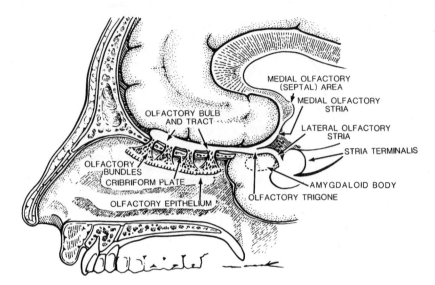

Fig. 18-2 Major features of the olfactory pathway. The olfactory system is comprised of the olfactory epithelium, bulbs, and tracts, together with olfactory areas of the brain. The olfactory epithelium is found in the roof of the nasal cavity, extending inferolaterally on the superior turbinate and inferomedially on the nasal septum. The olfactory bulb is the rostral enlargement of the olfactory tract; it is a bulbous structure that lies on the intracranial surface of the cribriform plate. The olfactory tract is the centrally projecting axons that convey olfactory information to the medial and lateral olfactory areas, which are the two main central projection areas of the rhinencephalon.

tory stria holds the central projection fibers that end in the medial olfactory area.

    b) The lateral olfactory area is the primary olfactory area. It consists of the cortex of the uncus, the anterior hippocampal gyrus, and part of the amygdaloid body.

  5) The more central connections of the olfactory system are a complex communications network that permits olfactory information to reach the autonomic centers for visceral responses, such as salivation in response to aromatic odors or nausea in response to exposure to noxious substances. Studying the specifics of these more central pathways will not help in any imaging context and therefore are omitted from this review.

2. Function and malfunction.

    a. The special sense of smell, or olfaction, is the single function subserved by the olfactory nerve.

    b. Loss of the sense of smell is referred to as *anosmia.*

    c. Olfactory hallucinations, in which phantom smells are experienced, may be the principal patient complaint when the lesion is centered in the medial temporal lobe.

3. MRI issues.

    a. Lesions affecting the sense of smell can be found anywhere along the course of the olfactory system.

    b. When anosmia is the principal patient complaint, the lesion usually is high in the nose, cribriform plate, floor of the anterior cranial fossa, or medial temporal lobe of the brain.

4. Lesions affecting the olfactory nerve.

    a. Lesions that cause malfunction of the olfactory nerve can be found anywhere along the olfactory pathway from the nose to the temporal lobe.

    b. Few of these lesions occur with any frequency. These include nasal polyposis, anterior cranial fossa meningioma, and temporal lobe astrocytoma.

    c. A more complete differential diagnosis can be found in Table 18-1.

C. Optic nerve (i.e., cranial nerve II) visual pathway.

1. Anatomy.

    a. The visual pathway is best considered in three parts: the optic nerves, optic chiasm, and retrochiasmal structures (Fig. 18-3).

       1) The retrochiasmal structures of the visual pathway include the optic tracts, lateral geniculate bodies, optic radiations, and visual cortex.

       2) The individual parts of the visual pathway can be visualized by either T1- or T2-weighted MRI.

2. Function and malfunction.

    a. Injury to the prechiasmal visual pathway (i.e., the pathway anterior to the optic chiasm) produces partial or complete monocular visual loss (i.e., scotoma).

    b. A lesion at the chiasm level classically produces bitemporal hemianopsia or heteronymous field defects (i.e., parts of both visual fields are affected).

    c. Retrochiasmal injury to the visual pathway usually creates homonymous hemianopsia (i.e., visual field defect restricted to a single side).

3. MRI issues.

    a. The visual pathway can be imaged thoroughly from the globe to the calcarine cortex with MRI using only the standard head coil, because it has only a small craniocaudad dimension.

    b. T1-weighted axial and coronal thin section (i.e., 2 to 3 mm) imaging from the chiasm anteriorly identifies structural lesions affecting the

Table 18-1 **Differential Diagnosis of Lesions Affecting the Olfactory Pathway**

Peripheral Conductive Area Lesions
Facial fracture involving cribriform plate
Sinonasal polyposis
Nasal tumor (esthesioneuroblastoma)
Cocaine abuse

Central Sensorineural Area Lesions
Congenital
   Kallmann's syndrome
      Combination of hypogonadotropic hypogonadism and anosmia secondary
         to agenesis of olfactory bulbs
Head trauma
   Multiple possible etiologies including:
      Shear injury at cribriform plate
      Olfactory bulb–tract contusion
      Contusion of the frontal and/or temporal lobe
Infection
   AIDS
Benign tumor
   Meningioma of planum sphenoidale
Malignant tumor
   Temporal lobe astrocytoma
Other central nervous system diseases
   Alzheimer's disease
   Parkinson's disease
   Huntington's disease
   Schizophrenia

optic nerve/sheath complex and the optic chiasm. If the axial images are angled along the course of the optic nerve as seen on the sagittal localization sequence, the entire nerve from the optic canal to the globe may be seen on one or two slices.

1) Fat saturation in conjunction with a contrast-enhanced T1-weighted, spin echo sequence removes the orbital fat signal, leaving enhancing lesions as conspicuous areas of high signal.

2) This technique is particularly useful in delineating optic nerve/sheath lesions such as optic neuritis (i.e., optic nerve) and meningioma (i.e., optic nerve sheath).

   c. T2-weighted axial images precisely delineate the retrochiasmal optic pathway and also help to characterize lesions seen on T1-weighted imaging.

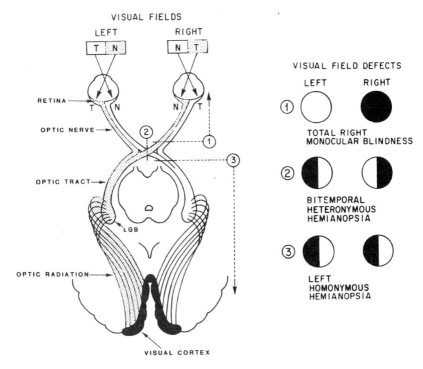

Fig. 18-3 Normal visual pathway. *Left,* Three principal lesions: prechiasmal (*1*), chiasmal (*2*), and retrochiasmal (*3*). *Right,* Corresponding visual field defects. (From Harnsberger HR: *Unlocking the brain stem, basal cisterns and skull base through MR imaging of the cranial nerves.* In Stark DD, Bradley WG, editors: *Syllabus. A categorical course in diagnostic radiology: MR imaging.* Radiological Society of North America, 1988. Used with permission.)

1) When fast spin echo sequences are substituted for T2-weighted, conventional spin echo sequences, fat saturation may be added to bring out areas of abnormal high signal in the orbital fat.
2) Although worthy substitutes for conventional spin echo T2-weighted sequences, fast spin echo sequences suffer because fat remains high signal if fat saturation does not accompany this pulse sequence.

   d. Other techniques that may enhance MRI scans of the visual pathway include:

1) Patients should be instructed to fix their gaze on a point during image acquisition. Blinking, eye motion, and tongue motion should be avoided if possible.

2) Dentures and any other intraoral removable hardware should be taken out before the MRI examination.
3) All make-up must be removed before imaging to avoid artifacts in the region of the globe.
4) Some institutions use oblique sagittal T1-weighted images along the optic nerve as part of their protocol.

4. Diseases affecting the visual pathway.
   a. Table 18-2 summarizes the unique differential diagnosis for lesions affecting the visual pathway, categorized as prechiasmal, chiasmal, and postchiasmal.
   b. Orbital lesions are discussed in the chapter covering the orbital area.
   c. The sellar and parasellar lesions that affect the chiasm are discussed in the chapter by this name in Osborn's *Handbook of Neuroradiology*.
   d. The parenchymal brain lesions that affect the retrochiasmal visual pathway also are discussed in the *Handbook of Neuroradiology*.

D. Oculomotor, trochlear, and abducens nerves (i.e., cranial nerves III, IV, and VI).

1. Movements of the eye are produced by the six extraocular muscles innervated by cranial nerves III, IV, and VI.
   a. Because these three cranial nerves are intimately associated both anatomically and functionally, they are discussed as a single unit.
   b. Normal anatomy and function of the individual cranial nerves are first reviewed, followed by imaging issues and diseases affecting this group.
2. Anatomy and function of the oculomotor nerve.
   a. The oculomotor nerve nuclear complex (i.e., oculomotor nucleus and associated paramedian parasympathetic, Perlia's, and Edinger-Westphal nuclei) is found in the motor column of the basal plate of the rostral midbrain at the level of the superior colliculi, wedged between the periaqueductal gray matter and the medial longitudinal fasiculus near the midline (Fig. 18-4A).

Table 18-2 Differential Diagnosis of Lesions Affecting the Visual Pathway

Prechiasmal Lesions
Optic nerve/sheath tumors
  Glioma
  Meningioma
  Neuroma of optic nerve sheath
Inflammatory lesions of optic nerve sheath
  Optic neuritis with or without multiple sclerosis
  Orbital pseudotumor
  Sarcoidosis   (*continued*)

Table 18-2   (*continued*)

Other nonneoplastic lesions of optic nerve sheath
  Toxoplasmosis
  Tuberculosis
  Graves' disease
  Hematoma
  Papilledema
  Optic nerve drusen
Masses extrinsic to the optic nerve
  Congenital
    Hemangioma
    Lymphangioma
    Epidermoid
    Dermoid
Lesions of orbital muscles
  Graves' disease
  Pseudotumor
Lesions of bony orbit
  Fibrous dysplasia
Malignant tumor
  Metastatic tumor
  Lymphoma
  Myeloma
  Rhabdomyosarcoma
  Lacrimal gland tumor
Paranasal sinus lesions
  Polyposis
  Mucocele
  Subperiosteal abscess
  Sinus tumor

Chiasmal Lesions
  Rathke's cleft cyst
  Pituitary adenoma
  Chiasmal glioma
  Craniopharyngioma
  Parasellar meningioma
  Internal carotid artery aneurysm

Retrochiasmal Lesions
  Cavernous angioma with or without hemorrhage
  Arteriovenous malformation
  Infarct
  Brain stem neoplasm: glioma, metastasis
  Multiple sclerosis

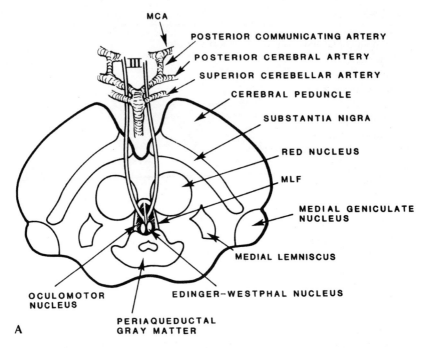

MCA

POSTERIOR COMMUNICATING ARTERY

POSTERIOR CEREBRAL ARTERY

SUPERIOR CEREBELLAR ARTERY

CEREBRAL PEDUNCLE

SUBSTANTIA NIGRA

RED NUCLEUS

MLF

MEDIAL GENICULATE NUCLEUS

MEDIAL LEMNISCUS

OCULOMOTOR NUCLEUS

EDINGER–WESTPHAL NUCLEUS

PERIAQUEDUCTAL GRAY MATTER

A

Fig. 18-4 **A**, Transverse section through the superior colliculus illustrating the primary internal features of the upper midbrain. Observe cranial nerve III arising from its nucleus in the dorsal paramedian midbrain tegmentum, then coursing through the red nucleus and substantia nigra to exit the midbrain into the interpeduncular cistern. The cisternal third nerve courses between the posterior cerebral and the superior cerebellar arteries and passes in close proximity to the posterior communicating artery. *MCA*, Middle cerebral artery; *MLF*, medial longitudinal fasciculus. (From Harnsberger HR: *Unlocking the brain stem, basal cisterns and skull base through MR imaging of the cranial nerves.* In Stark DD, Bradley WG, editors: *Syllabus. A categorical course in diagnostic radiology: MR imaging.* Radiological

(continued)

    b. From the dorsally located nuclear complex, the oculomotor fascicles course ventrally through the red nucleus, substantia nigra, and medial cerebral peduncle to exit the anterior midbrain in the interpeduncular cistern (Fig. 18-4*A*).

    c. The cisternal third nerve passes between the posterior cerebral artery and the superior cerebellar artery, then courses anteriorly just inferior to the posterior communicating artery.

    d. Once it enters the roof of the cavernous sinus, the third nerve remains the most cephalad of the nerves in this structure, remaining just superolateral to the cavernous internal carotid artery (Fig. 18-4*B*).

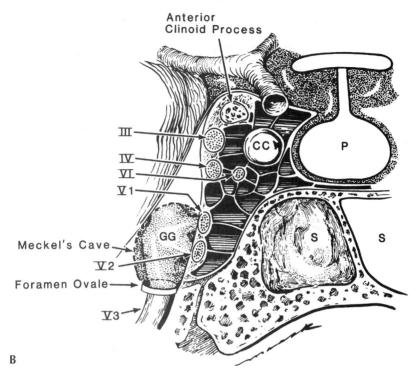

Anterior
Clinoid Process

III

IV
VI
V1

Meckel's Cave

V2

Foramen Ovale

V3

CC

P

GG

S

S

B

Fig. 18-4 (*continued*)   Society of North America, 1988. Used with permission.) **B**, Coronal view of the cavernous sinus area depicting the approximate location of the cranial nerves associated with this structure. Cranial nerve III is the most superior of the cavernous sinus cranial nerves. Cranial nerve IV is lateral to cranial nerve VI, which is the only centrally located nerve in the cavernous sinus. The first division of the trigeminal nerve (i.e., cranial nerve V_1) is considered within the cavernous sinus, while branch V_2 is not. Instead, branch V_2 is within a dural sleeve on the inferolateral aspect of the cavernous sinus. Branch V_3 obviously is not within the cavernous sinus at any point along its intracranial course.

     e. The superior orbital fissure transmits the oculomotor nerve into the orbit, where it innervates the superior, medial, and inferior recti; levator palpebrae; and inferior oblique muscles (Fig. 18-5).
       1) Parasympathetic fibers traveling with the nerve go to the ciliary ganglion of the orbit, which controls pupillary sphincter function and accommodation (i.e., ciliary muscle).
3. Anatomy and function of the trochlear nerve.
     a. The trochlear nuclei are located in the midline of the same basal plate motor column as the oculomotor nerve, just caudal to the third nerve nuclear complex (Fig. 18-6).

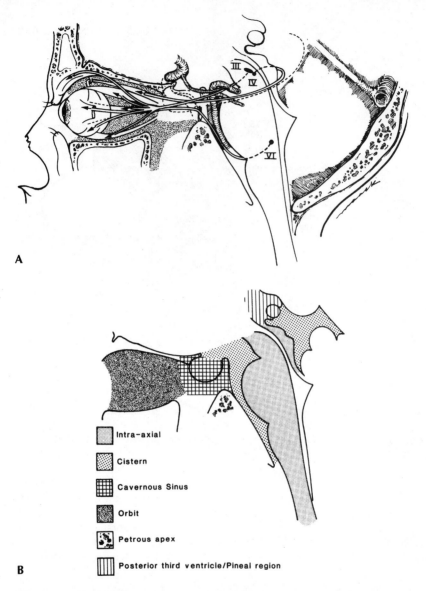

A

B

- ▨ Intra-axial
- ░ Cistern
- ▦ Cavernous Sinus
- ▓ Orbit
- ▨ Petrous apex
- ▥ Posterior third ventricle/Pineal region

Fig. 18-5 **A**, Cranial nerve III, IV, and VI origins and muscular innervations. Cranial nerves III, IV, and VI provide all motor innervation to the extraocular muscles of the eye. Cranial nerves III and IV have their origins in the midbrain, while cranial nerve VI nuclear origins can be found in the lower pons. All three nerves pass through a portion on the prepontine cistern before passing through the cavernous sinus and on into the orbit through the superior orbital fissure. **B**, Sagittal view showing the key anatomic areas to inspect in a patient undergoing imaging for extraocular muscle malfunction. The general clinical complaint in such a patient often is diplopia. (From Digre KB: Neuro-radiologic evaluation of supranuclear and infranuclear disorders of eye movement. *Ophthalmol Clin North Am*, in press, 1994. Used with permission.)

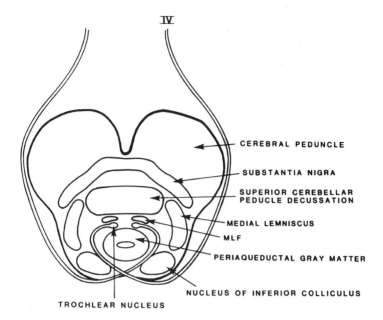

IV

CEREBRAL PEDUNCLE

SUBSTANTIA NIGRA

SUPERIOR CEREBELLAR
PEDUCLE DECUSSATION

MEDIAL LEMNISCUS

MLF

PERIAQUEDUCTAL GRAY MATTER

NUCLEUS OF INFERIOR COLLICULUS

TROCHLEAR NUCLEUS

Fig. 18-6   View through the inferior colliculus depicting the important internal features of the midbrain at this level. Observe cranial nerve IV decussation before its emergence from the dorsal midbrain. *MLF,* Medial longitudinal fasciculus. (From Harnsberger HR: *Unlocking the brain stem, basal cisterns and skull base through MR imaging of the cranial nerves.* In Stark DD, Bradley WG, editors: *Syllabus. A categorical course in diagnostic radiology: MR imaging.* Radiological Society of North America, 1988. Used with permission.)

b. From their nuclear site just ventral to the aqueduct, the trochlear nerve fascicles loop dorsal and caudal around the cerebral aqueduct and into the rostral anterior medullary velum where they decussate.

c. The fourth nerve proper emerges from the dorsal midbrain just caudal to the inferior colliculus.

d. The cisternal course of the fourth nerve is similar to that of the third nerve. It also passes between the posterior cerebral artery above and the superior cerebellar artery below after it courses around the lateral pons.

e. The nerve then passes forward on the free edge of the tentorium and penetrates the dura, entering the cavernous sinus just inferior to the oculomotor nerve.

f. The trochlear nerve finally leaves the cavernous sinus via the superior orbital fissure, entering the orbit and providing motor innervation to the superior oblique muscle (Fig. 18-5).

4. Anatomy and function of the abducens nerve.
   a. The abducens nucleus is located in the pontine tegmentum (Figs. 18-7 and 18-8) near the midline, just ventral to the fourth ventricle.
   b. Axons of the facial nerve (i.e., cranial nerve VII) loop around the abducens nucleus, creating a bulge in the floor of the fourth ventricle called the *facial colliculus* (Fig. 18-7).
   c. Axons of the abducens nucleus course anterioinferiorly through the pontine tegmentum, emerging from the brain stem at the ventral aspect of the pontomedullary junction.
   d. The cisternal abducens nerve ascends anterior to the belly of the pons to pierce the dura covering the posterior sphenoid bone at Dorello's canal (Fig. 18-8).
   e. The nerve then continues forward to enter the cavernous sinus. It enters the orbit through the superior orbital fissure, penetrating the lateral rectus muscle that it supplies (Fig. 18-5).
5. Imaging issues of cranial nerves III, IV, and VI.
   a. When considering imaging issues of the third and fourth cranial nerves, it is imperative that the sixth (i.e., abducens nerve) be in-

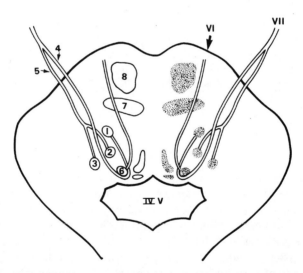

Fig. 18-7   Diagram of the axial lower pons illustrating the nuclei and courses of the abducens (VI) and facial (VII) nerves. *1,* Motor nucleus of facial nerve; *2,* superior salivatory nucleus; *3,* solitary nucleus; *4,* motor root of facial nerve; *5,* intermediate nerve; *6,* abducens nucleus; *7,* medial lemniscus; *8,* corticospinal tract. (From Harnsberger HR: *Unlocking the brain stem, basal cisterns and skull base through MR imaging of the cranial nerves.* In Stark DD, Bradley WG, editors: *Syllabus. A categorical course in diagnostic radiology: MR imaging.* Radiological Society of North America, 1988. Used with permission.)

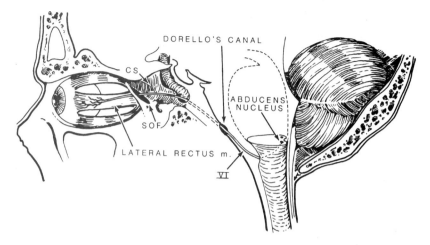

Fig. 18-8 Sagittal depiction of the abducens nerve from its nuclear origins to its orbital insertion. The abducens nuclei are found in the lower pontine tegmentum. Axons from the nuclei descend as they run anteriorly through the pons to emerge as the abducens nerve at the anterior pontomedullary junction. From there the abducens nerve ascends in the prepontine cistern to pierce the dura in the posterior wall of the sphenoid bone at Dorello's canal. It then runs anteriorly through the cavernous sinus (*CS*) and superior orbital fissure (*SOF*) to penetrate the medial surface of the lateral rectus muscle.

cluded because of its shared orbital functions and similar course through the cisterns, cavernous sinus, and superior orbital fissure.

b. Cranial neuropathies involving nerves III, IV, and VI are most simply approached by dividing the deficits into complex (i.e., nonisolated) and simple (i.e., isolated) groups based on clinical presentation.

1) Complex III, IV, and VI cranial neuropathy.

a) Complex III, IV, and VI cranial neuropathy is localized to the brain stem when dysfunction of one or more of these nerves occurs in conjunction with malfunction of other brain stem structures.

b) Any of the intraaxial lesions of the brain stem can cause these types of symptom complexes. The principal patterns of midbrain involvement of cranial nerves III, IV, or VI are listed in Table 18-3.

c) When complex III, IV, and VI neuropathy occurs without associated "brain stem symptoms," the lesion is found in the anterior basilar cistern, cavernous sinus, superior orbital fissure, or orbital apex.

Table 18-3   Complex Cranial Neuropathy with Associated Brain Stem Symptoms

Symptom Complex	Location of Lesion
Syndrome of Weber Ipsilateral III Contralateral hemiparesis	III fascicles/crus cerebri
Claude's syndrome Ipsilateral III Contralateral hemiparesis and ataxia	III fascicles/crus cerebri Red nucleus
Millard-Gubler syndrome Ipsilateral VI and/or VII Contralateral hemiparesis	Ventral pons affecting the VI fascicles/corticospinal tract
Abducens nucleus lesion Ipsilateral gaze paralysis VII palsy	Abducens nucleus/facial colliculus
Intranuclear ophthalmoplegia Paresis of ipsilaterial abduction during conjugate eye movement	Medial longitudinal fasciculus

    d) Characteristic symptom patterns based on anatomic grouping of the cranial nerves that may help localize these nonisolated lesions outside the midbrain are listed in Table 18-4.

  2) Simple III, IV, and VI cranial neuropathy.

    a) Simple or isolated III, IV, and VI cranial neuropathies often signal the presence of unique disease depending on the cranial nerve involved (Table 18-5).

  3) Isolated oculomotor neuropathy.

    a) In the case of isolated third nerve palsy the initial clinical presentation dictates whether imaging will be performed and which method will be used.

Table 18-4   Complex Cranial Neuropathy Without Associated Brain Stem Symptoms

Symptom Complex	Lesion Location
V, VI, VII, and VIII palsies	Cerebellopontine angle cistern or petrous apex
III, IV, V_1, V_2, V_3, and VI palsies	Anterior basilar cistern (retrocavernous area)
III, IV, V_1, V_2, and VI palsies	Posterior to midcavernous sinus
III, IV, V_1, and VI palsies	Anterior cavernous sinus/superior orbital fissure

Table 18-5   Imaging Issues in Isolated III, IV, and VI Cranial Nerve Palsy

Age > 40 Years (Vasculopathic Age)

Third cranial nerve palsy

Pupillary sparing (History of diabetes with or without hypertension)

Follow-up clinically versus MRI with MRA

If palsy continues to spare the pupil, imaging may not be performed, because the clinician has that presumed microvascular infarct is cause

If palsy evolves to affect the pupil, perform immediate MRI with MRA. If mass or neuritis is found, stop. If negative, perform an immediate angiogram to look for a posterior communicating aneurysm

Pupillary involvement

MRI with MRA. If mass or neuritis is found, stop. If negative, perform an immediate angiogram to look for aneurysm

Nontraumatic fourth or sixth cranial nerve palsy

No radiographic work-up in patients with diabetes or hypertension, unless disease progresses to nonisolated neuropathy or patient has known primary tumor, making metastasis a concern. Presumed microvascular infarct

Age < 40 Years (Nonvasculopathic Age)

Congenital third, fourth, or sixth cranial nerve palsy presumed to result from in utero insult or birth trauma

Nontraumatic acquired third nerve palsy

Age < 14 years

Follow-up clinically

Remains as isolated sixth nerve palsy, presumably from benign viral cause. No imaging

Progressive neurologic findings. MRI for mass lesion diagnosis

Young adult (age 15 to 40 years)

Clinical evaluation of patient for multiple sclerosis, hypertension, and collagen vascular disease

MRI to look for multiple sclerosis, infarct, vasculitic changes, and so on

---

b) In a patient over 40 years of age (i.e., old enough to have vasculopathic cranial neuropathy) isolated third nerve palsy with pupillary sparing may be followed with close clinical observation. Imaging may or may not be performed initially because of the assumption that the lesion results from microvascular infarction (depending on the bias of the referring physician). This is particularly true if the patient has diabetes or hypertension.

Q#1

c) In the case of isolated third nerve palsy with loss of pupillary function, MRI with MRA is performed initially to exclude mass lesions and to screen for aneurysm. If MRI does not explain the loss of third nerve function, angiography is performed immediately to search for a posterior communicating artery aneurysm.

d) Comment. The explanation for pupillary fiber damage from a posterior communicating artery aneurysm is that the pupillary fibers are in the superficial aspect of the third nerve, precisely where the average posterior communicating artery aneurysm projects. Microvascular infarction, however, involves the vessel supplying the core of the nerve with relative sparing of the peripheral pupillary fibers. If the angiogram is negative, T2-weighted MRI of the midbrain and coronal, contrast-enhanced, T1-weighted images of the anterior basilar cistern, cavernous sinus, and orbital apex are recommended to exclude other structural lesions.

4) Isolated trochlear neuropathy.
   a) Simple trochlear nerve palsy most commonly is secondary to trauma.
   b) The principal theories to explain the predisposition of the trochlear nerve to traumatic injury include contusion of the anterior medullary velum, where the nerve decussates, or cisternal fourth nerve segment injury by the free edge of the tentorium.
   c) Nontraumatic trochlear nerve palsy results primarily from microvascular infarction or tumor.

5) Isolated abducens neuropathy.
   a) Isolated abducens palsy is the most common ocular motor nerve palsy.
   b) In determining whether to image and what to look for in simple abducens nerve palsy, the age of the patient is the pivotal historical feature.
   c) In patients younger than 14 years of age clinical follow-up to guarantee that the palsy remains isolated is recommended. If it does remain isolated, the palsy probably is postviral, benign, and does not require imaging. If symptoms progress to include other neurologic findings, MRI of the brain stem is used to search for a brain stem glioma.
   d) Multiple sclerosis, hypertension, and collagen vascular disease must be ruled out as potential causes in young adults (age, 15 to 40 years) with isolated sixth nerve palsy.
   e) In patients older than 40 years clinical evaluation to rule out hypertension and diabetes is undertaken first. If the results of

this work-up are negative, MRI to look for a brain stem or peripheral cause is recommended (Table 18-5).

f)   When the lateral rectus muscle is infiltrated by a lesion such as pseudotumor or real tumor, the patient may present as if a neurogenic abducens neuropathy is present. Scanning shows a mass within the lateral rectus. Mechanical limitation of movement presumably is the cause of this clinical confusion.

E. Trigeminal nerve.

1. Introduction.
   a. The trigeminal nerve is the largest of the cranial nerves and has both sensory and motor functions.
   b. This nerve is associated with the first branchial arch and innervates the structures that derive from the first arch.
   c. Specifically, the trigeminal nerve mediates sensation to the scalp, face, and ectodermally derived mucous membranes of the nasal cavity, sinuses, and mouth.
      1) Motor innervation is seen in the mandibular division (i.e., cranial nerve V_3) only. The four muscles of mastication as well as the anterior belly of the digastric, mylohyoid, tensor tympani, and tensor palati muscles are all innervated by cranial nerve V_3.

2. Normal anatomy.

Q#2
   a. Four brain stem nuclei contribute to the trigeminal nerve (Fig. 18–9).
      1) Mesencephalic nucleus. Proprioception from the face.
      2) Main sensory nucleus. Tactile sensation from the face.
      3) Motor nucleus. Motor innervation of the muscles of mastication, tensor palatini and tensor tympani muscles, and the mylohyoid and anterior belly of the digastric muscles.
      4) Spinal nucleus. Pain and temperature from the face.
   b. These nuclei predominantly lie in the tegmentum of the lateral pons along the anterolateral aspect of the fourth ventricle at the level of the root entry zone of the trigeminal nerve (Fig. 18-9).

Q#2
      1) From this area of the pons the mesencephalic nucleus projects cephalad into the midbrain to the level of the inferior colliculus, and the spinal nucleus extends caudally to the level of the second cervical vertebrae (Fig. 18-9).
   c. Preganglionic segment and Meckel's cave.
      1) The trigeminal nerve emerges from the lateral pons at a point referred to as the *root entry zone*. A large sensory root and a smaller motor root emerge together at this point.

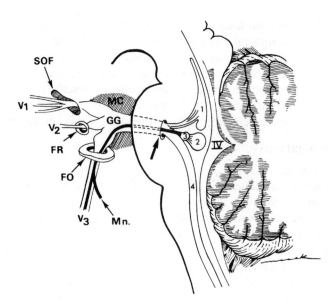

Fig. 18-9 Normal intracranial portion of the trigeminal nerve. Four brain stem nuclei contribute to the trigeminal nerve: mesencephalic nucleus (*1*), principal sensory nucleus of cranial nerve V (*2*), main motor nucleus (*3*), and spinal nucleus (*4*). Fibers from these nuclei coalesce to exit the lateral pons at the root entry zone (*arrow*). The segment of the trigeminal nerve from the root entry zone to the gasserian ganglion (*GG*) is referred to as the *preganglionic segment*. IV, Fourth ventricle; *FO*, foramen ovale; *FR*, foramen rotundum; *MC*, Meckel's cave; *Mn*, masticator nerve; *SOF*, superior orbital fissure. (From Hardin CW, Harnsberger HR: The radiographic evaluation of trigeminal neuropathy. *Semin Ultrasound CT MR* 8:214–239, 1987. Used with permission.)

2) This common sensorimotor trunk is known as the *preganglionic segment* and runs anteriorly and superiorly through the prepontine cistern.

3) The main trunk then enters Meckel's cave through the porus trigeminus (i.e., entrance to Meckel's cave). The nerve carries a dural covering with it into Meckel's cave. The leptomeninges also follow the nerve, resulting in a subarachnoid space filled with cerebrospinal fluid surrounding the nerve and ganglion within Meckel's cave, referred to as the *trigeminal cistern*.

4) The gasserian ganglion (also called the *trigeminal* and *semilunar ganglion*) lies in Meckel's cave and contains the cell bodies of the afferent sensory fibers, excluding those that mediate proprioception. This ganglion lies in the anterior–inferior aspect of

Meckel's cave; it occupies only 10% of this space. The ganglion normally enhances on T1-weighted, enhanced MRI.

d. Peripheral branches.

Q#3

1) Distal to the gasserian ganglion the trigeminal nerve trifurcates into its three principal branches: the ophthalmic (i.e., V_1), maxillary (i.e., V_2), and mandibular (i.e., V_3) nerves (Figs. 18-9 and 18-10).

2) The ophthalmic division courses in the lateral wall of the cavernous sinus, exiting the skull base through the superior orbital fissure.

   a) Within the orbit it subdivides into three major branches: the lacrimal, frontal, and nasociliary nerves. These branches ramify and provide sensory innervation to the scalp, forehead, nose, and globe.

3) The maxillary division travels near the crease formed between the lateral dural wall and skull base along the lateral margin of the cavernous sinus, exiting the skull base through the foramen rotundum (Fig. 18-4*B*).

   a) After passing through the foramen rotundum, the nerve enters the roof of the pterygopalatine fossa, where it gives off several branches, including the zygomatic, pterygopalatine, and superior alveolar nerves.

   b) The main trunk of branch V_2 continues anteriorly as the infraorbital nerve, entering the orbit through the inferior orbital fissure. This nerve travels anteriorly within the infraorbital groove, in the floor of the orbit, and emerges onto the face through the infraorbital foramen.

   c) Branch V_2 supplies sensory innervation to the middle third of the face (i.e., cheek) and the maxillary (i.e., upper) teeth.

4) The mandibular division of the trigeminal nerve does not transverse the cavernous sinus. Instead, it runs along the skull base and exits through the foramen ovale.

   a) The motor root bypasses the gasserian ganglion and joins branch V_3 as it exits the skull base through the foramen ovale.

Q#4

   b) Branch V_3 is the only major branch of the trigeminal nerve that carries both sensory and motor fibers.

   c) As branch V_3 plunges through the foramen ovale of the skull base, it immediately enters the nasopharyngeal masticator space.

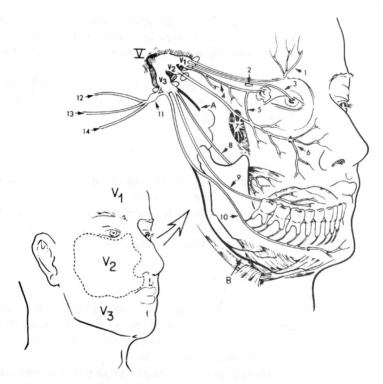

Fig. 18-10   A, Extracranial ramifications of trigeminal nerve. Sensory branches are numbered; major motor branches are lettered. V₁: *1*, Frontal nerve; *2*, ciliary ganglion; *3*, nasociliary nerve; *4*, lacrimal nerve. V₂: *5*, Zygomatic nerve; *6*, infraorbital nerve; *7*, pterygopalatine ganglion. V₃: *8*, Buccal nerve; *9*, lingual nerve; *10*, inferior alveolar nerve; *11*, otic ganglion; *12*, nerve to parotid gland; *13*, nerve to tensor palatini muscle; *14*, nerve to tensor tympani muscle. *A*, Masticator nerve; *B*, mylohyoid nerve. *Inset*, Sensory distribution of the three divisions of the trigeminal nerve. (From Hardin CW, Harnsberger HR: The radiographic evaluation of the trigeminal neuropathy. *Semin Ultrasound CT MR* 8:214–239, 1987. Used with permission.)

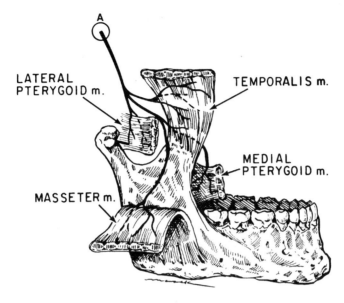

Fig. 18-10   (*continued*)

d) Branch V_3 then divides into several sensory branches: the buccal, auriculotemporal, inferior alveolar, and lingual nerves.
e) The inferior alveolar nerve enters the mandibular foramen in the ramus of the mandible and travels through the mandibular canal to emerge on the chin at the mental foramen.
f) The sensory branches of cranial nerve V_3 supply sensation to the lower third of the face, tongue, floor of the mouth, and jaw.
g) In addition to the sensory branches, V_3 has two motor branches: the masticator nerve, and the mylohyoid nerve.

Q#4

h) The masticator nerve enters the masticator space to supply motor innervation to the masseter, temporalis, and the medial and lateral pterygoid muscles (Fig. 18-10*B*).
i) The mylohyoid nerve supplies the mylohyoid and anterior belly of the digastric muscles in the floor of the mouth (Fig. 18-10*A*).

3. Trigeminal neuropathy.
    a. Symptoms of trigeminal nerve injury.

1) The clinical presentation of trigeminal nerve disease depends on the division affected.
2) Because all three divisions of the trigeminal nerve have sensory function, patients may complain of pain, burning, itching, or numbness in any region innervated by any of the three divisions.
3) If branch V_3 is primarily involved, patients may complain of weakness in chewing (i.e., muscles of mastication) or decreased hearing because of serous otitis media secondary to eustachian tube dysfunction from malfunction of the tensor palatini muscle.
4) Tic douloureux (i.e., trigeminal neuralgia).
   a) Characterized by lancinating pain down the course of the second or third division of the trigeminal nerve. Usually has trigger points or trigger events.

   b. Signs of trigeminal nerve injury.
1) Physical findings vary with division affected. A decreased sense of pain, touch, or temperature in any division of cranial nerve V can be seen.
2) When branch V_1 is primarily affected, the corneal reflex (which tests the integrity of the V_1 afferent sensory fibers from the cornea) via the ciliary branches of the nasociliary nerve (i.e., V_1 branch) may be diminished or absent.
3) When branch V_3 is affected, the muscles of mastication may be weakened or atrophic. Serous otitis media also may be noted.
4) The specificity of many of these symptoms and signs as indicators for structural disease involving the trigeminal nerve is variable.
   a) Intrinsic lesions of the trigeminal nerve may occur with normal trigeminal nerve function and symptoms resulting from compression of the adjacent structures.
   b) Facial pain is the least specific symptom, but the character of this pain may be an important clue to the presence of a lesion. Progressive symptoms, numbness, and motor abnormalities are ominous findings and strongly suggest a structural lesion.

4. Imaging issues of the trigeminal nerve.
   a. Excellent imaging of the trigeminal nerve can be accomplished with either CT or MRI, with the exception of detecting the more subtle, intraaxial brain stem and cisternal lesions.
1) CT is blind to these lesions. If available, MRI is the imaging method of choice when a structural lesion of the trigeminal nerve is suspected.
   b. MRI protocol.
1) The routine MRI protocol is designed to cover the entire trigeminal nerve, with the exception of the distal aspect of branch V_3.

2) Axial and coronal thin section (i.e., 3–5 mm), high-resolution sequences are required. Axial scans must cover the area from the hard palate below to the top of the sella above in all cases.

3) If branch V_3 is involved, a second axial T1-weighted sequence that covers to the inferior tip of the mandible prevents the radiologist from missing lesions involving the inferior alveolar nerve.

4) Coronal T1-weighted scans should span the dorsal brain stem posteriorly to the anterior face anteriorly. A T2-weighted, whole brain, axial sequence also is required to evaluate the trigeminal nerve completely for intraaxial disease.

5) Is contrast needed? Routine use of MRI contrast with T1-weighted images has resulted from the observation that contrast can help to diagnose trigeminal neuritis and other more subtle lesions involving the trigeminal nerve.

c. Trigeminal nerve and masticator space.

1) A common imaging error occurs when a tumor of the deep facial masticator space is identified and it is forgotten that the mandibular division of cranial nerve V provides a path for perineural tumor to transverse the skull base and become intracranial.

2) The extracranial part of the tumor then is incompletely treated, and "early intracranial recurrence" is diagnosed in the region of Meckel's cave.

3) To avoid this pitfall the imager needs only to think of the masticator space mass and branch V_3 as a single imaging problem.

Q#5

a) Complete imaging of branch V_3 to the proximal level of the root entry zone of the trigeminal nerve must be completed whenever a tumor is discovered that involves the masticator space or mandible.

d. Motor atrophy of the trigeminal nerve (Table 18-6).

1) CT or MRI findings of motor atrophy secondary to branch V_3 injury may be missed or misinterpreted by the uninitiated radiologist.

2) Atrophy resulting from branch V_3 injury is seen as two distinct patterns, depending on whether the involvement is distal or proximal along the course of V_3.

a) The distal portion of branch V_3 is between the takeoff of the masticator nerve from the main trunk of V_3 and the origin of the mylohyoid nerve from the inferior alveolar nerve. If injury to the nerve is distal, only the muscles innervated by the mylohyoid nerve (i.e., anterior belly of the digastric and mylohyoid muscles) are affected.

Table 18-6   Motor Atrophy of the Trigeminal Nerve

Proximal V_3 Atrophy (Masticator and Mylohyoid Nerves)
Masseter muscle
Temporalis muscle
Medial pterygoid muscle
Lateral pterygoid muscle
Anterior belly of digastric muscle
Mylohyoid muscle

Distal V_3 Atrophy (Mylohyoid Nerve Only)
Anterior belly of digastric muscle
Mylohyoid muscle

b) If the injury is proximal to the masticator nerve takeoff, then all muscles innervated by V_3 will be affected, including the muscles of mastication. Motor atrophy is recognized by loss of normal side-to-side symmetry, with the muscles on the affected side demonstrating decreased volume and increased fat.

e. Tic douloureux (i.e., trigeminal neuralgia).

1) Tic douloureux is characterized by sharp, short bursts of excruciating pain in the distribution of cranial nerves V_2 and V_3.

2) The cause of this disease is controversial, but the predominant theory suggests that vascular compression of the root entry zone of the trigeminal nerve is responsible.

3) Treatment initially is medical. If the disease is unresponsive to medical treatment, surgical intervention is used.

4) MRI with MRA is recommended before surgery both to rule out a structural lesion as the cause and to search for the offending ectatic or aberrant vessel.

   a) At times the vessel is too small to be visualized with MRI, even when using flow sensitive imaging techniques.

   b) A negative MRI scan does not preclude surgical intervention.

   c) In a center that performs vascular loop surgery, approximately 25% of patients imaged before surgery will show a nonvascular loop as the cause for the tic. For example, multiple sclerosis or benign cisternal tumor (e.g., schwannoma, epidermoid, lipoma) may be identified on MRI scans.

5) During surgery, decompression of an abnormal vessel (if one is found) is completed. If no vessel is discovered, selective rhizotomy of the affected division is performed.

Table 18-7   Differential Diagnosis of the Trigeminal Nerve

IntraAxial (Brain Stem)
Arteriovenous malformation
Cavernous angioma
Infarct
Brain stem neoplasm
  Glioma
  Metastasis
Multiple sclerosis

Cisternal (Preganglionic Segment)
Trigeminal neuritis
Sarcoidosis
Vascular compression
  Superior cerebellar artery
  Anterior inferior cerebellar artery
  Vertebrobasilar arteries or branches
  Cisternal veins
Aneurysm
Arteriovenous fistula
Compression by local tumor
  Meningioma
  Trigeminal or acoustic neuroma
  Epidermoid
Tumor
  Trigeminal schwannoma or neurofibroma
  Perineural malignancy

Meckel's Cave
Arachnoid cyst
Tumor
  Meningioma
  Trigeminal neuroma
  Perineural malignancy

Cavernous Sinus/Skull Base
Cavernous internal carotid aneurysm
Tumor
  Schwannoma or neurofibroma
  Meningioma
  Invasive pituitary tumor
  Perineural tumor on branches V_1, V_2, or V_3
  Hematogenous metastasis
Skull base neoplasm
  Primary: chordoma, chondroma, chondrosarcoma
Fibrous dysplasia

(*continued*)

Table 18-7   *(continued)*

Extracranial

Maxillary sinusitis (branch V_2)

Mandibular osteomyelitis (branch V_3)

Masticator space abscess (branch V_3)

Primary neurogenous neoplasm

  Neurofibroma

  Schwanomma

  Malignant schwannoma

Other local primary neoplasm

  Squamous cell carcinoma

  Lymphoma

  Adenoid cystic carcinoma

  Mucoepidermoid carcinoma

SUGGESTED READING

Braffman BJ, Zimmerman RA, Rabischong P: Cranial nerves III, IV, and VI: a clinical approach to the evaluation of their dysfunction. *Semin Ultrasound CT MR* 8:185–213, 1987.

Brazis PW: Localization of lesions of the oculomotor nerve: recent concepts. *Mayo Clin Proc* 66:1029–1035, 1991.

Brazis PW: Palsies of the trochlear nerve: diagnosis and localization: Recent concepts. *Mayo Clin Proc* 68:501–509, 1993.

Burger LJ, Kalvin NH, Smith JL: Acquired lesions of the fourth cranial nerve. *Brain* 93:567–574, 1970.

Carpenter MB: *Core text of neuroanatomy*. Baltimore, 1978, Waverly Press.

Daniels DL, Kneeland JB, Shimakawa, et al: MR imaging of the optic nerve and chiasm. *Radiology* 152:79–83, 1984.

Daniels DL, Pech P, Pojunas KW, et al: Trigeminal nerve: correlation with MR imaging. *Radiology* 159:577–583, 1986.

Depper MH, Truit CL, Dreisbach JN, et al: Isolated abducens nerve palsy: MR imaging findings. *Am J Roentgenol* 160:837–841, 1993.

Flannigan BD, Bradley WG, Mazziotta JC, et al: Magnetic resonance imaging of the brain stem: normal structure and basic functional anatomy. *Radiology* 154:375–383, 1985.

Gilman S, Winans SS: *Manter and Gatz's essentials of clinical neuroanatomy and neurophysiology*. Philadelphia, 1982, FA Davis.

Hardin CW, Harnsberger HR: The radiographic evaluation of trigeminal neuropathy. *Semin Ultrasound CT MR* 8:214–239, 1987.

Harnsberger HR: Cranial nerve imaging. *Semin Ultrasound CT MR* 8:163–313, 1987.

Hershey BL, Peyster RG: Imaging of cranial nerve II. *Semin Ultrasound CT MR* 8:164–184, 1987.

Hutchins L, Harnsberger HR, Hardin CW, et al: The radiologic assessment of trigeminal neuropathy. *AJNR* 10:1031–1038, 1989.

Hutchins L, Harnsberger HR, Jacobs J et al: Trigeminal neuralgia (Tic Douloureux): MR imaging assessment. *Radiology* 175:837–841, 1990.

Kalovidouris A, Mancuso AA, Dillon WP: A CT-clinical approach to patients with symptoms related to the V, VII, IX–XII cranial nerves and cervical sympathetic plexus. *Radiology* 151:671–676, 1984.

Keane JR: Fourth nerve palsy: historical review and study of 215 inpatients. *Neurology* 43:2439–2443, 1993.

Kwan ES, Laucella M, Hedges TR, et al: A clinico-neuroradiologic approach to third cranial nerve palsies. *AJNR* 8:459–468, 1987.

Laine FJ, Braun IF, Jensen ME, et al: Perineural tumor extension through the foramen ovale: evaluation with MR imaging. *Radiology* 174:65–71, 1990.

Li C, Yousem DM, Doty RL, et al: Neuroimaging in patients with olfactory dysfunction. *Am J Roentgenol* 162:411–418, 1994.

Mark AS, Blake P, Atlas SW, et al: Gd-DTPA enhancement of the cisternal portion of the oculomotor nerve on MR imaging. *AJNR* 13:1463–1470, 1992.

Pansky B: The neuroanatomic basis of face pain. The fifth (trigeminal) nerve. *Postgrad Med* 776:101–111, 1984.

Peyster RG, Hoover ED: *Computerized tomography in orbital disease and neuroophthalmology.* Chicago, 1984, Year Book Medical Publishers.

Rucker CW: The courses of paralysis of the third, fourth, and sixth cranial nerves. *Am J Ophthalmol* 61:1293–1298, 1966.

Ruff RL, Weiner SN, Leigh RJ: Magnetic resonance imaging in patients with diplopia. *Invest Radiol* 21:311–319, 1986.

Rush JA, Younge BR: Paralysis of the cranial nerves III, IV, and VI: cause and prognosis in 1,000 cases. *Arch Ophthalmol* 99:76–79, 1982.

Samii M, Jannetta P: *The cranial nerves: anatomy, pathology, pathophysiology, diagnosis, and treatment.* New York, 1981, Springer-Verlag.

Suzuki M, Takashima T, Kadoya M, et al: MR imaging of olfactory bulbs and tracts. *AJNR* 10:955–957, 1989.

Tash RR, Sze G, Leslie DR: Trigeminal neuralgia: MR imaging features. *Radiology* 172:767–770, 1989.

Yousem DM, Atlas SW, Grossman RI, et al: MR imaging of Tolosa-Hunt syndrome. *AJNR* 10:1181–1184, 1989.

19

The Lower Cranial Nerves

CRITICAL IMAGING QUESTIONS:
THE LOWER CRANIAL NERVES

1. What are the three special functions of the facial nerve other than movement of the muscles responsible for facial expression? How can these functions be used to localize a lesion topographically along the length of the facial nerve?
2. What is the typical appearance of the facial nerve when affected by Bell's palsy on T1-weighted, enhanced MRI scans?
3. What are you looking for when you image a patient with hemifacial spasm under consideration for possible exploratory surgery of the cerebellopontine angle?
4. Name the principal components of the acoustic pathway. What is the major decussation of this pathway? Where is it found?
5. Describe a method allowing the imager to divide the vagus nerve into halves to expedite imaging in a patient with hoarseness.
6. What are the symptoms of a proximal vagus nerve lesion? What are the symptoms of a distal vagus nerve lesion?
7. Why is MRI a better choice for imaging in most patients with signs or symptoms that suggest cranial neuropathy?
8. If the hypoglossal nerve is injured and no lesion found in the brain stem, cisterns, or skull base, how far below the skull base must the examination extend so that a clinically occult lesion is not missed?

Answers to these questions are found in the text beside the question number (Q#) in the margin.

THE LOWER CRANIAL NERVES (VII–XII)

A. Introduction.

1. The twelve cranial nerves are subdivided into upper (i.e., cranial nerves I through VI) and lower (i.e., cranial nerves VII through XII) groups to simplify the task of relearning this material.
2. This chapter reviews the lower cranial nerves, with specific attention given to:
   a. Normal anatomy.
   b. Function and dysfunction.
   c. Imaging problems unique to each nerve.
3. Cranial nerves VII (i.e., facial nerve) and VIII (i.e., vestibulocochlear nerve) are discussed first. Both nerves exit the lower pons, cross the cerebellopontine angle, and enter the temporal bone through the internal auditory canal. As a result, the two nerves can be considered a subset of the lower cranial nerve group (Table 19-1).
   a. Cranial nerve VIII is covered at great length in Chapter 20. In this chapter only the salient teaching points will be reviewed.
4. Cranial nerves IX (i.e., glossopharyngeal), X (i.e., vagus), and XI (i.e., spinal accessory) compose a second subset of the lower cranial nerve group because of their common medullary nuclear origins, mutual exit through the jugular foramen (Table 19-1), and travel through the nasopharyngeal carotid space.
   a. Of this subgroup the vagus nerve is by far the most important to the imager, because it has such complex functions and malfunctions. This handbook concentrates on an imaging approach to patients with vagal neuropathy.
5. Cranial nerve XII (i.e., hypoglossal nerve) is best considered alone because of its unique nuclear origin, skull base exit, and peripheral function.

Table 19-1   Skull Base Passages of the Lower Cranial Nerves

Cranial Nerve	Skull Base Passage
Facial nerve	Internal auditory canal (anterior–superior portion)
	Stylomastoid foramen
Vestibulocochlear nerve	Internal auditory canal
Superior vestibular branch	Posterior–superior portion
Inferior vestibular branch	Posterior–inferior portion
Cochlear branch	Anterior–inferior portion (modiolus)
Glossopharyngeal nerve	Jugular foramen (pars nervosa)
Vagus nerve	Jugular foramen (pars vascularis)
Spinal accessory nerve	Jugular foramen (pars vascularis)
Hypoglossal nerve	Hypoglossal canal

B. Facial nerve (i.e., cranial nerve VII).

1. Normal anatomy (Figs. 19-1 and 19-2*A,B,C*).

   a. Global perspective.

   1) The facial nerve is comprised of a larger motor root and a smaller sensory root (i.e., nervus intermedius) (Fig. 19-2*A,B*).

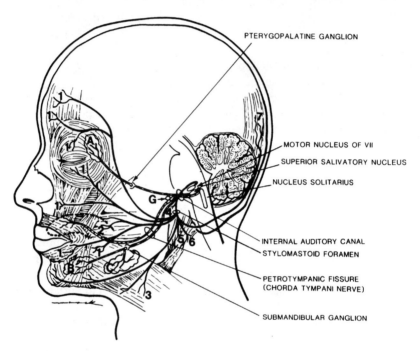

PTERYGOPALATINE GANGLION

MOTOR NUCLEUS OF VII

SUPERIOR SALIVATORY NUCLEUS

NUCLEUS SOLITARIUS

INTERNAL AUDITORY CANAL

STYLOMASTOID FORAMEN

PETROTYMPANIC FISSURE
(CHORDA TYMPANI NERVE)

SUBMANDIBULAR GANGLION

Fig. 19-1 The three major components of the facial nerve. The branchial motor component (*solid line*), which arises from the motor nucleus in the pontine tegmentum, supplies motor innervation to the muscles of facial expression: (*1*); the buccinator (*2*), platysma (*3*), stapedius (*4*), and stylohyoid (*5*) muscles; posterior belly of the digastric muscle (*6*); and the occipitalis muscle (*7*). The visceral motor, or parasympathetic, component (*dashed line*) arises from the superior salivatory nucleus of the pontine tegmentum, supplying autonomic fibers that control the function of the lacrimal (*A*), sublingual (*B*), and submandibular (*C*) glands of the face. The special sensory component (*dotted line*) carries information from the taste buds of the anterior two thirds of the tongue. Fibers of this component first run with the lingual nerve, then separate from it to enter the temporal bone as the chorda tympani nerve. The cell bodies of the special sensory component are located in the geniculate ganglion (*G*). The fibers terminate in the solitary nucleus of the of the pontomedullary tegmentum. (From Harnsberger HR: *Unlocking the brain stem, basal cisterns and skull base through MR imaging of the cranial nerves.* In Stark DD, Bradley WG, editors: *Syllabus. A categorical course in diagnostic radiology: MR imaging.* Radiological Society of North America. Used with permission.)

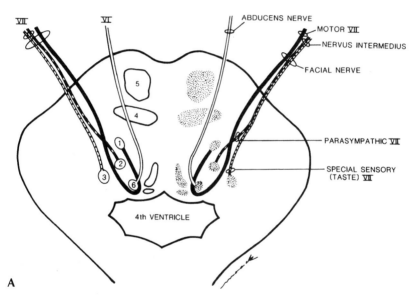

Fig. 19-2   **A**, Axial perspective of the lower pons illustrating the nuclei and rootlets of the intramedullary and cisternal portions of the facial nerve. The branchial motor portion (*solid line*) of the facial nerve, which is the largest portion, originates in the motor nucleus (*1*) in the pontine tegmentum. This fiber group loops dorsally around the abducens nucleus (*6*), then turns to exit the ventrolateral pons at the pontomedullary junction. The nervus intermedius contains the visceral motor, or parasympathetic, fibers (*dashed line*), which supply stimulation to the lacrimal, submandibular, and sublingual glands, and special sensory fibers (*dotted line*) that convey taste information from the anterior two thirds of the tongue. Although the main motor component and the nervus intermedius are closely approximated along their course, the nervus intermedius is bounded by its own distinct fascial sheath. *2*, Superior salivatory nucleus; *3*, solitary nucleus; *4*, medial

(*continued*)

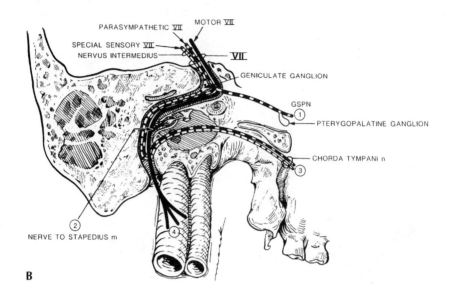

B

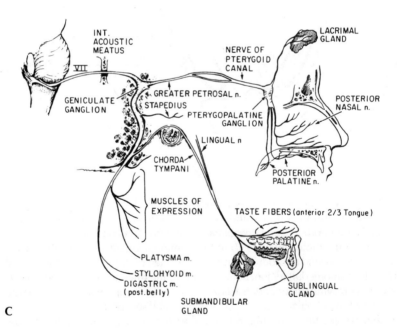

C

Fig. 19-2 (*continued*)   lemniscus; *5*, corticospinal tract. **B,** Facial nerve components as they interact in the temporal bone. The branchial motor portion (*solid line*) leaves a single branch (*2*) to the stapedius muscle in its midmastoid section before continuing into the face to innervate the muscles of facial expression (*4*). The parasympathetic portion (*dashed line*) branches at the anterior genu to sup-

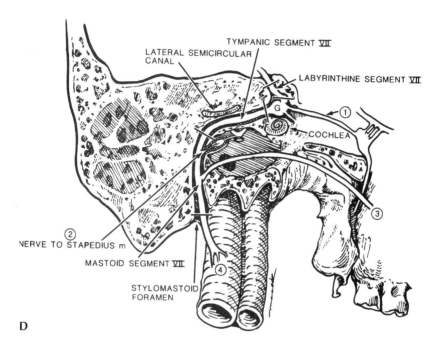

TYMPANIC SEGMENT VII
LATERAL SEMICIRCULAR CANAL
LABYRINTHINE SEGMENT VII
G
COCHLEA
①
③
② NERVE TO STAPEDIUS m
MASTOID SEGMENT VII
④
STYLOMASTOID FORAMEN

D

ply the lacrimal gland (*1*) via the greater superficial petrosal nerve (*GSPN*) before continuing as part of the chorda tympani nerve to supply secretomotor function to the submandibular and sublingual glands. The special sensory fibers (*dotted line*) constitute the major part of the chorda tympani nerve. These fibers convey taste both from the anterior two thirds of the tongue (*3*) and centrally. Their cell bodies are concentrated at the anterior genu of the facial nerve as the geniculate ganglion. **C**, Special functions of the peripheral facial nerve in topographic order. *1*, Lacrimation (greater superficial petrosal nerve); *2*, stapedius reflex (stapedius nerve); *3*, anterior two thirds of tongue taste (chorda tympani facial nerve). (From Disbro MA, Harnsberger HR, Osborn AG: Peripheral facial nerve dysfunction. *Radiology* 155:659–663, 1985. Used with permission.) **D**, Sagittal view of the facial nerve as it traverses the temporal bone. The first intratemporal segment is the labyrinthine segment. At the anterior geniculate ganglion (*G*) the nerve turns abruptly in a posterior direction to become the tympanic segment (*horizontal segment*). Note that much of the tympanic segment passes just under the lateral semicircular canal. When it reaches the posterior genu, the nerve turns inferiorly to become the mastoid segment (*descending segment*). *1*, Greater superficial petrosal nerve; *2*, nerve to stapedius muscle; *3*, chorda tympani nerve; *4*, main motor trunk of the facial nerve.

2) The motor root innervates the muscles of facial expression, stapedius, platysma, and posterior belly of the digastric muscles (Table 19-2).

Table 19-2   Motor Innervation by Individual Cranial Nerve

Cranial Nerve	Muscles	Muscle Function
Facial nerve	Muscles of facial expression	Facial expressions
	Buccinator	Keeps fluid from pooling in vestibule of mouth
	Posterior belly of digastric	Mouth opening, chin retraction
	Platysma	Facial expression
	Anterior scalp	Facial expression
	Stylohyoid	Retracts and elevates hyoid bone
	Stapedius	Acoustic damping
Glossopharyngeal nerve	Stylopharyngeus	Laryngopharynx elevator
Vagus nerve	Muscles of soft palate excluding tensor palati	Flap valve, can block oropharynx or nasopharynx
	Pharnygeal constrictors Superior Middle Inferior	Swallowing
	Cricothyroid	Speech, prevents aspiration
	Endolaryngeal muscles	
Spinal accessory nerve	Sternocleidomastoid	Head movement
	Trapezius	Scapular rotation
Hypoglossal nerve	Intrinsic tongue muscles	Change tongue shape
	Extrinsic tongue muscles Genioglossus Hyoglossus Styloglossus	Change tongue position
	Geniohyoid	
	Thyrohyoid (strap muscle)	Laryngeal depression
	Other strap muscles through ansa cervicalis	

3) The nervus intermedius contains:
   a) General visceral efferent secretomotor fibers (i.e., parasympathetic fibers) to the lacrimal, submandibular, and sublingual glands (Fig. 19-2*A,B*).
   b) Special visceral afferent fibers conveying taste from the anterior two thirds of the tongue.

b. Nuclear origins (Fig. 19-2*A*).
  1) The motor nucleus is a nuclear column in the ventrolateral pontine tegmentum.
  2) The superior salivatory nucleus in the pons is the site of origin of the parasympathetic fibers, which terminate in and stimulate both the lacrimal gland and the sublingual and submandibular glands.
  3) The nucleus solitarius (i.e., solitary nucleus) is the end point of the fibers that convey taste sensation from the anterior two thirds of the tongue. The cell bodies of these fibers are found in the geniculate ganglion, which is found in the geniculate fossa of the temporal bone.

c. Course.
  1) Motor fibers of the facial nerve loop dorsally around the sixth nerve nucleus in the lower pons (Fig. 19-2*A*), then course ventrolaterally to exit the area as the more anterior nerve bundle of the cerebellopontine angle. The intermediate nerve fibers usually join the motor root of the facial nerve just as they exit the brain stem.
   a) The more posterior nerve bundle in the cerebellopontine angle is the vestibulocochlear nerve.
  2) After entering the internal auditory canal, cranial nerve VII lies in the anterosuperior quadrant of the fundus of the canal. The nerve follows a circuitous path through the temporal bone (Fig. 19-2*B*), exiting the skull base through the stylomastoid foramen.
  3) The extracranial facial nerve runs anterolaterally into the substance of the parotid gland, passing superficial to the retromandibular vein.
   a) The nerve begins to subdivide into multiple, extracranial branches shortly after leaving the temporal bone, as it first enters the substance of the parotid gland.

d. Branches (Fig. 19-2*C,D,E*).

Q#1

1) Greater superficial petrosal nerve.
   a) This nerve branches from the main trunk of the facial nerve at the geniculate ganglion. It courses anteromedially along the anterior margin of the temporal bone.

 b) The nerve carries parasympathetic fibers subserving the function of lacrimation.
 c) Injury to this branch is manifested as impairment of ipsilateral lacrimation.
2) Stapedius nerve.
 a) The stapedius nerve branches in the high mastoid segment of the facial nerve.
 b) The nerve provides motor innervation to the stapedius muscle.
 c) Injury to this branch is manifested as hyperacusis.
3) Chorda tympani nerve.
 a) This nerve branches from cranial nerve VII just before its exit from the stylomastoid foramen. It courses across the middle ear cavity to exit the anterior temporal bone.
 b) The nerve carries fibers of taste from the anterior two thirds of the tongue. These fibers travel with the lingual branch of the mandibular division of the trigeminal nerve.
 c) Injury to this nerve results in loss of taste sensation in the anterior two thirds of the tongue and of parasympathetic stimulation of the submandibular and sublingual glands.
 e. Vascular supply.
1) Circumneural arteriovenous plexus.
 a) The circumneural arteriovenous plexus is a lush arterial–capillary–venous plexus that supplies the vascular needs of the facial nerve.
 b) The plexus has three components. Its anterior portion comes from an arterial branch of the middle meningeal artery. The middle portion is supplied by an arterial branch off the ascending pharyngeal artery. The posterior portion is supplied by the stylomastoid artery, which arises from the occipital artery.
2) The least well-vascularized portion of the intratemporal facial nerve is the labyrinthine segment.
3) Given the lush nature of facial nerve vascular supply provided by the circumneural arteriovenous plexus, it is not surprising that spotty, asymmetric, mild enhancement of the facial nerve normally is seen on T1-weighted, enhanced MRI scans through the temporal bone.
4) This normal, spotty, mild enhancement should not be confused with the intense, holoneural, intratemporal facial nerve enhancement commonly seen in association with Bell's palsy (discussed later).
2. Clinical manifestations of facial nerve injury.
 a. The term *peripheral facial nerve paralysis* implies injury to the facial nerve from the level of the brain stem nucleus to its motor end

plates in the face. All of the ipsilateral muscles of facial expression are paralyzed in a peripheral injury.

    1) In comparison, the term *central facial nerve paralysis* refers to a supranuclear injury that manifests itself as paralysis of the contralateral muscles of facial expression with sparing of the forehead muscles.

  b. Within the spectrum of peripheral facial nerve injuries, if the lesion is proximal to the geniculate ganglion, the three special functions of lacrimation, sound dampening, and taste will be absent. See section 3 in this chapter for further discussion.

3. Imaging issues.

  a. Whenever the temporal bone or the patient is imaged because of peripheral facial nerve paralysis, the entire facial nerve canal *must* be visualized and inspected radiographically.

  b. During imaging of facial nerve paralysis with either CT or MRI, the most common error is to complete an unfocused brain scan without attempting to localize the lesion along the course of the facial nerve. The scan is judged normal, with the occult lesion remaining undiagnosed in the temporal bone or parotid gland.

  c. A lesion affecting the facial nerve should be localized precisely to one of the following segments:

    1) Intraaxial segment. Facial nerve nucleus and tracts within the lower pons.

    2) Cerebellopontine angle–internal auditory canal segment. Facial nerve spanning its root exit from the pons to its exit from the fundus of the internal auditory canal.

    3) Labyrinthine segment. Short segment curling anteriorly over the top of the cochlea. Terminates in the anterior genu (i.e., geniculate ganglion).

    4) Tympanic segment. Facial nerve from the anterior to posterior genu. Along this segment the nerve travels just under the lateral (i.e., horizontal) semicircular canal in the medial wall of the tympanic cavity.

    5) Mastoid segment. Facial nerve from the posterior genu to the stylomastoid foramen.

    6) Parotid segment. Extracranial segment of the facial nerve dividing the parotid gland into superficial and deep lobes.

Q#1

  d. The facial nerve has four major functions that may be used to localize topographically a lesion along its course (Fig. 19-2). From central to peripheral these functions are:

    1) Lacrimation (via greater superficial petrosal nerve).

2) Stapedius reflex. Sound dampening.
3) Anterior two thirds of tongue taste (via chorda tympani nerve to lingual nerve to oral tongue).
4) Muscles of facial expression.
  e. Generalizations that allow focused imaging along the facial nerve include:
    1) First, decide if the lesion is central (i.e., supranuclear) or peripheral. If peripheral, the following issues are considered.
    2) If cranial nerve VI also is involved with peripheral nerve VII, the lower pons is the site of the lesion (i.e., VII circles the sixth nerve nucleus on its way out of the brain stem). (Fig. 19–2A).
    3) If cranial nerve VIII also is involved, the cerebellopontine angle–internal auditory canal area needs careful inspection.
    4) If the first three functions are variably involved with an isolated peripheral nerve VII, a temporal bone lesion should be suspected.
    5) Finally, if nerve VII is involved by itself with preservation of the three special functions, extracranial nerve VII (i.e., intraparotid) is implicated.
4. Lesions.
  a. Lesions of the brain stem (i.e., pons) and cerebellopontine angle cistern that cause peripheral facial nerve paralysis are not unique to the facial nerve. Intraaxial and cisternal lesions also cause cranial neuropathy depending on their anatomic location.
    1) The best description of the intraaxial and cisternal lesions causing facial nerve paralysis is in Chapter 20, where they are reviewed relative to vestibulocochlear neuropathy.
    2) Brain stem and cisternal lesions are summarized in Tables 19-3 and 19-4, respectively.
  b. Lesions causing peripheral facial nerve paralysis and found within the temporal bone and parotid space are thoroughly discussed in Chapters 16 and 4, respectively.
  c. Table 19-5 summarizes the unique lesions of the temporal bone and parotid space that cause peripheral facial nerve paralysis.
  d. Bell's palsy.
    1) One lesion of particular importance in facial nerve imaging is Bell's palsy. Whether and when to image patients with peripheral facial nerve paralysis hinges on a complete understanding of typical and atypical Bell's palsy. For this reason a complete discussion of this lesion is included here.
    2) Clinical presentation.
      a) Acute onset of peripheral facial nerve paralysis involving the muscles of facial expression and variably involving the three special functions of the peripheral facial nerve.

**Table 19-3   Differential Diagnosis of Brain Stem Lesions Causing
Cranial Neuropathy**

Tumor
   Chiasmal–hypothalamic glioma (II)*
   Primary brain stem glioma
   Metastatic tumor
   Lymphoma
   Syringobulbia (V, IX–XII)

Inflammatory
   Multiple sclerosis (II, V, VII, VIII)
   Amyotrophic lateral sclerosis (IX–XII)
   Abscess
   Acute disseminated encephalomyelitis

Vascular
   Arteriovenous malformation
   Cavernous angioma
   Stroke
   Posterior inferior cerebellar artery (VIII–XI)

Miscellaneous
   Trauma (IV)
   Hemorrhage

*Cranial nerves in parentheses particularly tend to be affected by that particular lesion.

   b) The natural course of untreated Bell's palsy is complete
remission in 70% of cases. Complete and permanent facial
palsy in Bell's palsy is extremely rare, and this should trigger
a search for another underlying etiology (i.e., MRI of the
facial nerve).

3) Pathophysiology.

   a) The most accepted hypothesis suggests that Bell's palsy
results from viral infection of the facial nerve.

   b) Herpes simplex I and varicella-zoster are the most common
causative agents.

   c) Reactivation of a dormant virus in the geniculate ganglion,
which is the location of cell bodies for the anterior two thirds
of tongue taste, is a pathogenic mechanism consistent with
numerous observations regarding this disease.

   d) In the meager pathologic material available, a cellular inflammatory infiltrate of the facial nerve, some degree of neural
degeneration, and hypervascularity have been observed.

Table 19-4   Differential Diagnosis of Cisternal Lesions Causing Cranial Neuropathy

Inflammatory
Granulomatous meningitis
   Sarcoidosis
   Tuberculosis or bacterial

Vascular
Vertebrobasilar dolichoectasia
Arteriovenous fistula with venous verix
Vertebral artery aneurysm
Posterior inferior cerebellar artery aneurysm (VI)*
Anterior inferior cerebellar artery aneurysm (VII, VIII)
Posterior communicating artery aneurysm (III)
Microvascular infarct (III, IV, VI)

Tumor
Meningioma
Schwannoma, neurofibroma (VIII)
Epidermoid (VIII)
Perineural tumor spread (V)

Miscellaneous
Trauma (IV)
Subarachnoid hemorrhage

*Cranial nerves in parentheses particularly tend to be affected by that particular lesion.

   e) Facial nerve dysfunction appears to result from an entrapment neuropathy, which in turn results from neural edema within the tight confines of the osseous facial nerve canal.
   f) Compression of the facial nerve within the bony canal may disrupt nerve function either by vascular congestion with ischemia or by impairment of axoplasmic flow.
4) Imaging issues.
   a) The typical patient with acute onset of peripheral facial nerve paralysis (i.e., Bell's palsy) need not undergo radiographic examination in the initial phase of the illness. Imaging of this common malady is not cost-effective, because the yield of positive results is extremely low.
   b) Only when recovery is not occurring and decompressive surgery is anticipated should contrast-enhanced MRI be performed. In this setting, the exam is done to exclude other possible etiologies and to look for typical MRI features confirming the diagnosis of Bell's palsy.

Table 19-5   Peripheral Facial Nerve Paralysis

Intraaxial
  See Table 19-3

Extraaxial
  Cerebellopontine angle–internal auditory canal (see Table 19-4)

Intratemporal
  Trauma
    Fracture through nerve VII canal
  Tumor
    Primary cholesteatoma (epidermoid)
    Paraganglioma
    Hemangioma
    Facial nerve schwannoma
    Adenomatous tumor
    Metastasis
  Inflammation
    Bell's palsy
    Otitis media
    Malignant otitis externa
    Cholesterol granuloma

Extracranial (Parotid Space)
  Trauma
    Forceps delivery
    Penetrating trauma
    Parotid surgery
  Tumor
    Primary parotid malignancy
    Metastatic tumor
  Inflammation
    Malignant otitis externa

Miscellaneous
  Möbius' syndrome
  Diabetes mellitus
  Myasthenia gravis
  Hyperparathyroidism

  c) Patients with atypical Bell's palsy should be examined with
      enhanced MRI to look for a clinically occult cause of the
      paralysis. Atypical Bell's palsy is defined as persistent (i.e.,
      > 4 months), progressive, or recurring peripheral facial nerve
      paralysis. Associated symptoms signaling involvement of
      other cranial nerves also indicate atypical Bell's palsy.

    d) Axial and coronal enhanced, fat-saturated, thin-section (i.e., 3 mm), contiguous T1-weighted MRI scans of the IAC–temporal bone area form the mainstay of imaging during atypical Bell's palsy. Whole-brain, T2-weighted images looking for intraaxial causes such as multiple sclerosis also must be done. The lower axial T2-weighted images as well as the coronal postcontrast images will give sufficient parotid information in most cases.

Q#2

5) MRI appearance in Bell's palsy.
    a) Diffuse, intense enhancement of the facial nerve from the apex of the internal auditory canal (i.e., premeatal segment) to the stylomastoid foramen is the rule in Bell's palsy. Note that enhancement usually is particularly well seen in the labyrinthine segment, an area that normally never enhances.
    b) Enhancement should be asymmetric toward the side of the facial nerve paralysis. It should not in any way be nodular. If nodular enhancement is seen, other tumor-based differential diagnoses must be considered.
    c) Contrast this appearance to the mild, patchy enhancement often normally seen along the facial nerve secondary to the normal circumneural arteriovenous plexus. Normal enhancement of the facial nerve does not occur within the apex of the internal auditory canal (i.e., premeatal segment) or within the labyrinthine segment of the intratemporal facial nerve canal.

Q#3

  e. Hemifacial spasm.
    1) Clinical features.
      a) Hemifacial spasm is a disease of middle and later life. It is characterized by involuntary, paroxysmal, painless contractions of muscles innervated by the facial nerve.
      b) Patients failing conservative management undergo surgical visualization of the root exit zone of the facial nerve, with surgical displacement of the compressive vessel.
    2) Pathophysiology.
      a) Less than 2% of hemifacial spasms result from tumor or arteriovenous fistula/malformation. This number may be much higher in medical centers that perform surgical correction of vascular loop syndromes.
      b) Compression of the facial nerve root exit zone on the caudal brain stem by loops of otherwise normal appearing vessels is

the most frequent cause of hemifacial spasm. Pulsatile compression is thought to cause focal demyelination at the junction between the central and peripheral myelin, leading to increased neuronal discharge in the facial nucleus via ephaptic (i.e., nonsynaptic nerve impulse transmission via direct membrane to membrane contact) transmission and/or antidromic (i.e., retrograde nerve impulse transmission) stimulation.

   c) Primary offending arteries include the vertebral, posterior inferior cerebellar (PICA) and anterior inferior cerebellar (AICA) arteries.

3) Imaging issues in hemifacial spasm.

   a) MRI with MRA is the recommended imaging tool in patients with hemifacial spasm.

   b) MR technique should include:

      i) Whole-brain, T2-weighted imaging. This excludes multiple sclerosis and other intraaxial causes.

      ii) MRA focused on the posterior fossa. This should be done before contrast. Source images need to be reviewed as well as the reconstruction of projectional MRA. Source images display better than projectional images the vessel relationship to the facial nerve bundle in the cerebellopontine angle cistern.

      iii) Axial and coronal postcontrast, fat-saturated, T1-weighted images focused to the internal auditory canal and temporal bone. These sequences look for cisternal, temporal bone, and parotid lesions that initially may present as hemifacial spasm.

4) MRI findings in hemifacial spasm.

   a) Rarely, an intraaxial (e.g., multiple sclerosis), cisternal (e.g., schwannoma), intratemporal (e.g., hemangioma), or extracranial (e.g., parotid malignancy) disorder will present as hemifacial spasm. In all cases these causes must be sought so that the image inspection process does not overly focus on the root exit zone in the cerebellopontine angle cistern.

   b) MRA source images best display the offending artery. MRA projection images help to assess the complex architecture of the vertebrobasilar system.

   c) In my experience the most common finding on MRI with MRA in patients with hemifacial spasm is a tortuous vertebral artery swinging up into the cerebellopontine angle cistern, with the ipsilateral PICA artery actually making contact with the root exit zone of the facial nerve.

    d) Any of the arteries of the vertebrobasilar system, however, can be the culprit. The vertebral artery, PICA, AICA, PICA–AICA complex, and even the basilar artery itself have been implicated.

C. Vestibulocochlear nerve (i.e., cranial nerve VIII).

1. Comment.
    a. The vestibulocochlear nerve is covered at great length in Chapter 20.
    b. Only the major points of interest are emphasized here.
2. Normal anatomy.
    a. Nuclear origins of the auditory component.
        1) Dorsal and ventral cochlear nuclei are found on the lateral aspect of the inferior cerebellar peduncle (i.e., restiform body).
        2) These two nuclei receive axons from neurons, with their cell bodies in the spinal ganglion found in the modiolus of the cochlea.
    b. Nerve course.
        1) After leaving the cochlea, the auditory axons traverse the internal auditory canal in the anteroinferior quadrant.
        2) The vestibulocochlear nerve then crosses the cerebellopontine angle cistern at the posterior nerve bundle (i.e., cranial nerve VII is anterior) to enter the brain stem at the junction of the medulla and pons.
        3) As the entering nerve fibers pierce the brain stem, they bifurcate, making synapses with both cochlear nuclei.
2. Normal anatomy of the acoustic pathway.
    a. The acoustic pathway traditionally is divided along the lines of sensorineural hearing loss, into sensory (i.e., cochlear) and neural (i.e., retrocochlear) components.
    b. The sensory portion is comprised of the cochlea alone.
    c. The neural portion is by far the more complex, involving multiple components as it passes from the cochlea to the temporal lobe (Fig. 19-3).

Q#4

    d. The major pieces of the neural portion, from distal to proximal, include:
        1) Vestibulocochlear nerve.
        2) Ventral and dorsal cochlear nuclei.
        3) Trapezoid body. Major decussation of the acoustic pathway, found in the pontine tegmentum.
        4) Lateral lemniscus.
        5) Inferior colliculus.

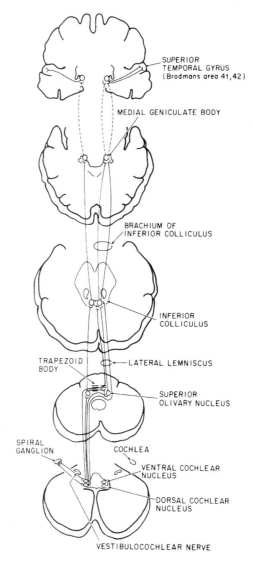

Fig. 19-3   Composite of the complete acoustic pathway from the cochlea to the superior temporal gyrus. Note that the major decussation is at the level of the pons through the trapezoid body. (From Armington WG, Harnsberger HR, Smoker WRK, et al: Normal and diseased acoustic pathway: evaluation with MR Imaging. *Radiology* 167:509–515, 1988. Used with permission.)

       6) Medial geniculate body.

       7) Superior temporal gyrus.

3. Clinical manifestations of acoustic pathway injury.

    a. Sensorineural hearing loss and tinnitus (i.e., ringing or roaring in the ear) are the principal symptoms of injury to nerve VIII.

    b. If unilateral sensorineural hearing loss is present, the injury has occurred somewhere between the cochlea and the cochlear nuclei of the brain stem.

    c. Unilateral involvement of the auditory pathway above the cochlear nuclei usually causes bilateral sensorineural hearing loss, with that loss being greater in the ear contralateral to the side of the lesion.

    d. Cortical acoustic pathway lesions, which rarely cause disruption of auditory function, may cause auditory agnosia (i.e., sounds are perceived but interpretation is impaired).

4. Imaging issues in sensorineural hearing loss.

    a. Audiometric testing now is sensitive enough to localize the lesion causing sensorineural hearing loss to either the sensory or neural component of the acoustic pathway.

    b. When the lesion is suspected to be in the sensory (i.e., cochlea) component, MRI and CT both are suggested as the preferred imaging method. See Chapter 20 for further discussion.

    c. When the lesion is suspected to be in the neural (i.e., retrocochlear) region, MRI is the undisputed procedure of choice.

5. Vestibulocochlear nerve lesions.

    a. For complete discussion of the lesions that cause sensorineural hearing loss, see Chapter 20.

    b. For complete differential diagnosis of lesions that cause sensorineural hearing loss, see Table 20-1.

D. Glossopharyngeal nerve (i.e., cranial nerve IX)

1. Normal anatomy.

    a. Nuclear origins.

       1) The glossopharyngeal nuclei are in the upper and middle medulla (Fig. 19-4).

       2) Motor fibers originate in the nucleus ambiguus.

       3) Sensory fibers terminate in the tractus solitarius.

       4) Parasympathetic fibers originate in the inferior salivatory nucleus.

    b. Nerve course.

       1) The glossopharyngeal nerve leaves the lateral medulla in the postolivary sulcus, passes through the basal cistern as the IX–X–bulbar XI nerve complex, then diverges alone into the more anterior pars nervosa of the jugular foramen.

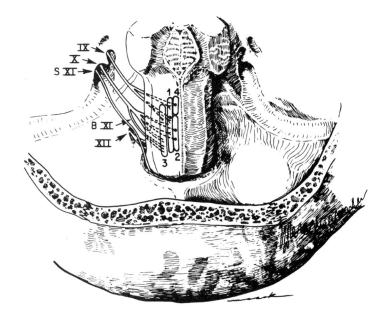

Fig. 19-4   Normal medullary origins and cisternal courses of the glossopharyn-geal (*IX*), vagus (*X*), spinal accessory (*XI*), and hypoglossal (*XII*) nerves. Note that the glossopharyngeal nerve passes through the more anterior part of the jugular foramen (pars nervosa), while the vagus and spinal accessory nerves pass through the more posterior pars vascularis. The hypoglossal nerve passes through its own foramen, the hypoglossal canal, more inferiorly. *1*, Solitary nucleus; *2*, dorsal motor nucleus of tenth cranial nerve; *3*, nucleus ambiguus; *4*, salivatory nucleus; *BXI*, bulbar root of eleventh cranial nerve; *SXI*, spinal root of eleventh cranial nerve. (From Jacobs JM, Harnsberger HR, Lufkin RB, et al: CT and MRI in the eval-uation of vagal neuropathy. *Radiology* 164:97–102, 1987. Used with permission.)

    2) Cranial nerve IX exits the jugular foramen in the anterior nasopharyngeal carotid space, curving forward around the lat-eral side of the stylopharyngeus muscle to terminate in the pos-terior sublingual space at the floor of the mouth (Fig. 19-5).

  c. Nerve branches.

    1) The glossopharyngeal nerve has five distinct branches.

      a) Tympanic branch (i.e., Jacobsen's nerve). Sensory to middle ear and bony eustachian tube; parasympathetic to parotid gland.

      b) Stylopharyngeus branch. Motor to the stylopharyngeus mus-cle (Table 19-2).

      c) Sinus nerve. Supplies the carotid sinus and carotid body (i.e., pressor and chemoreceptors).

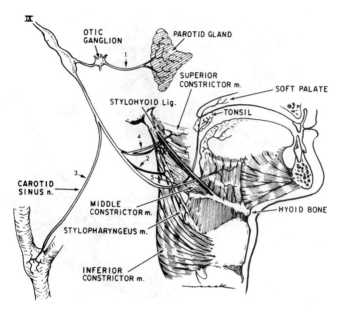

Fig. 19-5 Extracranial branches of the glossopharyngeal nerve (*IX*). After passing through the jugular foramen, the glossopharyngeal nerve continues in the nasopharyngeal carotid space, then diverges anteroinferiorly. Note that this nerve only has one motor innervation. As a result, injury to the nerve cannot be detected easily through recognition of a motor atrophy pattern in the extracranial head and neck. *1*, Tympanic branch; *2*, stylopharyngeal motor branch; *3*, sinus nerve; *4*, pharyngeal branches; *5*, lingual branch. (From Remley K, Harnsberger HR, Smoker WRK, et al: CT and MRI in the evaluation of glossopharyngeal, vagal, and spinal accessory neuropathy. *Semin Ultrasound CT MR* 8:284–300, 1987. Used with permission.)

       d) Pharyngeal branches. Sensory to the posterior oropharynx and soft palate (i.e., afferent limb of gag reflex).

       e) Lingual branch. Sensory and taste to posterior one third of the tongue.

2. Clinical manifestations of injury to nerve IX.

    a. Isolated glossopharyngeal neuropathy is exceedingly rare. Injury to this nerve usually is associated with vagus nerve injury.

    b. If the glossopharyngeal nerve alone is injured, the following symptoms and signs result:

       1) Otalgia. Referred pain along the tympanic branch to the ear.

       2) Dysphagia. Stylopharyngeus muscle dysfunction.

       3) Tachycardia and bradycardia, hypotension. Sinus nerve dysfunction.

     4) Loss of afferent limb of the gag reflex. Pharyngeal and lingual branch dysfunction.

     5) Loss of taste to posterior one third of the tongue. Lingual branch dysfunction.

3. Imaging issues.

  a. MRI is the method of choice for imaging cranial nerve IX.

  b. Because both the ninth nerve nuclei are mostly shared with the tenth nerve and the cisternal ninth nerve usually is conjoined with the tenth and bulbar eleventh nerves, glossopharyngeal nerve imaging essentially is the same as imaging the proximal tenth nerve.

     1) Refer to section *E3c* and *d* for a discussion of imaging proximal vagal neuropathy.

4. Glossopharyngeal nerve lesions.

  a. The pathologic processes affecting the glossopharyngeal nerve also affect the proximal vagus nerve.

  b. See section *E2b* and Table 19-6.

E. Vagus nerve (i.e., cranial nerve X).

1. Normal anatomy.

  a. Nuclear origins.

     1) The vagus nerve has three nuclear columns in the upper and middle medulla (Fig. 19-4).

     2) Vagal motor fibers to the muscles of the pharynx and larynx originate from the nucleus ambiguus.

     3) Vagal sensory fibers end in the tractus solitarius. The cell bodies of these fibers are in the vagal superior and inferior nodosal ganglion, in the nasopharyngeal carotid space near the skull base.

     4) Parasympathetic secretomotor fibers originate from the dorsal motor nucleus.

  b. Nerve course.

     1) The vagus nerve leaves the lateral medulla in the retroolivary sulcus and traverses the basal cistern conjoined to the ninth and bulbar eleventh cranial nerves to enter the more posterior pars vascularis of the jugular foramen with the spinal eleventh cranial nerve.

     2) After exiting the jugular foramen, the nerve plunges "like a plumb line" along the posterolateral aspect of the carotid artery to the aortopulmonic window of the mediastinum on the left and to the clavicle on the right (Fig. 19-6).

     3) The right recurrent laryngeal nerve turns cephalad around the right subclavian artery, whereas the left recurrent nerve turns cephalad by looping through the aortopulmonic window (Fig.

Table 19-6   Differential Diagnosis of Vagal Neuropathy

Proximal Lesions (Complex IX–XII)
- Intramedullary (nuclear)
  - See Table 19-3
- Cisternal
  - See Table 19-4
- Jugular foramen/suprahyoid carotid space
  - Vascular
    - Jugular vein thrombosis
    - Carotid artery aneurysm
    - Internal carotid artery dissection
  - Inflammatory
    - Malignant otitis externa
    - Carotid space abscess
  - Tumor, benign
    - Paraganglioma
    - Schwannoma, neurofibroma
    - Meningioma
  - Tumor, malignant
    - Nasopharyngeal carcinoma
    - Skull base metastasis
    - Non-Hodgkin lymphoma
    - Rhabdomyosarcoma (pediatric population)

Distal Lesions (Isolated X)
- Infrahyoid neck
  - Miscellaneous
    - Penetrating trauma
    - Thyroid or parathyroid surgery
  - Vascular
    - Jugular vein thrombosis
  - Inflammatory
    - Carotid space abscess
  - Tumor, benign
    - Schwannoma, neurofibroma
    - Thyroid goiter, adenoma, or colloid cyst
  - Tumor, malignant
    - Squamous cell carcinoma, primary or nodal
    - Thyroid malignancy
    - Non-Hodgkin lymphoma
- Mediastinum (*left* isolated X only)
  - Inflammatory
    - Mediastinitis
  - Vascular
    - Aortic arch aneurysm
    - Cardiomegaly
  - Tumor, malignant
    - Bronchogenic carcinoma
    - Non-Hodgkin lymphoma
    - Mediastinal metastasis

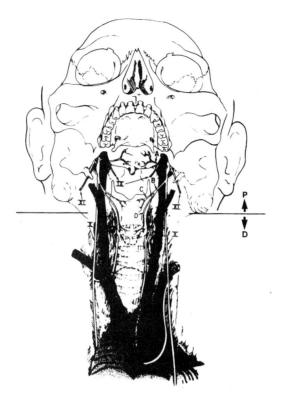

Fig. 19-6 Extracranial portion of vagus nerve and associated cranial nerves IX and XI. The vagus nerve is best considered from an imaging viewpoint as a proximal segment (*Arrow P*) and a distal segment (*Arrow D*). The proximal segment stretches from the brain stem nuclei to the oropharyngeal carotid space. The distal segment is from the oropharyngeal carotid space to the aortopulmonic window on the left and to the cervical thoracic junction on the right. The distal segment also includes the recurrent laryngeal nerve in the tracheoesophageal grooves. Note that the glossopharyngeal nerves (*IX*) and the spinal accessory nerves (*XI*) diverge from the carotid space in the low nasopharynx. Proximal vagal branches: *A*, pharyngeal plexus; *B*, superior laryngeal nerve; *C*, internal laryngeal nerve; *D*, external laryngeal nerve. Distal vagal branch: *E*, recurrent laryngeal nerve. (From Jacobs JM, Harnsberger HR, Lufkin RB, et al: CT and MRI in the evaluation of vagal neuropathy. *Radiology* 164:97–102, 1987. Used with permission.)

19-6). Both reach the larynx via the tracheoesophageal groove.
   c. Vagus nerve branches relevant to head and neck imaging (Table 19-2, Fig. 19-6).
    1) Proximal vagus branches.

a) Pharyngeal plexus. Motor to soft palate (except the tensor tympani muscle) and superior and middle constrictor muscles. Efferent limb of the gag reflex.

b) Superior laryngeal nerve divides into the internal and external laryngeal nerves.

c) Internal laryngeal nerve. Sensory to the hypopharynx and larynx above the true vocal cords.

d) External laryngeal nerve. Motor to inferior constrictor muscle and cricothyroid muscle.

2) Distal vagal branches.

a) Recurrent laryngeal nerve. Motor to inferior constrictor muscle and endolaryngeal muscles. Vocal cord function.

2. Clinical manifestations of vagus nerve injury.

 a. Clinical evidence of vagus nerve injury is best divided into proximal and distal symptom complexes. Injury to the vagus nerve above the hyoid bone produces proximal symptoms; injury distal to the hyoid bone produces distal symptoms.

 b. Proximal injury (above the hyoid bone).

1) With a proximal injury multiple cranial nerves (i.e., IX, X, XI, XII) are involved.

2) Oropharyngeal symptoms are present because of pharyngeal plexus malfunction. These symptoms include:

a) Absent efferent limb of the gag reflex.

b) Uvular deviation away from side of lesion.

3) Endolaryngeal symptoms resulting from recurrent laryngeal nerve malfunction include:

a) Hoarseness.

b) Aspiration from vocal cord malfunction.

c) Dysphagia in cervical esophagus.

 c. Distal injury (below hyoid bone).

1) A distal injury will involve only the vagus nerve and create isolated vagus nerve symptoms, including:

a) No oropharyngeal symptoms, because the pharyngeal plexus is not involved (Fig. 19-6).

b) Endolaryngeal symptoms only.

3. Imaging issues.

 a. All patients with vagus nerve malfunction have some degree of hoarseness. Physical examination includes visualization of the vocal cords. If a larger vocal cord tumor is seen, CT or MRI is used to stage the squamous cell carcinoma.

1) If the vocal cords are normal and no palpable lesion is found in the neck, the occult lesion should be grouped into one of two

separate imaging groups (i.e., proximal or distal) based on results of remaining the clinical examinations.

Q#5

b. Placing each lesion into a proximal or distal imaging group allows the radiologist to split the neck examination into halves—from medulla to hyoid bone (i.e., proximal group), and from hyoid bone to mediastinum (i.e., distal group)—shortening the CT or MRI study.

Q#6

c. This grouping of lesions is easily accomplished using the following criteria:
1) Proximal group (i.e., lesion above hyoid bone).
   a) Complex vagal neuropathy (i.e., cranial nerve IX, X, XI, XII).
   b) Oropharyngeal signs or symptoms.
      i) Abnormal gag reflex.
      ii) Uvular deviation to normal side.
      iii) Absent cough reflex.
   c) Hoarseness from vocal cord dysfunction.
   d) Aspiration from vocal cord dysfunction.
2) Distal group (i.e., lesion below hyoid bone).
   a) Isolated vagal neuropathy manifested as hoarseness and aspiration secondary to vocal cord dysfunction.
   b) Absent oropharyngeal signs.
   c) Normal cough reflex.

d. Proximal lesions are best imaged with MRI of the suprahyoid carotid space, skull base, and basal cisterns.
1) MRI is the preferred imaging method for proximal vagal neuropathy because of its superior sensitivity to skull base, cisternal, and brain stem lesions.
2) The MRI technique can be completed entirely within the head coil in most patients. T2-weighted, whole-brain images are the most sensitive to brain stem disease. T1-weighted images both without and with contrast (plus fat saturation) best delineate the lesions of the basal cisterns, skull base (i.e., jugular foramen), and suprahyoid carotid space.

e. Distal lesions require a different approach, depending on which side is affected by vagus nerve malfunction.
1) If the lesion is a distal left vagal neuropathy, a chest radiographic examination is performed first to rule out any obvious mediastinal cause of the vocal cord malfunction (Table 19-6).
   a) A negative chest radiograph does not preclude proceeding to CT, because occult malignancy is still a distinct possibility.

      b) Transaxial imaging of the distal vagus nerve from the hyoid bone to the aortopulmonic window should be undertaken with CT.

      c) CT has an advantage over MRI in this area. Artifacts may result on MRI scans from respiratory motion, coil reach problems associated with the transition from neck to chest, and bulk susceptibility artifacts associated with the significant change in volume between the neck and chest.

      d) CT performed with maximum intravascular contrast best delineates the many normal vessels from lesions in this area. Contiguous axial 5-mm slices are sufficient.

   2) In the case of distal right vagal neuropathy, transaxial imaging from the hyoid bone to the cervicothoracic junction is the first step in the work-up. Either CT or MRI is adequate to this task.

   3) When inspecting scans of patients suspected of having a distal vagal neuropathy, remember that the two most important areas to look at are the carotid space (i.e., main vagus trunk) and tracheoesophageal groove (i.e., recurrent laryngeal nerve).

      a) On the left, the scan and the inspection must be carried to the aortopulmonic window.

      b) On the right, the scan and the inspection must reach only as far as the cervical–thoracic junction.

4. Lesions.

   a. Lesions that cause vagal neuropathy can be subdivided into proximal and distal groups.

   b. The proximal group can be subdivided further by anatomic area, into brain stem, cistern, and jugular foramen–suprahyoid carotid space lesions.

     1) Brain stem and cisternal lesions are generic in that they can injure any cranial nerve depending on the area of the brain stem or cistern in which they arise (Table 19-3).

      a) Intraaxial and cisternal lesions are discussed at length in Chapter 20.

      b) Suprahyoid carotid space lesions are thoroughly discussed in Chapter 5.

   c. The distal group of lesions causing distal vagal neuropathy are discussed in Chapter 9. Those sections on the infrahyoid carotid space and the visceral space cover the anatomy and lesions of the main vagal trunk and recurrent laryngeal nerves, respectively.

   d. A final word about the so-called "idiopathic vagal neuropathy." When I first started into the area of head and neck radiology, idiopathic vagal neuropathy was thought to be a common explanation for vagus nerve dysfunction.

1) In a recent article on this subject, Terris and coworkers (1992) reviewed 1019 cases of vagal neuropathy both reported in the literature and seen in their practice, with the group labeled as idiopathic constituting approximately 14% of this group.
2) Certainly, an intensive search for a cause of an unexplained vagal neuropathy is warranted given this low statistic.

F. Spinal accessory nerve (i.e., cranial nerve XI).

1. Normal anatomy.
   a. Nuclear origins.
      1) Two distinct origins exist for the spinal accessory nerve (Figs. 19-4, 19–7).

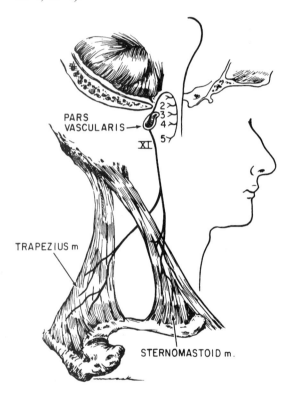

Fig. 19-7 Spinal accessory nerve (*XI*). The spinal portion of cranial nerve XI receives fibers from cervical levels 1 through 5, ascends through the foramen magnum, and exits the skull base through the pars vascularis of the jugular foramen. Its extracranial branches supply motor fibers to the sternomastoid and trapezius muscles. (From Remley K, Harnsberger HR, Smoker WRK, et al: CT and MRI in the evaluation of glossopharyngeal, vagal, and spinal accessory neuropathy. *Semin Ultrasound CT MR* 8:284–300, 1987. Used with permission.)

2) Medullary origin (bulbar or accessory). Motor fibers begin in the nucleus ambiguus of the upper medulla, then join the vagus nerve to innervate the endolaryngeal muscles through the recurrent laryngeal nerve.
3) Spinal origins (external). Motor fibers arise from the anterior horn cells of the first five cervical cord segments. These fibers coalesce to form the spinal part of the spinal accessory nerve. They ultimately innervate the trapezius and sternocleidomastoid muscles in the neck.

b. Nerve course.
1) The spinal root emerges from the lateral cervical cord and ascends through the foramen magnum to leave the skull via the posterior portion of the pars vascularis of the jugular foramen (Fig. 19-7).
2) The nerve exits the skull base into the nasopharyngeal carotid space only to diverge quickly posterolaterally and descend along the medial aspect of the sternocleidomastoid muscle. It then continues across the posterior triangle of the neck and terminates in the trapezius muscle.

c. Nerve branches of the spinal root.
1) The main nerve trunk divides into two terminal motor branches to supply the trapezius and sternocleidomastoid muscles (Table 19-2).

2. Clinical manifestations of injury to nerve XI.
a. Injury to the spinal accessory nerve anywhere along its course results in shoulder drop and inability to lift the arm.
b. The most common cause of isolated injury to nerve XI is radical neck dissection. When the mechanism is not neck dissection, nerve XI usually is injured along with some combination of nerves IX, X, and XII.

3. Imaging issues.
a. Injury to nerve XI will be seen as a loss of volume (i.e., atrophy) of the ipsilateral sternocleidomastoid and trapezius muscles.
b. The levator scapulae muscle hypertrophies and enlarges in response to spinal accessory neuropathy. This enlarged but normal muscle may be mistaken for tumor if the radiologist is unaware of this normal pseudomass.

Q#7
c. Imaging of nerve XI is similar to imaging of the ninth, proximal tenth, and twelfth nerves, with the exception of its most distal ramification into the posterior cervical space (i.e., posterior triangle). If no mass is palpable in this region, MRI should be performed if pos-

sible because of its sensitivity to intraaxial lesions of the medulla and its ability to visualize directly cranial nerves in the basal cisterns.

4. Lesions.
   a. Lesions affecting the spinal accessory nerve are similar to those causing proximal vagal neuropathy.

G. Hypoglossal nerve (i.e., XII).

1. Normal anatomy.
   a. Nuclear origins.
      1) The hypoglossal nerve originates in the hypoglossal nucleus, which is paramedian in the floor of the fourth ventricles (Fig. 19-8A).
      2) The two paired, hypoglossal nuclear columns run in the floor of the fourth ventricle for almost the entire length of the medulla. The bulge made by the nucleus into the fourth ventricle is the hypoglossal eminence.
   b. Nerve course.
      1) Nerve root fibers course anterolaterally from the hypoglossal nucleus just lateral to the medial lemniscus, traversing the inferior olivary nucleus to exit the medulla as the hypoglossal nerve in the preolivary sulcus.
      2) The hypoglossal nerve then passes through the premedullary cistern as multiple rootlets in close proximity to the vertebral artery to enter the hypoglossal canal.
      3) After passing through the skull base in the hypoglossal canal, the nerve dives caudally in the nasopharyngeal carotid space.
      4) Just inferior to the mastoid tip the hypoglossal nerve swings anteriorly, deep to the posterior belly of the digastric muscle, and continues forward to enter the posterior portion of the sublingual space of the oral cavity.
         a) Within the sublingual space, the nerve ramifies to supply motor innervation to both the intrinsic and extrinsic muscles of the tongue (Fig. 19-8B).
         b) Note that this nerve loops inferiorly to the level of the hyoid bone before ascending to the tongue.
   c. Nerve function and malfunction (Table 19-2).
      1) Cranial nerve XII supplies motor innervation to:
         a) Intrinsic tongue muscles (i.e., longitudinal, transverse, vertical).
         b) Extrinsic tongue muscles, which include the genioglossus, geniohyoid, hyoglossus, and styloglossus muscles.
      2) The C1 nerve root rides on the hypoglossal nerve before diverging to help supply motor innervation to the geniohyoid and thyrohyoid muscles.

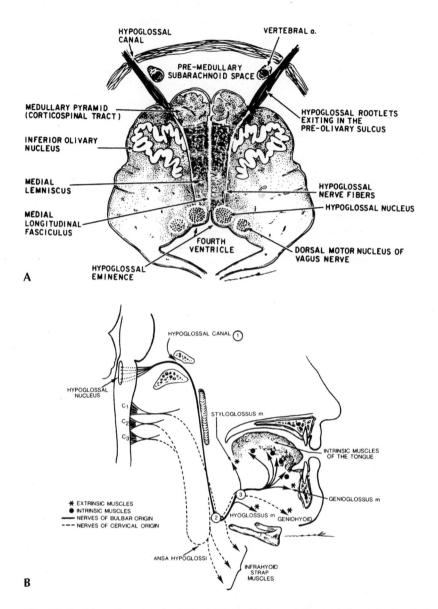

Fig. 19-8 Hypoglossal nerve (*XII*). **A,** Cross-section of the medulla at the level of the hypoglossal nucleus. The hypoglossal nucleus sits in the floor of the fourth ventricle. The nerve fibers project anteriorly through the medulla to emerge in the preolivary sulcus. Note the proximity of the cisternal portion of the hypoglossal nerve to the vertebral artery. The combination of multiple rootlets and vertebral artery movement makes the cisternal portion of the hypoglossal nerve difficult to see on T1-weighted MRI scans. **B,** Hypoglossal nerve and its peripheral connections. Observe the communication of the peripheral hypoglossal nerve with the fibers from the first cervical nerve. Also note that the ansa hypoglossi is formed by fibers of the first three cervical nerves. (From Smoker WRK, Harnsberger HR, Osborn AG: The hypoglossal nerve. *Semin Ultrasound CT MR* 164:301–312, 1987. Used with permission.)

3) The C1 nerve root also combines with the C2 and C3 roots to form the ansa hypoglossi nerve. This nerve provides motor innervation to the infrahyoid strap muscles (Fig. 19-8*B*).

d. Clinical manifestations of injury to nerve XII.

1) Deviation of the tongue toward the side of the lesion on protrusion.
2) Tongue atrophy, including both the intrinsic and extrinsic muscles after 4 to 6 weeks of serious hypoglossal nerve injury.
3) Fasciculations of the tongue muscles in the first 6 weeks after serious hypoglossal nerve injury.
4) Dysarthria.

e. Imaging issues.

1) Imaging of proximal cranial nerve XII is similar to imaging nerves IX, proximal X, and XI in that the nerve comes from a nucleus in the medulla, traverses the basal cistern, and travels in the nasopharyngeal carotid space.
2) MRI is the preferred imaging method because of its sensitivity to small brain stem lesions and its ability to see into the basal cisterns.
3) Direct visualization of the cisternal twelfth nerve usually is not possible with MRI, because it is partially wrapped around the vertebral artery and comprised of multiple small rootlets at this level.
4) The extracranial twelfth cranial nerve is equally well examined by CT or MRI. In the face of a palpable mass, either method can be used.

Q#8

a) Remember that the hypoglossal nerve loops as far caudal as the hyoid bone before ascending to the tongue musculature. Therefore any study of the extracranial twelfth nerve must extend inferiorly to the level of the hyoid bone.

H. Brain stem and basal cistern lesions.

1. Throughout the discussion of lesions affecting the individual cranial nerves, brain stem and basal cistern lesions have been purposefully omitted, because they for the most part are common to all of the cranial neuropathies.
2. Tables 19-3 and 19-4 summarize lesions that occur in the brain stem and cisterns that may result in isolated or complex cranial neuropathies.
3. In some instances particular cranial nerves are affected by specific brain stem or cistern lesions as indicated in parenthetic entries in Tables 19-3 and 19-4.

SUGGESTED READING

Armington WG, Harnsberger HR, Smoker WRK, et al: Normal and diseased acoustic pathway: evaluation with MR imaging. *Radiology* 167:509–515, 1988.

Bernardi B, Zimmerman RA, Savino PJ, et al: Magnetic resonance tomographic angiography in the investigation of hemifacial spasm. *Neuroradiology* 35:606–611, 1993.

Carpenter MB: *Core text of neuroanatomy.* Baltimore, 1988, Waverly Press.

Chusid JG: *Correlative neuroanatomy and functional neurology,* ed 19. Los Altos, Calif., 1985, Lange Medical Publications.

Daniels DL, Czervionke LF, Millen SJ, et al: MR imaging of facial nerve enhancement in Bell palsy or after temporal bone surgery. *Radiology* 171:807–809, 1989.

Daniels DL, Herfkins R, Koehler PR, et al: Magnetic resonance imaging of the internal auditory canal. *Radiology* 151:105–108, 1984.

Daniels DL, Millen SJ, Meyer GA, et al: MR detection of tumor in the internal auditory canal. *AJNR* 8:249–252, 1987.

Daniels DL, Williams AL, Haughton KVM: Jugular foramen: anatomic and computed tomographic study. *Am J Roentgenol* 142:153–158, 1984.

Disbro MA, Harnsberger HR, Osborn AG: Peripheral facial nerve dysfunction: CT evaluation. *Radiology* 155:659–663, 1985.

Flannigan BD, Bradley WG, Mazziotta JC, et al: Magnetic resonance imaging of the brainstem: normal structure and basic functional anatomy. *Radiology* 154:375–383, 1985.

Gebarski SS, Telian SA, Niparko JK: Enhancement along the normal facial nerve in the facial canal: MR imaging and anatomic correlation. *Radiology* 183:391–394, 1992.

Gentry LR, Jacoby CG, Turski PA, et al: Cerebellopontine angle-petromastoid mass lesions: comparative study of diagnosis with MR imaging and CT. *Radiology* 162:513–520, 1987.

Gilman S, Newman SW: *Manter and Gatz's essentials of clinical neuroanatomy and neurophysiology,* ed 7. Philadelphia, 1987, FA Davis.

Hans JS, Huss RG, Benson JE, et al: MR imaging of the skull base. *J Comput Assist Tomogr* 8:944–952, 1984.

Harnsberger HR: Cranial nerve imaging. *Semin Ultrasound CT MR* 8:163–313, 1987.

Harnsberger HR, Dillon WP: Major motor atrophic patterns in the face and neck: CT evaluation. *Radiology* 155:665–670, 1985.

Hirsch WL, Kemp SS, Martinez AJ, et al: Anatomy of the brain stem: correlation of in vitro MR images with histologic sections. *AJNR* 10:923–928, 1989.

Jacobs CJM, Harnsberger HR, Lufkin RB, et al: CT and MRI in the evaluation of vagal neuropathy. *Radiology* 164:97–102, 1987.

Kalvoridouris A, Mancuso AA, Dillon WP: A CT-clinical approach to patients with symptoms related to the V, VII, IX-XII cranial nerves and cervical sympathetic plexus. *Radiology* 151:671–676, 1984.

Kumar A, Maudelonde C, Mafee MF: Unilateral sensorineural hearing loss: analysis of 200 consecutive cases. *Laryngoscope* 96:14–18.

Lo WWM, Solti-Bohman LG: High-resolution CT of the jugular foramen: anatomy and vascular variants and anomalies. *Radiology* 150:743–747, 1984.

Mafee MF: Acoustic neuroma and other acoustic nerve disorders: role of MRI and CT. Analysis of 238 cases. *Semin Ultrasound CT MR* 8:256–283, 1987.

Mafee MF, Kumar A, Valvassori GE, et al: CT in the evaluation of the vestibulocochlear nerves and their central pathways. *Radiol Clin North Am* 22:45–66, 1984.

Mafee MF, Selis JE, Yannias DA, et al: Congenital sensorineural hearing loss. *Radiology* 150:427–434, 1984.

Martin N, Sterkers O, Mompoint D, et al: Facial nerve neuromas: MR imaging. *Neuroradiology* 34:62–67, 1992.

Mokri B, Schievink WI, Olsen KD, et al: Spontaneous dissection of the cervical internal carotid artery: presentation with lower cranial nerve palsies. *Arch Otolaryngol Head Neck Surg* 118:431–435, 1992.

New PFJ, Bachow TB, Wismer GL, et al: MR imaging of the acoustic nerves and small acoustic neuromas at 0.6 T: prospective study. *AJNR* 6:165–170, 1985.

Pozzo GD, Mascalchi M, Fonda C, et al: Lower cranial nerve palsy due to dissection of the internal carotid artery: CT and MR imaging. *J Comput Assist Tomogr* 13:989–995, 1989.

Remly K, Harnsberger R, Smoker WRK, et al: CT and MRI in the evaluation of glossopharyngeal, vagal, and spinal accessory neuropathy. *Semin Ultrasound CT MR* 8:284–300, 1987.

Sammi M, Jannetta PJ: *The cranial nerves*. New York, 1981, Springer-Verlag.

Schwaber MK, Larson TC, Zealer DL, et al: Gadolinium-enhanced magnetic resonance imaging in Bell's palsy. *Laryngoscope* 100:1264–1269, 1990.

Shpizner BA, Holliday RA: Levator scapulae muscle asymmetry presenting as a palpable neck mass: CT evaluation. *AJNR* 14:461–464, 1993.

Smoker WRK, Harnsberger R, Osborn AG: The hypoglossal nerve. *Semin Ultrasound CT MR* 8:301–312, 1987.

Soo KC, Hamlyn Pj, Pegington J, et al: Anatomy of the accessory nerve and its cervical contributions in the neck. *Head Neck Surg* 9:111–115, 1986.

Tash R, DeMerritt J, Sze G, Leslie D: Hemifacial spasm: MR imaging features. *AJNR* 12:839–842, 1991.

Teresi L, Lufkin R, Wortham D, et al: MR imaging of the intratemporal facial nerve using surface coils. *AJNR* 8:49–54, 1987.

Teresi LM, Kolin E, Lufkin RB, et al: MR imaging of the intraparotid facial nerve: normal anatomy and pathology. *Am J Roentgenol* 148:995–1000, 1987.

Teresi LM, Lufkin R, Nitta K, et al: MRI of the facial nerve: normal anatomy and pathology. *Semin Ultrasound CT MR* 8:240–255, 1987.

Terris DJ, Arnstein DP, Nguten HH: Contemporary evaluation of unilateral vocal cord paralysis. *Otolaryngol Head Neck Surg* 107:84–90, 1992.

Tien R, Dillon WP, Jackler RK: Contrast-enhanced MR imaging of the facial nerve in 11 patients with Bell's palsy. *AJNR* 11:735–741, 1990.

Valvassori GE, Morales FG, Palacios E, et al: MR of the normal and abnormal internal auditory canal. *AJNR* 9:115–119, 1988.

20

Sensorineural Hearing Loss with Emphasis on the Cerebellopontine Angle and Inner Ear

CRITICAL IMAGING QUESTIONS: SENSORINEURAL HEARING LOSS WITH EMPHASIS ON THE CEREBELLOPONTINE ANGLE AND INNER EAR

1. Name the major components of the central acoustic pathway.
2. What are two intralabyrinthine lesions that cannot be diagnosed with temporal bone CT scans?
3. What are the most important morphologic features to observe when analyzing a lesion of the cerebellopontine angle?
4. Why do 15% of acoustic neuromas cause acute onset of sensorineural hearing loss?
5. What two possible explanations are there for observing "cystic areas" associated with an acoustic neuroma?

Answers to these questions are found in the text beside the question number (Q#) in the margin.

THE VESTIBULOCOCHLEAR CRANIAL NERVE

A. Introduction.

1. The discussion of the vestibulocochlear nerve combines the imaging issues of sensorineural hearing loss with those issues of the cerebellopontine angle and inner ear lesions.
2. Lesions of the cerebellopontine angle statistically are the most responsible for unilateral sensorineural hearing loss. Many other disease processes cause hearing loss, however, especially lesions within the bony and membranous labyrinth of the inner ear and pontomedullary brain stem.
    a. Anatomic areas to consider when evaluating a patient for sensorineural hearing loss include (Table 20-1):
      1) Labyrinthine lesions (bony or membranous labyrinth)
      2) Cisternal lesions (cerebellopontine angle–internal auditory canal [CPA-IAC])
      3) Intraaxial lesions (primarily in the pons–high medullary brain stem)
3. This chapter reviews the acoustic pathway with special emphasis on the vestibulocochlear cranial nerve. Specific attention is given to:
    a. Normal anatomy of the acoustic pathway.
    b. Pathophysiology of lesions causing sensorineural hearing loss.
    c. Imaging problems unique to the vestibulocochlear nerve.

B. The vestibulocochlear nerve (i.e., cranial nerve VIII).

1. Normal anatomy of the vestibulocochlear nerve.
    a. This handbook approaches anatomy of the vestibulocochlear nerve from the periphery to the center, because this is the direction that information flows along the acoustic pathway.
    b. The vestibulocochlear nerve has two distinctive parts: the vestibular part (i.e., balance), and the cochlear part (i.e., hearing). This chapter concentrates on the cochlear part.
      1) The vestibular part of the vestibulocochlear nerve seldom provides the impetus for imaging. In fact, when vertigo, dizziness, or imbalance are imaged, especially in the older population, the MRI scan usually is normal.
    c. Cochlear nerve course.
      1) After leaving the spiral ganglion of the cochlea, the auditory axons traverse the IAC in the anterior–inferior quadrant (Figs. 20-1 and 20-2). The facial nerve is just above the cochlear nerve in the anterior–superior quadrant (Fig. 20-2). Near the fundus these two nerves are separated from one another by the crista falciformis (i.e., the transverse crest that divides the fundus of the internal auditory canal into superior and inferior fossa).

Table 20-1   Lesions Causing Sensorineural Hearing Loss

Sensory Causes (Cochlear Lesions)
Congenital
    Mondini malformation (cochlear dysplasia)
    Michel's deformity (inner ear aplasia)
    Vestibular aqueduct syndrome
Inflammatory/other
    Labyrinthitis
    Labyrinthine ossificans
    Paget disease
    Cochlear otosclerosis
Trauma
    Temporal bone fracture
    Hemorrhage into membranous labyrinth
Tumor
    Labyrinthine schwannoma (cochlear or vestibular)
    Temporal bone tumor eroding into labyrinth
        Paraganglioma
        Hemangioma
        Adenomatous tumor of vestibular aqueduct

Neural Causes (Retrocochlear Lesions)
Extraaxial lesions (cerebellopontine angle–internal auditory canal)
    Benign tumor
        Acoustic neuroma
        Meningioma
        Epidermoid
        Paraganglioma
    Malignant tumor
        Metastases
        Non-Hodgkin lymphoma
    Vascular
        Arteriovenous malformation
        Vertebrobasilar dolichoectasia
        Aneurysm
    Inflammatory
        Granulomatous meningitis (TB, sarcoid)
        Cysticercosis
    Congenital
        Arachnoid cyst
Intraaxial (brain-stem) lesions
    See Table 20-4

2) At approximately the porus acusticus both the superior and inferior vestibular nerve join together with the cochlear nerve to become the vestibulocochlear nerve bundle (Fig. 20-3).

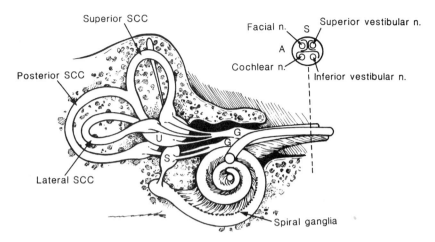

Superior SCC

Facial n. S Superior vestibular n.

A

Cochlear n.

Inferior vestibular n.

Posterior SCC

Lateral SCC

U

G

G

S

Spiral ganglia

Fig. 20-1 Normal anatomy of the inner ear. The inner ear structures can be divided into two functional groups; the balance-related and the hearing-related structures. Hearing-related structures include the snail-shaped cochlea, spiral ganglia, and cochlear nerve. The balanced-related group includes the superior, posterior, and lateral semicircular canals (*SCC*); the utricular (*U*) and saccular (*S*) portions of the vestibule; vestibular ganglion (*G*); and the superior and inferior vestibular nerves. A cross-section of the apex of the internal auditory canal is provided in the upper right. *A*, Anterior; *S*, superior.

    3) The vestibulocochlear nerve then crosses the CPA cistern at the posterior nerve bundle (i.e., the facial nerve is anterior) to enter the brain stem at the junction of the medulla and pons.

    4) The entering nerve fibers bifurcate as they pierce the brain stem, making synapses with both the dorsal and ventral cochlear nuclei (Fig. 20-3).

  d. Nuclei of the auditory component of nerve VIII

    1) Dorsal and ventral cochlear nuclei are found on the lateral surface of the inferior cerebellar peduncle (i.e., restiform body). It is not possible to resolve these nuclei, but their location now can be determined accurately by looking at high-resolution T1- or T2-weighted axial images and identifying the inferior cerebellar peduncle contour (Fig. 20-3).

    2) These two nuclei receive axons from neurons with their cell bodies in the spiral ganglion, found just inside the modiolus of the cochlea.

2. Normal anatomy of the acoustic pathway.

  a. The acoustic pathway is traditionally divided along the lines of sensorineural hearing loss into two parts: the sensory part (i.e., cochlear), and the neural (i.e., retrocochlear) parts.

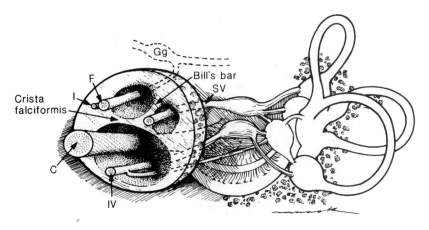

Fig. 20-2 Normal anatomy of the fundus of the internal auditory canal, showing the relationships commonly found between the cranial nerves in the internal auditory canal. The facial nerve (*F*) and nervus intermedius (*I*) are found in the anterior–superior quadrant, the cochlear nerve (*C*) in the anterior–inferior quadrant, the superior vestibular nerve (*SV*) in the posterior–superior quadrant, and the inferior vestibular nerve (*IV*) in the posterior–inferior quadrant. The crista falciformis is a horizontal bony strut that cleaves the fundus of the internal auditory canal into halves. It can be seen routinely on high-resolution CT or MRI scans of the inner ear in the coronal plane. Bill's bar, a vertical bony ridge separating the facial nerve from the superior vestibular nerve, is a surgical landmark not usually seen on any imaging. *Gg*, Geniculate ganglion of the facial nerve.

    b. The sensory portion is comprised of the complex structures within the cochlea itself.

    c. The neural portion is by far the most complex, involving multiple components as it passes from the cochlea to the superior temporal gyrus of the temporal lobe of the brain (Fig. 20-4).

Q#1

    d. The major pieces of the neural portion of the acoustic pathway, from distal to proximal, include (Figs. 20-3 and 20-4):

       1) Cochlear nerve.

       2) Vestibulocochlear nerve (i.e., cranial nerve VIII).

       3) Dorsal and ventral cochlear nuclei.

       4) Trapezoid body.

       5) Lateral lemniscus.

       6) Inferior colliculus.

       7) Medial geniculate body.

       8) Superior temporal gyrus.

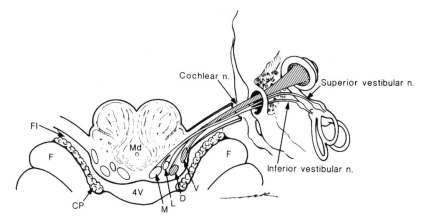

Fig. 20-3   Normal vestibular and cochlear nuclei in the lateral margin of the inferior cerebellar peduncle of the brain stem. This axial drawing of the upper medulla (*Md*) shows the medial (*M*) and lateral (*L*) vestibular nuclei relative to the dorsal (*D*) and ventral (*V*) cochlear nuclei. Both nuclear groups are nestled in the lateral aspect of the inferior cerebellar peduncle. Other normal structures included are the lateral foramen Lushka (*Fl*) of the fourth ventricle (*4V*), choroid plexus (*CP*) protruding into the cerebellopontine angle, and the cerebellar flocculus (*F*).

     e. The trapezoid body serves as the major decussation of the acoustic pathway.
        1) Few auditory fibers from the cochlear nuclei ascend directly into the ipsilateral lateral lemniscus.
        2) Any lesion proximal to the trapezoid body decussation will manifest itself primarily as contralateral hearing loss. Unilateral hearing loss also will be present but less prominent.
3. Clinical manifestations of acoustic pathway injury
     a. Hearing loss and tinnitus (i.e., ringing or roaring in the ear) are the principal symptoms of injury to nerve VIII.
     b. If unilateral sensorineural hearing loss is present, the injury has occurred somewhere between the membranous labyrinth of the cochlea and the cochlear nuclei of the inferior cerebellar peduncle of the brain stem.
     c. Unilateral involvement of the auditory pathway above the cochlear nuclei usually causes bilateral sensorineural hearing loss, which is greater in the ear contralateral to the side of the lesion.
     d. Cortical acoustic pathway lesions, which rarely cause disruption of auditory function, may give an auditory agnosia (i.e., sounds are perceived but interpretation is impaired).
4. Imaging issues in sensorineural hearing loss.

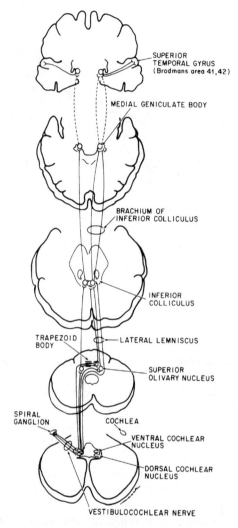

Fig. 20-4   Composite drawing of complete acoustic pathway from the cochlea to the superior temporal gyrus. Note that the major decussation is at the level of the pons through the trapezoid body. Lesions from the level of the cochlear nuclei on the surface of the restiform body outward to the membranous labyrinth present with unilateral sensorineural hearing loss. When the lesion is intraaxial and above the trapezoid body decussation, hearing loss is bilateral but asymmetrically worse on the side opposite the lesion. The more proximal along the acoustic pathway the lesion, the more difficult to implicate it as the cause of the patients hearing loss. (From Armington WG, Harnsberger HR, Smoker WRK, et al: Normal and diseased acoustic pathway: evaluation with MR imaging. *Radiology* 167:509–515. Used with permission.)

a. Audiometric testing now is sensitive enough to localize the lesion causing sensorineural hearing loss to either the sensory or the neural component of the acoustic pathway.

b. When the lesion is suspected to be located in the cochlea (i.e., sensory component), MRI with contrast and CT are approximately equal in their ability to diagnose the main differential diagnostic considerations (Table 20-1).

    1) Congenital lesions of the membranous labyrinth can be seen as abnormalities in the fluid spaces seen on MRI or in the bony labyrinth shape on CT scans.

    2) CT is the better tool if cochlear otosclerosis, Paget disease, or trauma is suspected. Little is known about the sensitivity of MRI to the diagnosis of otosclerosis or Paget disease. MRI is blind to the linear fractures and pneumolabyrinth that may be present in trauma with resultant hearing loss.

    3) MRI alone will diagnose labyrinthitis or intralabyrinthine tumor on contrast-enhanced, T1-weighted MRI. CT will see nothing when these entities are present.

    4) Either MRI or CT can diagnose labyrinthine ossificans. CT may have a slight edge because of the experience that exists with making the diagnosis with this modality. Early reports suggest MRI may be able to show fibrous obliteration of the membranous labyrinth; CT will show nothing in such a case.

    5) The best tool for imaging cochlear-level pathology may vary by specific pathology. At times it may be necessary to do both examinations.

c. When the lesion is suspected to be located in the retrocochlear (i.e., neural) region of the acoustic pathway, MRI is the procedure of choice.

    1) T1-weighted, high-resolution MRI scans of the CPA area are obtained to evaluate for acoustic neuroma or other CPA lesions.

    2) T2-weighted MRI scans of the remaining intraaxial auditory pathway are obtained during the same examination to exclude brain-stem tumor, stroke, or multiple sclerosis as a cause of the patient's hearing loss.

    3) Contrast-enhanced, T1-weighted MRI scans are completed when both nongadolinium T1- and T2-weighted images are normal. This is to look for the very small (i.e., < 4 mm) intracanalicular acoustic neuroma and other causes of hearing loss such as membranous labyrinthitis.

    4) Thin section, high-resolution, fast spin echo images focused to the CPA-IAC are beginning to make the diagnosis of CPA mass

lesions (i.e., acoustic neuroma, meningioma, epidermoid) without use of MRI contrast. This technique also is opening up the arena of inner ear morphologic abnormalites. More research must be done with this alternative, but the initial experience with this technique is encouraging.

5. Pathology affecting the cochlea.
   a. MRI and cochlear lesions.
      1) Standard head MRI sequences are absolutely useless when evaluating the bony and membranous labyrinth. If no custom imaging is done for this area, then CT scans of the temporal bone are by far the better tool. However, if 3-mm, contiguous imaging of the IAC and inner ear is done with the head coil or the TMJ coil, it is possible to make virtually all of the diagnoses seen in Table 20-1.
      2) Details of the specific lesions listed in Table 20-1 are beyond the scope of this chapter. Inner ear lesions listed in Table 20-1 are thoroughly discussed in the chapter covering the temporal bone.

Q#2

      a) Contrast-enhanced MRI is the only way that radiologists can diagnose membranous labyrinthitis and primary intralabyrinthine tumor (i.e., vestibular and cochlear schwannoma).
      b) The most advanced high-resolution techniques in MRI of the inner ear are beginning to change our understanding of congenital lesions such as the Mondini spectrum lesions as well as the large vestibular aqueduct syndrome. For details regarding this subject, see the inner ear section of the temporal bone chapter.
      3) Clearly, MRI has an important role in the diagnosis of labyrinthine pathology. It is just a question of how hard radiologists are willing to push this technology.

6. Pathology affecting the vestibulocochlear nerve (Tables 20-2 through 20-4).
   a. MRI and CPA Lesions.
      1) General comments.
         a) With the emergence of MRI, the lesions of the CPA must be considered from two separate viewpoints. The first is the traditional CPA mass differential diagnosis (Table 20-2), and the second is by the MRI appearance (Table 20-3).
      2) MRI appearance of CPA lesions.
         a) Observations regarding the MRI appearance of lesions in the CPA region now are well developed for the more common ones of this area, but these are only sparsely reported for the more uncommon diseases.

Table 20-2   Differential Diagnosis of CPA Mass

Neoplasm, Extraaxial
Acoustic neuroma
Meningioma
Epidermoid
Metastasis
Paraganglioma
Chordoma
Other neuroma

Neoplasm, Intraaxial
Pedunculated brain stem glioma
Metastasis
Choroid plexus papilloma
Ependymoma
Medulloblastoma
Cystic cerebellar astrocytoma
Cerebellar hemangioblastoma

Vascular Lesions
Arteriovenous malformation
Aneurysm
Vertebrobasilar dolichoectasia

Inflammatory Lesions
Granulomatous meningitis
Cysticercosis

Congenital Lesions
Lipoma
Arachnoid cyst

Pseudomasses
Cerebellar flocculus
Choroid plexus
Jugular tubercle
Prominent AICA
High jugular bulb

Q#3

b) The best way to approach the radiologic evaluation of a CPA lesion is to rely on the anatomic and morphologic guidelines previously used in imaging this area with CT. These include whether the lesion is intraaxial or extraaxial, if it is dural based, and if it is tubular (i.e., vascular) or globular (i.e., tumor).

Table 20-3   Major Imaging Features of Acoustic Neuroma, Meningioma, and Epidermoid Tumors of the Cerebellopontine Angle

Tumor Type	Tumor Appearance	MRI Appearance
Acoustic neuroma	"Ice cream in a cone"	T1- and T2-weighted signal approximates gray matter
	Acute angle to T-bone margin	T1-weighted signal with contrast shows enhancement
	Centered on porus acusticus	Cystic component (15%)
Meningioma	"Mushroom head shape"	T1- and T2-weighted signal approximates gray matter
	Obtuse angle to T-bone margin	T1-weighted signal with contrast shows enhancement
	Eccentric to porus acusticus	Susceptibility affect on GRE images. May have associated edema in adjacent brain on T2-weighted images
Epidermoidoma	Conforms to shape of the space of origin. May invaginate the adjacent brain stem	T1-weighted signal is hypointense to brain but not as hypointense as CSF. T2-weighted signal may be as high as CSF. T1-weighted signal with contrast shows no enhancement

CSF, cerebrospinal fluid.

       i)   Intraaxial lesions are a completely different group from the extraaxial lesions.

      ii)   In extraaxial tumors, the shape alone often will reveal the specific diagnosis, regardless of the signal characteristics (Table 20-3).

    3)   The following section discusses the lesions mentioned in Table 20-3. Where possible, the MRI appearance of the lesion is described.

  b. Congenital CPA Lesions.

    1)   Arachnoid Cyst.

      a)   Clinical presentations. Causes symptoms as a result of compression of adjacent structures. In the posterior fossa an

Table 20-4   Differential Diagnosis of Brain Stem Lesions

Tumors
Primary brain stem glioma
Ependymoma
Metastatic tumor
Lymphoma

Inflammatory Lesions
Multiple sclerosis
Encephalitis
Abscess

Vascular Lesions
Arteriovenous malformation with or without hemorrhage
Cavernous angioma with hemorrhage
Stroke
PICA CVA (Wallenburg's Syndrome)
Pontine perforators

Miscellaneous
Trauma
Hemorrhage
Syringobulbia

arachnoid cyst may act like a mass lesion, causing hydrocephalus by compressing the aqueduct or outlets of the fourth ventricle. Hearing loss usually is not part of the presenting symptomatology in CPA arachnoid cyst.

b) Pathology. Forms from cerebrospinal fluid collecting in a split or duplication in the arachnoid membrane. Most frequently found in the sylvian, parasagittal, and convexity regions. Less frequently seen in the CPA, incisura, suprasellar, and fourth ventricular regions.

c) CT features. Hypodense (i.e., uniform cerebrospinal fluid density) collections with well-defined, smooth, and often angular margins. The margins of the lesion do not enhance. One half of these cysts produce smooth erosion of adjacent bone.

d) MRI features. Same structural attributes as on CT scans, with the hallmark that fluid within the cyst shows signal intensity similar to cereobrospinal fluid (i.e., low intensity on T1-weighted scans and high intensity on T2-weighted scans). Also, the fluid within the cyst will not demonstrate any of the flow-related phenomenon seen in the adjacent cerebrospinal fluid.

   c. Extraaxial tumor of the CPA.
      1) Acoustic neuroma.
         a) This is the most common CPA mass.

Q#4

         b) Clinical presentation. Salient clinical complaint is sen-
            sorineural hearing loss. Other symptoms include tinnitus,
            dizziness, gait disturbance, and headaches. Fifteen percent of
            cases present with acute onset of hearing loss, probably
            because of hemorrhage into the tumor.

Q#5

         c) Pathology. The tumor usually arises from the sheath of the
            vestibulocochlear nerve. Most commonly seen in patients 50
            to 70 years of age. Five percent have associated arachnoid
            cysts; 10% to 15% have associated cystic necrosis within the
            tumor associated. When bilateral, the patient has neurofibro-
            matosis type II.
         d) CT features. Homogeneous, uniformly enhancing mass in
            the IAC and/or CPA depending on size. Calcification is
            absent. Forms an acute angle with the temporal bone. Less
            commonly the acoustic neuroma will demonstrate partial or
            total internal low density secondary to tumor necrosis.
         e) MRI features. Contrast-enhanced T1-weighted scan shows a
            hyperintense mass centered in the CPA over the IAC, with
            IAC extension. Cerebrospinal fluid hypointensity acts as a
            natural contrast agent to identify the tumor. Associated fluid
            intensity areas may be seen within the tumor (i.e., necrosis)
            or adjacent to the tumor (i.e., arachnoid cyst).
         f) Additional imaging features. The acoustic neuroma will take
            on different shapes depending on its size. If it is small (i.e.,
            0.5–1.5 cm), it takes on the shape of the IAC and remains
            intracanalicular. When medium size (i.e., 1.5–3 cm), it looks
            like an "ice cream cone" with the intracanalicular compo-
            nent as the cone and the CPA component as the ice cream.
            When large (i.e., > 3 cm), it will have a large CPA compo-
            nent that compresses the adjacent middle cerebellar pedun-
            cle of the brain stem.
      2) Meningioma.
         a) This is the second most common CPA mass.
         b) Clinical presentation. Varies depending on location of the
            meningioma. Often found incidentally in an asymptomatic
            patient. Cranial nerves V, VII, and VIII are variably affected
            depending on the tumor size and actual location.

    c) Pathology. Benign tumor thought to arise from meningothelial cells of the arachnoid villi. Seen in patients 40 to 60 years of age, with a 2:1 ratio of females to males. Only 10% of cases occur in the posterior fossa.

    d) CT features. Densely enhancing, sessile CPA mass adjacent to but usually not centered over the IAC. Calcification may be present. Hyperostosis of adjacent temporal bone is possible, but IAC extension is extremely rare. Forms a obtuse angle with the temporal bone.

    e) MRI features. Variable. Most typical appearance is isointense to gray matter on all unenhanced sequences; 85% enhance strongly with MRI contrast. When densely fibrous or calcified, it may be hypointense on T2-weighted images. A thin rim of low intensity may separate the tumor from adjacent brain (i.e., cerebrospinal fluid cleft or dura). Dural tail of thickened meninges in continuity with the mass is seen in 60% of cases. Enlargement of the adjacent signal void from nearby bone indicates hyperostosis.

    f) Comment. More important than the density (CT) or signal characteristics (MRI) of meningioma is the lesion location and shape in making this radiologic diagnosis.

3) Epidermoidoma.

    a) Clinical presentation. CPA epidermoid usually occurs in patients from 20 to 50 years of age. Symptoms at presentation vary with the location of the mass. Symptoms usually appear late in the course of disease and result from compression.

    b) Pathology. Epidermoidoma is a congenital neoplasm resulting from intracranial or intraosseous inclusions of ectoderm occurring during early fetal life. At surgery epidermoid is "the beautiful tumor," appearing as a glistening, pearly-white mass in the cistern. Three sites of occurrence have been reported: the fourth ventricle, the basal cisterns including the CPA, and the petrous temporal bone.

        i) Epidermoidoma contains a combination of keratin debris shed from a lining of squamous epithelium and solid cholesterin. The exact proportions of these two components determines the signal seen on MRI scans.

    c) CT features. Homogenous, low-density mass often taking the shape of the region where found. Does not change density with enhancement.

    d) MRI features. When keratin debris predominates, the epidermoidoma is hypointense on T1-weighted and hyperintense on T2-weighted scans. This is the most common signal characteristic. When the solid cholesterin component predominates, the tumor will be hyperintense on T1-weighted imaging. Rim enhancement or no enhancement occurs with contrast-enhanced T1-weighted imaging. Usually the intensity is sufficiently different from cerebrospinal fluid to make these lesions easily seen. The intensity signal fills the cistern, conforming to the shape allotted it, and appears to be "burrowing" into the adjacent brain stem.

   e) Comment. Again, signal characteristics are less important in the diagnosis of epidermoid than its shape and appearance. A lesion of the CPA that conforms to the shape of the cistern and appears to be burrowing into the adjacent brain stem is an epidermoid.

4) Other rare CPA extraaxial tumors.

   a) Paraganglioma, chordoma, non-Hodgkin lymphoma, and metastasis are rare causes of extraaxial tumors of the CPA, which are identified by their site of origin and CT/MRI appearances.

   b) Paraganglioma involving the CPA-IAC is centered in the jugular foramen, welling up from this site of origin. Therefore they are large lesions possessing the standard MRI features of paraganglioma (i.e., flow voids, intense contrast enhancement, adjacent bone invasion).

   c) Chordoma is centered in the adjacent clivus and only involves the CPA-IAC when large. Their very destructive appearance and clival origin are highly suggestive of this diagnosis.

   d) Non-Hodgkin lymphoma and metastatic tumor to the CPA-IAC may be indistinguishable. Bilaterality and other leptomeningeal or intra axial deposits may suggest these two possibilities to the radiologist if the patient history has not already done so.

d. Pseudomasses of the CPA.

1) Multiple normal structures traverse the CPA-IAC region of the basal cistern, including (Fig. 20-3):

   a) Cranial nerves V, VII, and VIII.

   b) Anterior inferior cerebellar artery.

   c) Choroid plexus protruding through the lateral recess of the fourth ventricle.

   d) Flocculus of the cerebellum.

   e) Jugular tubercle when prominent.

   f) High jugular bulb or jugular bulb diverticulum.

2) CPA-IAC pseudomasses.

a) Comment. When unusually prominent, these normal structures cause trouble during evaluation of the CPA. A radiologist aware of the variation in normal appearance of these structures, however, will have few problems in diagnosis. High-resolution MRI has made the problem of recognizing these structures far less troublesome.

b) Prominent anterior inferior cerebellar artery is seen as a looping flow void on MRI scans. As the velocity of flowing blood within this arterial structure is sufficiently rapid to create a signal void on conventional spin-echo sequences, contrast enhancement to confuse this arterial structure with a mass lesion does not occur.

c) Choroid plexus often protrudes through the lateral recesses of the fourth ventricle into the CPA. On MRI scans enhancing, bilateral, tear-shaped masses of the CPA are seen. They usually are sufficiently symmetric and characteristic in appearance to cause little trouble in interpretation.

d) The cerebellar flocculus is a lobule of the cerebellum normally projecting into the posterolateral aspect of the CPA. On MRI scans bilateral lobulation of the cerebellum that parallels brain intensity on T1- and T2-weighted scans is seen.

e) A prominent jugular tubercle once was a problem on CT imaging, because volume averaging of the tip of this structure could mimic an enhancing mass in the CPA. Because this occipital bone projection is low intensity on MRI scans, however, it does not cause a problem as in the CT days.

f) High jugular bulb or jugular bulb diverticulum may have slow, turbulent flow on contrast-enhanced, T1-weighted MRI. As a result, enhancing areas in the medial temporal bone just under or behind the internal auditory canal may be seen. Thankfully, T2-weighted images usually show no signal in this area. Sometimes T2-weighted imaging also shows signal associated with these normal venous structures. In such a case phase-contrast MRA or bone CT may be necessary to identify clearly these normal structures.

e. Vascular lesions of the CPA.

  1) Arteriovenous malformation.

    a) CT features. Dramatic enhancement of abnormal vessels without mass effect. Calcification may be present.

    b) MRI features: Racemose collection of abnormal vessels seen as multiple serpiginous flow voids. When hemorrhage has occurred, T1-weighted scan may show hyperintense areas of subacute blood (i.e., methemoglobin effect), while T2-

weighted scans may show hypointense areas of hemosiderin laden macrophages.

2) Aneurysm.

    a) Anterior inferior cerebellar artery usually is the diseased artery. Rare lesion.

    b) CT features. Oval to round, well-circumscribed mass in the CPA that at least in part is intensely enhancing. Linear calcification sometimes can be seen in the wall of the mass.

    c) MRI features. When the aneurysm is small and not thrombosed, an oval to round flow void is seen within the aneurysm. If thrombosis is present, increased signal intensity on T_1-weighted scans results from the methemoglobin in the thrombus. Giant aneurysms emit complex signal intensities secondary to flowing blood at different velocities and degrees of turbulence, thrombus in various stages of organization and age, and hemosiderin and calcium deposits.

3) Vertebrobasilar dolichoectasia or other vascular loops

    a) Vertebrobasilar dolichoectasia occurs when basilar and/or vertebral arteries are ectatic and tortuous.

    b) MRI features. Linear flow void in the location of the normal vertebrobasilar arterial system. The vertebrobasilar system may swing entirely into the CPA cistern, causing significant deformity of the facial and/or vestibulocochlear nerves.

    c) Comment. Hemifacial spasm may result from vertebrobasilar dolichoectasia or other vascular loops. Although not reported, cranial nerve VIII neuralgia probably can result from severe vertebrobasilar dolichoectasia or strategically placed vascular loops from other posterior fossa arterial branches. These patients usually present with a clinical picture of "atypical Meniere's disease" with episodic vertigo, nausea, vomiting, and intermittent roaring or ringing in the ear.

f. Inflammatory lesions of CPA-IAC.

1) Granulomatous meningitis.

    a) Pathology. Granulomatous meningitis is characterized by a thick exudate, perivascular inflammatory response, and granulation tissue.

    b) This process may result from bacterial, fungal, or tuberculous infection.

    c) When secondary to sarcoidosis, the optic chiasm, infundibulum, and pituitary gland also may be involved.

    d) CT features. Diffuse enhancement of the basal cisterns, including both CPA cisterns. If chronic or severe, communicating hydrocephalus is seen because of obliteration of the basal cisterns by inflammatory fibrosis.

  e) MRI features. MRI is relatively insensitive to diseases of the leptomeninges when performed without contrast. Contrast enhancement is necessary if leptomeningeal disease is suspected. Enhancing tissue may be seen thickening the leptomeninges or filling in the affected cistern.

 2) Cysticercosis.

  a) Pathology. Central nervous system involvement with cysticercosis is predominantly parenchymal and ventricular. Cisternal lesions are rare.

  b) CT features. Low-density cyst may be difficult to see in CPA. Indirect signs of CPA cistern widening or enlarged IAC may be all that is visible.

  c) MRI features. Cystic mass in the CPA cistern with slightly different T1- and T2-weighted signal characteristics than CSF. Rim or no enhancement.

g. Intraaxial tumor (Tables 20-2 and 20-4)

 1) Comment. Any of the following tumors, if large enough or pedunculated, can present at least in part as a CPA mass both clinically and radiographically. The age of the patient and the symptom complex can be very helpful in sorting through this group of tumors.

 2) Pedunculated brain stem (pontine) glioma.

  a) Clinical features. Tumor affects older children and young adults with progressive cranial nerve palsies (often bilateral), extremity weakness, and eventually respiratory insufficiency.

  b) CT features. Asymmetrically expanded brain stem with pedunculation into the adjacent CPA cistern. Hypodense on plain CT scans, with variable enhancement on enhanced CT. The fourth ventricle and CPA are compressed.

  c) MRI features. T1-weighted images show a hypo- to isointense mass compared to brain within the brain stem, with an exophytic component projecting into the CPA. T2-weighted images show the tumor and adjacent edema to be hyperintense. Contrast-enhanced T1-weighted images are variable but often show signal heterogeneity.

 3) Metastasis.

  a) Clinical features. Adult, usually with known primary tumor.

  b) CT features. Enhancing mass (sometimes ring enhancing) in the lateral brain stem, with an exophytic component extending into the CPA. When located in the cerebellar flocculus, it can appear to be "extra axial."

c) MRI features. T1-weighted images show a hypo- to isointense mass. T2-weighted images demonstrate a hyperintense mass. Contrast-enhanced T1-weighted images usually show moderate to intense enhancement. If multiple, the diagnosis of metastasis is suggested in the absence of a known primary tumor.

4) Ependymoma, lymphoma, medulloblastoma, choroid plexus papilloma, cystic cerebellar astrocytoma, and cerebellar hemangioblastoma are discussed by this series in the *Handbook on Neuroradiology*. These causes of CPA masses are sufficiently rare that they are not discussed in this chapter.

7. Pathology affecting the central acoustic pathway.
   a. The central acoustic pathway consists of the intraaxial components of the acoustic pathway, including:
      1) Dorsal and ventral cochlear nuclei.
      2) Trapezoid body.
      3) Lateral lemniscus.
      4) Inferior colliculus.
      5) Medial geniculate body.
      6) Superior temporal gyrus.
   b. Lesions affecting the inferior cerebellar peduncle will cause ipsilateral hearing loss in addition to the other brain stem related symptoms.
   c. Lesions proximal to the trapezoid body will cause bilateral hearing loss that is worse in the contralateral ear.
   d. Lesions involving the very proximal aspects of the central acoustic pathway (i.e., medial geniculate body, superior temporal gyrus) are difficult to link with the measured or reported hearing loss.
   e. A discussion of each major lesion affecting the central acoustic pathway is outside the focus of this chapter. The more common lesions are listed in Table 20-4.
   f. Brain stem tumors.
      1) Clinical presentation. Hearing loss usually is just one of many symptoms experienced by patients with any type of brain stem tumor. Multiple other cranial neuropathies, long tract signs, ophthalmoplegia, nausea, and vomiting are some of the other symptoms reported by such patients.
      2) Pathology. Statistically significant lesions include primary brain stem glioma, metastatic tumor, ependymoma, and lymphoma.
      3) Imaging features. Imaging features of glioma and metastatic tumor have been described previously.
   g. Inflammatory lesions affecting the brain stem.

1) Multiple sclerosis is the one inflammatory lesion found with any frequency during the search for causes of sensorineural hearing loss.
2) Imaging features. Periventricular multiple sclerosis plaques may be all that is found. Brain stem lesions may not be seen.
   a) Presumably, lesions affecting the central acoustic pathway in the brain stem are subradiologic.
h. Vascular lesions affecting the brain stem.
   1) Brain stem ischemia or stroke from occlusion of pontine perforators may present with a symptom complex that includes sensorineural hearing loss.
   2) Imaging features. MRI scans show focal high signal within the pons on T2-weighted images. In older people it is common to see diffuse, high signal on T2-weighted images in the pons, just like it is common to see periventricular "ischemic vascular markings." This should be distinguished from the more focal high signal associated with pontine CVA.
   3) In older patients who lose hearing in one ear asymmetrically, extensive periventricular high signal is seen on T2-weighted images, but nothing is seen on T1-weighted, contrast-enhanced images of the CPA-IAC.
      a) The presumed explanation in such cases is that the patient also has lost end-artery flow in the cochlear artery, resulting in ischemic damage to the hearing organ.

SUGGESTED READING

Armington WG, Harnsberger HR, Smoker WRK, et al: Normal and diseased acoustic pathway: evaluation with MR imaging. *Radiology*, 167:509–515, 1988.

Daniels DL, Herfkins R, Koehler PR, et al: Magnetic resonance imaging of the internal auditory canal. *Radiology* 151:105–108, 1984.

Daniels DL, Millen SJ, Meyer GA, et al: MR detection of tumor in the internal auditory canal. *AJNR* 8:249–252, 1987.

Gebarski SS, Tucci DL, Telian SA: The cochlear nuclear complex: MR location and abnormalities. *AJNR* 14:1311–1318, 1993.

Gentry LR, Jacoby CG, Turski PA, et al: Cerebellopontine angle-petromastoid mass lesions: comparative study of diagnosis with MR imaging and CT. *Radiology* 162:513–520, 1987.

Kumar A, Maudelonde C, Mafee MF: Unilateral sensorineural hearing loss: analysis of 200 consecutive cases. *Laryngoscope* 96:14–18, 1986.

Mafee MF: Acoustic neuroma and other acoustic nerve disorders: role of MRI and CT: analysis of 238 cases. *Semin Ultrasound CT MR* 8:256–283, 1987.

Mafee MF, Kumar A, Valvassori GE, et al: CT in the evaluation of the vestibulocochlear nerves and their central pathways. *Radiol Clin North Am* 22:45–66, 1984.

Mafee MF, Lachenauer CS, Kumar A, et al: CT and MR imaging of intra-labyrinthine schwannoma: report of two cases and review of the literature. *Radiology* 174:395–400, 1990.

Mafee MF, Selis JE, Yannias DA, et al: Congenital sensorineural hearing loss. *Radiology* 150:427–434, 1984.

Mark AS, Seltzer S, Harnsberger HR: Sensorineural hearing loss: more than meets the eye? *AJNR* 14:37–45, 1993.

Mueller DP, Gantz BJ, Dolan KD: Gadolinium-enhanced MR of the postoperative internal auditory canal following acoustic neuroma resection via the middle fossa approach. *AJNR* 13:197–200, 1992.

New PFJ, Bachow TB, Wismer GL, et al: MR imaging of the acoustic nerves and small acoustic neuromas at 0.6 T: prospective study. *AJNR* 6:165–170, 1985.

Smirniotopoulos JG, Yue NC, Rushing EJ: Cerebellopontine angle masses: radiologic-pathologic correlation. *RadioGraphics* 13:1131–1147, 1993.

Valvassori GE, Morales FG, Palacios E, et al: MR of the normal and abnormal internal auditory canal. *AJNR* 9:115–119, 1988.

Index

Page numbers followed by F indicate figures; page numbers followed by T indicate tables.

543

T

Technetium-99m radionuclide scanning, 180
Tempora fossa, 50
Temporal bone, (TB), 5F, 403–406, 403T,
    427–456
  diseased, 436–456
    external auditory canal, 436–439, 436T
    inner ear, 451–453, 452T
    lesions
      hearing loss, 446T
      pulsatile tinnitus, 447T
      vascular mass behind tympanic
        membrane, 448
    middle ear and mastoid, 439–451, 440T,
      otodystrophies of, 453–455
    trauma, 455–456
  normal, 427–435, 429F, 430F
    anatomy, 427–428
    external auditory canal, 428–429
    inner ear, 432–433
    middle ear, 429–432
    peripheral face nerve, 433–435, 435T
Temporalis muscle, 49T
Thallium-201 radionuclide scanning, 180
Third-branchial-cleft cysts, 205
Thrombophlebitis, 82, 184, 212
Thrombosis
  common carotid artery, 82
  jugular vein, 184
Thymic cysts, 218
Thyroglossal duct cyst, 201, 205–208, 207F
  infrahyoid paramedian type, 208F
  migration, 206F
  suprahyoid extension of, 139F
  visceral space of infrahyoid neck, 175
Thyroid
  adenoma, 219–220
    visceral space of infrahyoid neck, 177–178
  carcinoma, 221
    larynx, 226
    retropharyngeal space, 102
    visceral space of infrahyoid neck, 178,
      180
  colloid cyst, axial drawing, 218F
  cysts, 216
  lesions in visceral space of infrahyoid
    neck, 174, 176–177, 176T
  non-Hodgkin lymphoma, in visceral space
    of infrahyoid neck, 178
  notch, 226
  ophthalmopathy, 330
  tissue lesion,
    mucosal area of oral cavity, 127
    sublingual space of oral cavity, 131
Thyroiditis, 329
  acute, in visceral space of infrahyoid neck,
    181

Thyroiditis (*Continued*)
  subacute, in visceral space of infrahyoid
    neck, 181
Tic douloureux, 484
Tinnitus, lesions causing pulsatile, 447T
Tongue base, 121
  in oral cavity, 124
  tumors, 269
Tonsillar (peritonsillar) abscess of
    pharyngeal mucosal space, 42
Tornwaldt's cyst in pharyngeal mucosal
    space, 44
Tortuous carotid artery, in retropharyngeal
    space, 97, 98
Torus tubarius, 39
  suprahyoid neck and, 7
Transient ischemic attack, 82
Transpatial and multispatial disease
    processes, infrahyoid neck,
    194–196
Transverse cervical chain, 288
Transverse process, prominent in
    perivertebral space, 114
Trauma in extraconal orbit, 307T
Trauma
  conal and intraconal orbit, 306T
  optic nerve sheath, 305T
  orbit, 303T, 304T
  skull base, 415–416
  temporal bone, 455
Triangles of cervical neck, anterior and
    lateral drawings of, 152F
Triangles of infrahyoid neck, 152–154
Trigeminal nerve (V₃), 51, 272, 477–484,
    480T
  differential diagnosis, 485T–486T
  extracranial ramifications, 480F
  imaging issues, 482–483
  masticator space and, 483
  motor atrophy of, 483–484, 484T
  signs of injury, 482
  tic douloureux, 484
Tuberculosis, 195
Tuberculous adenitis, 184
Tularemia, 195
Tumors
  carotid space, 79T, 83–86, 86–87
  cerebellopontine angle, 532F, 534–536,
    539–540
  conal and intraconal orbit, 306T
  external auditory canal, 439
  extraconal orbit, 307T
  giant cell in perivertebral space, 116
  infrahyoid carotid space, 182T, 184–185
  infrahyoid perivertebral space, 193
  infrahyoid posterior cervical space, 186T,
    188